SLEEP ONSET

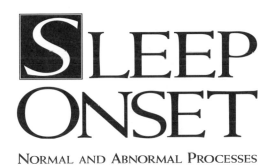

SLEEP ONSET

NORMAL AND ABNORMAL PROCESSES

Edited by Robert D. Ogilvie, PhD and John R. Harsh, PhD

AMERICAN PSYCHOLOGICAL ASSOCIATION

WASHINGTON, DC

Published by the
American Psychological Association
750 First Street, NE
Washington, DC 20002

Copies may be ordered from
APA Order Department
P.O. Box 2710
Hyattsville, MD 20784

In the UK and Europe, copies may be ordered from
American Psychological Association
3 Henrietta Street
Covent Gardens, London
WC2E 8LU England

Typeset in Minion by PRO-Image Corp., Techna Type Div., York, PA

Printer: Data Reproductions Corp., Rochester Hills, MI
Cover Designer: Supon Design Group, Washington, DC
Technical/Production Editor: Miria Liliana Riahi

Library of Congress Cataloging-in-Publication Data
Sleep onset : normal and abnormal processes / edited by Robert D. Ogilvie and
John R. Harsh.
    p.   cm.
    Includes bibliographical references and index.
    ISBN 1-55798-266-X
    1. Sleep—Stages. 2. Sleep—Psychological aspects. 3. Sleep—
Physiological aspects.   I. Ogilvie, Robert D., 1941–
II. Harsh, John R.
QP425.S6773   1994
612.8'21—dc20   94-41375
                                                                  CIP

British Library Cataloguing-in-Publication Data
A CIP record is available from the British Library.

Printed in the United States of America
First edition

We dedicate this book
to our wives
Margaret Ogilvie and Ann Harsh.

APA Science Volumes

APA expects to publish volumes on the following conference topics:

Changing Ecological Approaches to Development: Organism—Environment Mutualities
Converging Operations in the Study of Visual Selective Attention
Emotion, Disclosure, and Health
Maintaining and Promoting Integrity in Behavioral Science Research
Measuring Changes in Patients Following Psychological and Pharmacological Interventions
Perspectives on the Ecology of Human Development
Psychology of Industrial Relations
Psychophysiological Study of Attention
Stereotype Accuracy
Stereotypes: Brain–Behavior Relationships
Women's Psychological and Physical Health
Work Team Dynamics and Productivity in the Context of Diversity

As part of its continuing and expanding commitment to enhance the dissemination of scientific psychological knowledge, the Science Directorate of the APA established a Scientific Conferences Program. A series of volumes resulting from these conferences is produced jointly by the Science Directorate and the Office of Communications. A call for proposals is issued several times annually by the Science Directorate, which, collaboratively with the APA Board of Scientific Affairs, evaluates the proposals and selects several conferences for funding. This important effort has resulted in an exceptional series of meetings and scholarly volumes, each of which has contributed to the dissemination of research and dialogue in these topical areas.

The APA Science Directorate's conferences funding program has supported 33 conferences since its inception in 1988. To date, 21 volumes resulting from conferences have been published.

WILLIAM C. HOWELL, PHD
Executive Director

VIRGINIA E. HOLT
Assistant Executive Director

Contents

Contributors

Torbjorn Åkerstedt, Karolinska Institutet, Sweden

Donna A. Arand, Kettering Medical Center, Ohio

Roseanne Armitage, University of Texas Southwestern Medical Center at Dallas

Pietro Badia, Bowling Green State University, Ohio

Robin A. Battye, Carleton University, Canada

Michael H. Bonnet, Dayton VA Medical Center, Ohio

Roger Broughton, Ottawa General Hospital, Canada

Charles A. Czeisler, Brigham and Women's Hospital, Harvard University Medical School

Derk-Jan Dijk, University of Zurich, Switzerland

David Dinges, University of Pennsylvania

Jeanne F. Duffy, Brigham and Women's Hospital, Harvard Medical School

Thomas Fitch, University of Texas Southwestern Medical Center at Dallas

Simon Folkard, University of Swansea, Wales

Kazuhiko Fukuda, Fukushima University, Japan

John R. Harsh, University of Southern Mississippi

Joel Hasan, Tampere University Hospital, Finland

Mitsuo Hayashi, Hiroshima University, Japan

J. Allan Hobson, Harvard University Medical School

Tadao Hori, Hiroshima University, Japan

Angela Hudson, University of Texas Southwestern Medical Center at Dallas

Tamsin L. Kelly, Naval Health Research Center, California

Nancy Barone Kribbs, University of Pennsylvania

Heikki Lyytinen, University of Jyväskylä, Finland

Harvey Moldofsky, Toronto Hospital, Canada

Toshio Morikawa, Hiroshima Prefecture, Police Headquarters, Japan
Risto Näätänen, University of Helsinki, Finland
Paul Naitoh, Naval Health Research Center, California
Robert D. Ogilvie, Brock University, Ontario, Canada
Teresa Paiva, Centro de Estudos Egas Moniz, Hospital de Santa Maria, Portugal
Paula Pechacek, University of Texas Southwestern Medical Center at Dallas
Allan Rechtschaffen, University of Chicago
Agostinho Rosa, Instituto Superior Técnico, Lisbon, Portugal
Dean F. Salisbury, Harvard University Medical School
Sidney J. Segalowitz, Brock University, Ontario, Canada
Iain A. Simons, Brock University, Ontario, Canada
Robert Stickgold, Harvard University Medical School
Jane Storrie-Baker, Chedoke–McMaster Hospitals, Ontario, Canada
Diana Velikonja, University of Waterloo, Canada
Albert Wauquier, Texas Technical University
Wilse B. Webb, University of Florida
Kenneth P. Wright, Jr., Bowling Green State University, Ohio

Preface

In the past 10 to 15 years, the transition between wakefulness and sleep has become a focal point of the rapidly growing interest in normal and abnormal sleep. There are several reasons for this. Foremost among these is the recognition that going to sleep is not, as was once thought, a simple passive process attributable to reduced stimulation, but actually a multidimensional and active process governed by a host of endogenous and exogenous factors. How one moves from wakefulness, with all its psychological and physiological complexity, to the equally complex state of sleep is now a question of considerable interest. Another reason is the growing recognition that sleepiness is a too-readily accepted part of modern life. It has been known for some time that psychological functioning is impaired by loss of sleep; however, the suprisingly strong relationship between sleepiness and transportation accidents, reduced productivity and increased risk in the workplace, and lowered quality of day-to-day life has intensified the need for greater understanding. As a final example of the reasons for increased study of sleep onset, clinicians in the emerging field of sleep disorders medicine now know that disordered sleep is commonplace, and that sleep disorders nearly always involve a complaint of being unable to go to sleep or of being unable to avoid going to sleep. This and the knowledge that sleepiness can be an important symptom or a troublesome complication in the understanding, diagnosis, and treatment of many medical and psychiatric disorders add to the importance of the work in this area.

There were indications of worldwide interest in the sleep-onset period during the 1980s. At the European Sleep Research Society meetings held in Bologna, Italy, in 1982, several papers addressed subjective and objective indices of falling asleep. Also, the first symposium on sleep onset, held at the Sleep Research Society meeting in Seattle in 1985, attracted a large audience and enthusiastic discussion. By the end of the decade, research programs had been developed in many countries. It was at about this time that the editors of this volume began to consider ways of bringing together the work in this area. Nudged by Paul Naitoh, the editors approached potential contributors. The idea was greeted with unanimous approval; all recognized that it was time to collect current views from those active in this growing research area and to write the first book dealing exclusively with sleep onset. We are very pleased that the truly international nature of studies of sleep onset is reflected in this volume through the contributions of scientists from eight countries.

Equally gratifying was the response from potential sponsors. Our home universities, the University of Southern Mississippi and Brock University, both committed funds immediately. The Science Directorate of the American Psychological Association gave a firm commitment to the idea early in its development. Additional support was provided by the National Institute of Mental Health's (NIMH) Division of Neuroscience and Behavioral Science and by the Upjohn Company.

On behalf of the contributing authors, we would like to sincerely thank the host universities and sponsors. We are particularly grateful to the American Psychological Association for its support and guidance throughout this project. Dr. Isja Lederhendler at NIMH was especially supportive, and Marcia Jordan's editorial abilities were invaluable.

ROBERT D. OGILVIE
JOHN R. HARSH

Introduction:
A First Sketch

John R. Harsh and Robert D. Ogilvie

The process of falling asleep links our two most fundamental states, wakefulness and sleep. For the past several decades however, researchers have tended to ignore the wake-to-sleep transition, focusing rather on the states themselves. This volume begins to redress this imbalance. Theoretical models of sleep onset are presented along with original investigations of cognitive, behavioral, and physiological changes that occur as people enter the sleep state. The work of an international cast of researchers is presented. Before describing their efforts, we would like to say a few words about the reasons for the interest in this area of research.

WHY STUDY SLEEP ONSET?

Data from a variety of sources document a surprising incidence of sleepiness in modern society and also establish that sleepy individuals are unable to maintain normal daytime functioning and are at increased risk of being involved in an accident resulting in injury, or death, or property damage. Some of the following chapters, especially those by first authors Åkerstedt, Czeisler, Harsh, Kribbs, Webb, and Ogilvie, concern the determinants of sleepiness and of its cognitive and behavioral consequences.

It is also recognized that the inability to control sleep onset, i.e., the inability to go to sleep when sleep is desired or to stay awake when alertness is desired, may reflect psychological, medical, or sleep pathology. The chapters by first authors Armitage, Bonnet, and Paiva demonstrate that the study of sleep onset advances our understanding of both psychiatric and sleep-related disorders.

Finally, we know neither why nor how we fall asleep. The study of sleep has for the most part focused on measures obtained during established sleep, and many of the events and phenomena of sleep onset have been ignored. The chapters by first authors Åkerstedt, Czeisler, Webb, and Moldofsky concern the fundamental determinants of sleep onset, and those by first authors Badia, Hasan, Harsh, and Hori, provide insight into *how* sleep overtakes us.

WHAT IS SLEEP ONSET?

Most data presented in this volume support and elaborate the view, pointedly expressed by Rechtschaffen, that "there appears to be no hope of defining a specific behavioral or physiological point of sleep onset except by arbitrary criteria" (chapter 1, this volume, p. 7). The term sleep onset is described as changes in a host of physiologic, behavioral, and cognitive–mentational processes. These changes vary along dimensions that include degree and rate of change, temporal order, and dependence on other processes. Moreover, the timing and pattern of these changes vary across individuals and within individuals across time (see chapters by first authors Rechtschaffen, Moldofsky, Armitage, Bonnet, and Kribbs).

If there can be no sharply defined sleep-onset *point,* then there must be a sleep-onset *period*—a transition zone from wakefulness to sleep. When does this sleep-onset period begin? When does sleep-onset end and sleep begin? Again, different theoretical views and research tools suggest different beginning and end points for this transition zone. Sleep-related changes in event-related potentials (ERPs) may be evident, at times, before the appearance of behavioral and electroencephalographic (EEG) sleep indicators. At other times, wakefulness related ERPs may be evident in the presence of behavioral and EEG signs of sleep (see part 5, this volume). It has been suggested that underlying instigating processes that eventually lead to sleep onset may begin shortly after awakening (see models in the three chapters by first authors Åkerstedt, Rechtschaffen, and Webb). The sleep-onset period might conveniently be the accelerated or more acute sleep-onset phase beginning with relaxed drowsiness and terminating with the appearance of signs of established sleep (see the chapters by first authors Armitage, Badia, Harsh, Hasan, Hori, and Ogilvie).

Is there a need for a refined concept of "normal" or "complete" sleep? Such a concept might follow from an understanding of normal and abnormal sleep-onset processes and their relationship to learned behaviors, psychopathology, circadian rhythms, and so forth (see chapters by first authors Armitage, Fukuda, Moldofsky, Rechtschaffen, and others). Whether there are specific sleep-onset mechanisms is relevant to this issue. Some of the wakefulness-to-sleep changes are, or can be, abrupt (cognitive–mentational, behavioral, ERP, EEG, etc.) suggesting switchlike mechanisms. Sleep onset is subject to learning (see chapter 2), which suggests one or more specific processes. The notion that sleep onset can be viewed as a behavior provides a perspective, a methodology, and a terminology for addressing the question of what sleep onset is.

HOW TO STUDY SLEEP ONSET?

One way to address this issue is to examine the approaches and operational definitions used by the authors in this volume. Doing so reveals different definitions and levels of analysis. For example, Kribbs and Dinges offer a concept of functional sleep onset that is based on a person's inability to respond to a task that, only moments earlier, had been performed satisfactorily. Badia, Wright, and Wauquier provide a fine-grained EEG analysis of the end-point of sleep onset, studying single-Hertz changes in rapidly sampled EEG just before and after stable sleep patterns are established. With a similar physiological emphasis, Näätänen and Lyttinen suggest that the disappearance of the mismatch negativity component of the ERP at sleep onset could provide a physiological index of the first appearance of sleep. Chapters by Bonnet and Arand, Stickgold and Hobson, and Fukuda focus more on cognition, mentation, and subjective appreciation. Each of these chapters offers evidence of the variety of approaches currently used in the study of sleep onset. This variety is stimulating but also demonstrates a lack of standardization across laboratories and points to the need for caution when comparing findings.

Investigators differ in the conditions that they arrange for the study of sleep onset. Hori, Hayashi, and Morikawa studied natural sleep onset in normal university students to investigate the relationship between changing topographic EEG patterns and hypnagogic activity. Naitoh and Kelly used sleep-deprived subjects to establish that the contingent negative variation changes substantially as a function of degree of sleepiness. Armitage, Hudson, Fitch, and Pechacek showed that sleep-onset EEGs are different in depressed and normal people. As a final example, Bonnet and Arand manipulated arousal using agents such as caffeine and benzodiazepines and showed that doing so influenced both subjective and objective measures of sleep-onset latency. There are, of course, advantages and limitations associated with each of the above paradigms related to our lack of full understanding of the underlying processes and their dependence on learning, circadian variation, and so on.

ORGANIZATION OF THE BOOK

There are five parts to this volume. Part 1 contains overviews that address fundamental conceptual and methodological issues and provide perspectives on how the growing database might best be organized. Part 2 presents three predictive models of sleep onset and addresses their predictive validity and their usefulness. Part 3 involves behavioral, cognitive, and subjective changes at sleep onset, as seen through work conducted at four different laboratories. Part 4 consists of six papers examining EEG changes during sleep onset. Novel studies focus on moment-to-moment changes in EEG activity. Part 5 summarizes current ERP work, with each chapter providing a description of changes in ERP components that are unique to the sleep-onset period.

Part 1: Definitions, Problems, and Models

Rechtschaffen (chapter 1) addresses issues related to the definition of sleep onset. He describes a behavioral definition focusing on motor quiescence, reduced responsiveness to stimulation, stereotypic posture, and state reversibility, but also spells out the justification for and usefulness of defining sleep onset and sleep using physiological variables. No hope is given, however, for there being a nonarbitrary specification of the moment of sleep onset because available data indicate that sleep onset is gradual, that sleep-onset behaviors are not synchronized, and that there are large individual differences in the timing and synchrony of behavioral changes. The implications of these observations for the modeling of sleep onset are discussed. The asynchronies of sleep behaviors, it is suggested, may reflect multiple effector mechanisms modulated by active sleep generators.

Broughton (chapter 2) argues that models predicting sleep onset must reflect the complexity of the process if they are to be broadly applicable. Three aspects of sleep that are of apparent importance, but that have been neglected in the literature, are behavioral–cognitive aspects, circasemidian regulation, and phasic events. Behavioral and conditioning factors are significant because there is sufficient evidence to demonstrate their theoretical and clinical significance, but insufficient data to understand fully the underlying mechanisms. The circasemidian rhythm, he argues, accounts for a theoretically and practically important amount of the variance in sleep-onset behaviors, but cannot be accounted for by many prevailing models. The normal hyperexcitability of phasic motor, sensory, and EEG events during the sleep-onset period has barely begun to be explored either empirically or theoretically.

Moldofsky (chapter 3) cautions that sleep onset and sleep cannot be viewed in isolation from circadian patterns of immune, neuroendocrine, and thermal systems. A harmonious interrelationship of these systems may be important to the cause and function of sleep. Working within a homeostatic model, he discusses evidence for the existence of a long list of substances that researchers have found to be both immune activating and sleep promoting. Changes in these endogenous sleep substances can be clearly seen at or shortly after the beginning of sleep. Data from his laboratory indicate that citokines, such as IL-1, and aspects of peripheral immune cell function, such as NK cell activities, are importantly related to the wakefulness-to-sleep transition.

Part 2: Predictive Models

Webb (chapter 4) extends his earlier three-factor model of sleep to focus on the prediction of the onset of sleep. The principal parameters of the model are sleep demand, circadian timing, and behavioral facilitation or inhibition. How the model handles other important variables, including individual differences and age, is detailed, and evidence is presented that the model can predict sleep onset with considerable accuracy in a wide range of situations when the presence of moderator variables is taken into account.

Åkerstedt and Folkard (chapter 5), like Webb, have built a three-factor model for predicting alertness (subjective sleepiness) that extends from a two-factor model. In this chapter, the authors approach the problem of predicting–differentiating between intentional and unintentional sleep onset. Their model of alertness can be understood in terms of three processes: sleepiness (Process S), an exponential function of time since awakening; circadian factors (Process C), a sinusoidal function; and sleep inertia (Process W), observed most clearly after forced awakenings. They report high agreement between predicted and observed levels of sleepiness in both laboratory and work situations.

Czeisler, Dijk, and Duffy (chapter 6) explain the role of the supra-chiasmatic nucleus as the circadian pacemaker interacting with the wake–sleep cycle to influence cognitive activity and alertness. They discuss how this model accounts for variations in performance brought on by shiftwork and the lack of normal circadian timing cues. Their research involves separation of sleep-dependent and circadian factors and they specifically address how the interacting forces of the sleep–wake cycle and the endogenous circadian rhythm produce sustained alert wakefulness and monophasic sleep.

Part 3: Behavioral, Physiological, and Cognitive Changes

Kribbs and Dinges (chapter 7) use performance measures to demonstrate that when normal sleep is denied, sleep pressure is indexed both by an increased number of attempts to sleep and by accelerated sleep onset. These effects can be observed easily when using attention-based tasks. Understanding the relationship between sleepiness and performance depends on knowledge about the predictors and the underlying mechanisms.

Bonnet and Arand (chapter 8) provide preliminary evidence to support their notion that the perception of the time taken to fall asleep is influenced by physiological arousal during the sleep-onset period. This evidence is consistent with their hypothesis that insomnia or poor sleep is a physiological rather than a psychological phenomenon. When arousal is lowered by sleep deprivation, both objective and subjective sleep-onset latencies decrease, whereas the opposite occurs when arousal is increased by agents such as caffeine.

Stickgold and Hobson (chapter 9) used a sleep–wake monitoring device called the "Nightcap®", which monitors eye and body movement, to discriminate wakefulness from REM and non-REM (NREM) sleep. During the sleep-onset period, the device was programmed to awaken the sleeper after a brief period of ocular quiescence, previously established to be a time during which hypnagogic imagery appeared frequently. Taped mentation reports confirmed the predicted relationship between physiological and psychological events during the sleep-onset period. Further studies are planned to compare slow eye movement cessation with the development of hypnagogic imagery using home monitoring system.

Fukuda (chapter 10) provides an intriguing account of the differences in the reporting of sleep paralysis in sleep onset REM periods in normal people from several different cultures. It appears that the widely varying differences in the incidence of reported sleep paralysis are due more likely to cultural factors, such as whether there is a positive, popular term for the phenomenon (i.e., *kanashibari* in Japan or *Old Hag* in Newfoundland) versus a negatively evaluated medical term like *sleep paralysis,* than to racial factors—a hypothesis that seemed plausible at first.

Part 4: EEG Changes

Although there is heated discussion of whether period analysis or more traditional fast Fourier transform (FFT) analysis of EEG activity is more appropriate, chapters in this section show that both approaches yield useful distinctions among EEG events during the sleep-onset period.

Armitage, Hudson, Fitch, and Pechacek (chapter 11) conducted period analysis on EEG activity recorded during the wakefulness-to-sleep transition. They found that differences between unipolar depressed and normal people interacted with hemispheric differences such that, at sleep onset, asymmetries were greater in depressed than in normal participants. Beta and delta activity were elevated in depressed people immediately before sleep onset. The authors characterized these differences as being due to general interhemisphere dysregulation in depression. These authors are the first to report EEG differences between normal and abnormal sleepers at the onset of sleep.

Badia, Wright, and Wauquier (chapter 12) demonstrate that single-Hertz FFT analysis of ongoing EEG provides important information about EEG changes during the wake–sleep transition. The transition was characterized by large changes in activity in 3–4-Hz (increases) and 10-Hz (decreases) frequency bands. With 5-s epochs, many more fluctuations between wakefulness and sleep were noted than with 30-s epochs, suggesting that the shift from wakefulness to sleep is more abrupt than gradual. These abrupt changes were tracked better by changes in 3- and 4-Hz than in 10-Hz activity.

Hasan and Broughton (chapter 13) provide data from topographic mapping of the EEG during sleep onset. They have used a brain-mapping routine to synthesize information from 19 electrode sites, producing color-coded displays of changing frequencies over time. The authors demonstrate the superiority of this system over limited-site systems for detecting temporal and topographic differences or for moving changes in EEG power over time. Their data reveal a "high degree of complexity, diversity, and volatility of the EEG patterns from wakefulness through drowsiness, to Stage-2 sleep" (p. 231). Using the topographic system, they have identified differences between occipital and frontal alpha fluctuations at sleep onset, noted anterior changes in delta-wave activity, identified similarities between vertex sharp waves and the sawtooth waves of REM sleep, and commented on the distribution of spindle activity early in sleep.

Hori, Hayashi, and Morikawa (chapter 14) have also conducted topographical analyses to focus primarily on hypnagogic experiences as a function of EEG pattern. They used 12 electrode sites to assist in distinguishing among nine different EEG waveforms, which they used to make fine differentiations during the sleep-onset period (composed of relaxed wakefulness, Stage-1 and Stage-2 sleep). Behavioral and neurophysiological arousal was lower in Stage 1 than in relaxed wakefulness and lower again during Stage 2 as compared with late Stage 1. Their anterior/posterior EEG ratio holds promise as a sleep-onset index, changing dramatically between Stages 3 and 4 (in early Stage-1 sleep) of their nine-stage system. In Stages 3 to 9, hypnagogic imagery was significantly higher than in Stages 1 and 2, showing a peak at Stage 5 (theta suppression during Stage-1 sleep). They conclude that their research provides evidence for the uniqueness of the sleep-onset period—a period that is neither wakefulness nor sleep, and they agree with Hasan and Broughton that topographic analysis increases the resolving power of physiological indices.

Paiva and Rosa (chapter 15) used spectral analysis to compare EEG activity sampled immediately before spontaneous arousals from sleep with that obtained immediately afterward during the return to sleep in normal and dysthymic subjects. The clearest difference in EEG activity between groups occurred in delta activity, which rose more steadily after awakening in the normal subjects than in the moderately depressed dysthymic sleepers, perhaps reflecting a tendency for normal individuals to return to sleep more quickly than dysthymic individuals. The data were interpreted in relation to the significance of the difference in rhythmicities of phenomena in normal and disturbed sleep.

Ogilvie, Battye, and Simons (chapter 16) studied the relationships between EEG and ERP assessments of arousal during sleep onset and throughout the night. They did so by comparing frequently sampled, nearly simultaneous EEG and ERP measures. They predicted that the large variations in arousal level during sleep onset and beyond would be evidenced by high cross-domain correlations and factors. Instead, they found solid within-domain correlations and obtained interpretable but relatively weak cross-domain factors, indicating that changes in arousal occur more clearly within each of the two measurement domains than between them.

Part 5: ERP Changes

Salisbury (chapter 17) introduces the reader to the principles of ERP research and provides a context for this approach within the field of sleep research. The author presents a two-system hypothesis, which is a theoretical position accounting for both the similarities and differences in ERPs during wakefulness and sleep. Basically, the hypothesis proposes that many of the waking components of ERPs can still be observed during sleep, as are ERPs unique to sleep. These added elements are created primarily by the superimposition of the slow-wave components known as the K-complex. The implications for such dual processing during NREM sleep are explored.

Harsh (chapter 18) reports on a series of studies that examine P300 and N350 ERP components during the transition to sleep. Evidence is presented to show that, in subjects performing a routine oddball task, P300 disappears as behavioral responsiveness decreases and N350 emerges. The N350 is shown to be dependent on presleep instructions and also on the psychological characteristics of the experimental stimuli. An interpretation of these data is presented that focuses on inhibition of cortical activation. Data are presented showing differences in ERPs during the wake–sleep transition between good and poor sleepers and between individuals with differing information-processing styles during wakefulness.

Naitoh and Kelly (chapter 19), drawing upon their own findings and the work of others, argue that the sensitivity of the Multiple Sleep Latency Test (MSLT), a widely used measure of sleepiness, could be supplemented by obtaining an ERP measure, the contingent negative variation (CNV); during the MSLT period. Adding a physiological measure might minimize individual and situational factors that can lessen the value of the MSLT as currently used. The idea that the CNV can be used as a psychophysiological measure of sleepiness is supported by their data on CNV testing during sleep deprivation. So modified, the MSLT might provide a more valid estimate of sleepiness and sleep onset.

Näätänen (chapter 20) reviews sleep studies that have examined the mismatch negativity (MMN) potential. The MMN, a measure of automatic auditory sensory processing, decreases dramatically during drowsiness and is virtually absent at sleep onset, making it an interesting ERP component for those studying the transition to sleep. Näätänen argues that the absence of the MMN at sleep onset is an indication of the reduced cortical activation that occurs during sleep.

Segalowitz, Velikonja, and Storrie-Baker (chapter 21) point out that studies of arousal often confound attention and arousal. Their literature review leads them to conclude that the relationship between these two important concepts is not clearly established. The solution suggested is a series of complex investigations that eliminate the confounding by conducting experiments in which multiple levels of attention and arousal are created and studied interactively. The transition to sleep provides a context in which these interrelationships could be examined fruitfully.

The study of sleep-onset processes has really just begun. Although study of the chapters in this volume will undoubtedly raise many questions about fundamental empirical and theoretical issues and reveal many potentially serious methodological problems, it is clear that substantial progress has been made. There is now a greater understanding of the cognitive–mentational, behavioral, and physiological changes that occur as sleep approaches, and the ability to predict sleep onset, at least that of normal young adults, is impressive. Additionally, it is evident that abnormalities of sleep onset accompany disordered sleep and various types of psychopathology. The extent and the significance of the findings described in this volume are a clear indication that future work will yield greater understanding of normal and abnormal transitions between wakefulness and sleep states, in addition to providing answers to fundamental questions about how and why we go to sleep.

PART ONE

Definitions, Problems, and Models

1

Sleep Onset: Conceptual Issues

Allan Rechtschaffen

A ny specification of sleep onset requires first a definition of sleep. This definition is not to be confused with issues of sleep mechanisms or functions, which can logically be tackled only after sleep is identified. The scientific definition of sleep (like all scientific definitions) requires only that independent observers reach reasonable agreement on whether sleep is present or absent.

THE DEFINITION OF SLEEP

By which observables should sleep be defined? In a general sense, everyone knows what sleep is. There is no need to look it up in the dictionary. However, the criteria by which one recognizes sleep are not generally specified. For about 30 years, I have started a college class on sleep by asking "What is sleep?" Without fail, the initial response has been an embarrassed silence, sometimes followed by vague remarks about state of consciousness, brain waves, or brain activity. Then, I ask the students to imagine a friend sleeping on the other side of a room. They have no idea of the friend's state of consciousness, brain waves, or brain activity. What, then, makes them think that the friend is asleep? Then the answers start to come. The friend is lying down. There is very little movement. The friend does not respond to questions. Sometimes, a bright student even ventures that, because the friend eventually arises, moves, and responds to questions, the preceding state was sleep rather than death or coma. There we have the observations by which sleep has been known through the ages: stereotypic posture, reduced motility, reduced response to stimulation, reversibility. These are observations of behaviors.[1] By such behaviors, even my dog, who seeks my attention incessantly while I am awake, seems to know when I am asleep and leaves me alone at those times. Any scientific definition of sleep that ignores the behaviors by which sleep is generally known unnecessarily violates common understanding and invites confusion.

Subjective Awareness

For human sleep, one often adds the criterion of subjective awareness of prior sleep. Either through some sense of passage of time without sensory contact with the environment or by other sensations that have not been seriously studied, one can sense when one has been asleep. This sense may well be the most frequently used criterion in everyday life. Each of us knows when we awaken each morning that we have been asleep. For use as scientific data, the subjective experience must be objectified as a verbal report. These so-called *subjective reports* are behavioral indicators of presumed subjective experiences. We may not know how well the reports correspond to the experiences, but this is no different in principle from using any other observable as an indicator of unseen processes. Whether we use subjective reports to define sleep is a judgmental matter that, in practice, may depend on how well they correlate with the other criteria. Subjective reports do not always

---

[1]We have chosen to speak about the motor quiescence and diminished responsivity as *sleep behaviors*. Others have viewed this as a *lack* of behavior. Operationally, the two may be equivalent, but we have selected the former designation because changes during sleep may involve active inhibitory processes, implying behavior control rather than absence.

correlate with the other criteria, but, for that matter, the other criteria are not always well correlated with each other. This vexing problem will be discussed later.

Physiological Definitions of Sleep

The working sleep scientist rarely defines sleep by behaviors but by physiological patterns that include the electroencephalogram (EEG), electromyogram (EMG), and electrooculogram (EOG). If these physiological definitions are to reflect the common understanding of what sleep is, they must correlate highly with behavioral definitions of sleep. The physiological measures derive their value as indicators of sleep from their correlations with the behavioral criteria, not from any intrinsic ontological or explanatory superiority.

A small mind-experiment illustrates this point. Imagine that some day all the physiological mechanisms and functions of sleep become known. This knowledge reveals that the postures, motor quiescence, and decreased response to stimulation of sleep serve only to permit need-fulfilling physiological processes to proceed. The new knowledge also produces a drug that satisfies the function during behavioral wakefulness. Would we now define this behavioral wakefulness as sleep, or would we say that we have eliminated sleep? Probably the latter, simply because all the signs by which sleep was identified previously would now be absent. A scientist might define a new drug-induced physiological state that satisfies the need for sleep, but neither the scientist nor a layman would see any of the behaviors by which they had previously identified sleep. The absence of sleep would be defined by behavior for linguistic clarity—and that is reason enough.

Advantages of Physiological Measures

But why, if the definitional criteria are ultimately behavioral, should one ever use physiological measures to define sleep? There are several reasons:

1. Measuring the physiology is usually easier and less expensive than recording behavior continuously.
2. Physiological recordings may also provide information about the physiological causes and consequences of sleep.
3. Physiological recordings differentiate several stages of sleep, although it may be noted that a Stone-Age observer, sufficiently interested in the details of sleep behavior, could have, and perhaps did, differentiate rapid eye movement (REM) sleep from nonrapid eye movement (NREM) sleep 10,000 years ago by carefully observing the movement of the eyes under the closed lid, muscle twitches, irregular breathing, and, in men, penile erections.
4. Physiological recordings are important for studying uninterrupted sleep. If one attempted to define extended sleep by a failure of responses to repeatedly presented stimuli, one would risk either waking the subject, altering the sleep, or habituating the subject to the stimulation. One solution has been to preestablish correlations between behavioral criteria and physiological patterns and later infer the behavioral state from the *uninterrupted* physiological pattern alone.
5. Physiological measures can help describe the sequence of behavioral changes. When comparing responses to visual and auditory stimuli, one could present the two stimuli sequentially. But then, the first stimulus or the response to it might alter the response threshold for the second. However, one can make reasonable inferences about temporal relationships among sleep behaviors by first determining, on separate trials, the physiological correlates of the different behaviors. Later, the sequence of behavioral changes can be inferred from the uninterrupted progression of physiological changes.[2]

---

[2]Unfortunately, data are often presented as group averages per physiological stage, which could obscure stable but different sequential developments in different individuals.

PHYSIOLOGICAL CORRELATES OF SLEEP ONSET

Physiological progression of sleep onset in humans is generally recognized to be as follows: low-voltage, mixed-frequency EEG with high muscle tone and rapid eye movements (wakefulness); alpha-dominated EEG with reduced muscle tone and infrequent eye movements; alpha EEG with slow eye movements; mixture of alpha and low-voltage, mixed-frequency EEG with some slow components—usually with continuing slow eye movements (scored Stage 1 if alpha is less than 50% of record); same as preceding but with little or no alpha activity (Stage 1); appearance of 12–14-Hz sleep spindles (Stage 2).

Studies of physiological correlates of sleep onset behavior have produced some notable successes. For example, the most extensively studied sleep onset indicator, a decline in EEG alpha activity, has been related to a reported loss of awareness of the environment (Davis, Davis, Loomis, Harvey, & Hobart, 1937), failure to maintain muscle tone (Blake, Gerard, & Kleitman, 1939; Perry & Goldwater, 1987), decline in response to verbally presented materials (Simon & Emmons, 1956), increased visual separation threshold (Anliker, 1966), and inaccurate time perception (Anliker, 1963).

No Specific Point of Sleep Onset

Despite these and other significant relationships between behavioral sleep measures and physiological indicators, there appears to be no hope of defining a precise behavioral or physiological point of sleep onset, except by arbitrary criteria. This is not a new sentiment. It was expressed by Davis et al. (1937) in one of the earliest empirical studies of sleep onset; Kleitman (1963) said as much in the opening sentence of his chapter on sleep onset; and it has more recently been reiterated by Ogilvie and Wilkinson (1988). The following review of their and other rationales provides some insight on the sleep onset process.

Wake–Sleep Transitions Are Gradual

One major reason why a discrete point of sleep onset cannot be specified is that transitions from wakefulness to sleep are gradual. Observable gross motor behavior usually ceases before other sleep-related changes, but EMG recordings reveal more subtle motor changes. Jacobson, Kales, Lehmann, & Hoedemaker (1964) described a gradual decrease in tonus of all recorded head, neck, trunk, and limb muscles as subjects fell asleep. Litchman (1974) found a gradual decrease in precisely quantified mentalis EMG across the sleep-onset period.

Some studies have described categorical, stepwise failures of motor performance during the sleep-onset period, such as dropping an object held between the fingers (Blake et al., 1939; Ogilvie, Wilkinson, & Allison, 1989) or releasing a switch (Perry & Goldwater, 1987). However, given a gradual loss of muscle tone, sooner or later tonus will be insufficient for task success, and the point of categorical failure will depend partly on the tonus required for success on that specific task. In other words, the categorical performance failure is determined arbitrarily by a task parameter that ignores previous gradual changes. The task failures probably also involve failures of attention, which are not so dependent on tonus per se, but the failures of attention might also be gradual.

Studies have shown that responsivity to sensory signals decreases gradually during the transition from wakefulness to sleep (e.g., Anliker, 1966; Ogilvie & Simons, 1992; Ogilvie, Simons, Kuderian, MacDonald, & Rustenburg, 1991; Ogilvie & Wilkinson, 1984, 1988; Ogilvie et al., 1989; Simon & Emmons, 1956.) As in the case of muscle tone described earlier, it is possible to impose a discrete operational criterion on the continuum of response decline (e.g., a complete failure to respond as the end point of gradually decreasing reaction times), but this is a rather arbitrary definition of a point of sleep onset that ignores large behavioral changes preceding that point.

Subjective state also changes gradually over the sleep-onset period. Foulkes and Vogel (1965) showed that, as subjects progressed through the stages alpha with rapid eye movements, to alpha with slow eye movements, to Stage 1, and to Stage 2, there were progressive decreases in reports of controlling one's thoughts and images, awareness of being in the laboratory, and awareness that one was observing the contents of one's own mind. Reports of dreamlike activity increased progressively across the same stages. Agnew and Webb (1972) showed that reports of having slept increased progressively with the attainment of Stages 1, 2, and 3–4 during the test period.

Thus, changes in muscle tone, responsivity to external stimuli, and subjective reports all indicate gradual changes during the sleep-onset period. The gradual evolution of behavioral sleep over the sleep-onset period is probably a late phase in the gradual expression of sleep-instigating processes. In the cat, basal forebrain neurons show increased firing rates 10–15 s before the first sleep spindle (Szymusiak & McGinty, 1990). Ventral hippocampus spike potentials, which are more numerous in NREM sleep than in wakefulness or REM sleep, increase in frequency several minutes in advance of an NREM EEG (Hartse, Eisenhart, Bergmann, & Rechtschaffen, 1979). In fact, because the propensity to sleep increases with time awake, it is possible that sleep-instigating processes begin shortly after we wake up. The development of sleep-onset behaviors, as protracted as they are, probably reflect an acceleration of even longer term, sleep-instigating processes.

Sleep Onset Behaviors Not Synchronized

The second major reason why a precise moment of sleep onset cannot be established is that relevant behavioral changes are not entirely synchronized. For example, the decline in response to auditory stimulation appears to lag behind the decline in response to visual stimuli. Several studies have shown that response to auditory stimulation is fairly well preserved so long as alpha activity is not severely reduced (Ogilvie & Wilkinson, 1984; Ogilvie et al., 1989; Simon & Emmons, 1956). On the other hand, the ability to distinguish two light flashes presented in close proximity was severely reduced with even small reductions in integrated alpha activity (Anliker, 1966). Based on failures of visual fixation, Miles (1929) concluded that sleep was possible when the eyes were still open—certainly at a very early point in the sleep-onset process. In two subjects tested with their eyelids taped open, there was no recall of objects presented in front of the open eyes while alpha activity was still present but after slow eye movements had begun (Rechtschaffen & Foulkes, 1965).

Whereas muscle tone gradually decreases over the sleep-onset period, phasic twitches of the facial muscles increase during Stage 1 from the five preceding minutes, before subsiding again during the ensuing Stage 2 (Metz, Pivik, & Rechtschaffen, 1975). "Hypnic jerks" after sleep onset have also been recorded in animals (reviewed in Kleitman, 1963). Oswald (1959) reported that some subjects who were instructed to move rhythmically to music continued such movements even when clear EEG signs of sleep were present.

Whereas previously cited data indicated that responsivity to auditory stimuli was well preserved while the EEG record was dominated by alpha activity, Foulkes and Vogel (1965) reported increased sleep-like mental activity during the alpha-slow eye movement period. On the other hand, Agnew and Webb (1972) showed that reports of having slept were more closely associated with the prior occurrence of Stage 2 than of Stage 1, after responsivity to visual and auditory stimuli had been, presumably, substantially diminished.

Individual Differences in Sleep Onset

Not only are behavioral changes during the sleep-onset period asynchronous, but also there are large individual differences in when the changes occur. For example, in the Foulkes and Vogel (1965) study, although there were fairly progressive increases in dreamlike mental activity across the sleep-onset stages, there were great individual differences in when these changes appeared. Makeig and Inlow (1993) reported that the pattern of correspondence between EEG and behavioral lapses of alertness differed across individuals but remained stable within individuals across recording sessions. In one of the Ogilvie and Wilkinson studies (1988), the probability of response to a faint auditory signal in Stage 1 varied from 0.01 to 0.67 across subjects. There are also large individual differences in degree of behavioral synchrony: Phi coefficients expressing the relationship between response times to tones and failing to maintain pressure on a switch ranged from 0.04 to 0.60 across 10 subjects (Ogilvie et al., 1989).

The gradual changes in relevant behaviors, the asynchronies of behavioral changes, and the individual differences in sleep-onset behavioral patterns make it highly unlikely that we can ever define a specific point of sleep onset except by a somewhat arbitrary selection of defining criteria. Because physiological criteria derive their value from their correlations with behavioral changes, similar failures can be expected for physiological point definitions of sleep onset—not because we have the "wrong" physiological measures and not because of error of measurement, but simply because sleep just does not happen that way. Any attempt to integrate the several measures of sleep onset into a single comprehensive measure would amount to an abstraction that might not correspond to the changes in any single behavioral indicator.

SLEEP SCORING

What does this mean for the practical problem of how the sleep researcher or clinician scores physiological recordings of sleep? For scoring human sleep, attention is naturally directed to the widely used Rechtschaffen and Kales (1968) manual. The manual was constructed to standardize the scoring of about 850 pages of physiological recording per night by a manageable epoch system. (The possibility of successful point scoring is automatically precluded by within-epoch physiological variations intrinsic to the epoch system.) Stage 1 was designated as the first-appearing epoch of sleep based on empirical information then available about the physiological correlates of behavioral sleep. Now, 25 years later, it is appropriate to ask anew whether initial sleep is best described by Stage 1 or by an earlier or later stage. The asynchronies among behavioral criteria require that one set of criteria or another be chosen.

The solution, quite simply, is that one should choose the criteria that best capture the behavioral characteristics that one wishes to emphasize.

If the selected emphasis is on loss of vigilance, then one could designate a pre-Stage 1 pattern (e.g., alpha with slow eye movements) as sleep. (Certainly, one would not want to be chauffeured by someone in that state.) On the other hand, if one wanted to score sleep only when all the behavioral characteristics of sleep were well established, Stage 2 would be a better choice. This designation might also have functional value. In recent studies of sleep deprivation in rats (Everson, Bergmann, & Rechtschaffen, 1989), because attempts to sleep were frequent and because it was difficult to catch the very beginning of sleep episodes, low-voltage, NREM sleep, which is morphologically similar to human Stage 1, was regularly increased above baseline levels during the deprivation period. Nevertheless, this increase did not protect the rats against the physiological effects of sleep loss. Finally, if a scorer had no reason to emphasize one behavioral aspect of sleep over another, but wanted an indicator of beginning sleep that reflected substantial, albeit incomplete changes in all related behaviors, Stage 1 might serve as well as any other. The designation of different stages as sleep in different studies need not create chaos, so long as the physiological pattern is well described and labelled. (Happily, this is an approach already in use by some investigators.)

MODELS OF SLEEP ONSET

The common asynchronies of sleep onset are benign compared to less frequent but more dramatic asynchronies, such as sleep talking, sleep-walking, sleep paralysis, cataplexy, and REM-sleep movement disorder. The asynchronies do not fit well with the old concept that sleep occurs when generalized neural arousal falls below a certain critical value and response systems fail in synchrony.[3] To achieve a better fit, the model could be refined to postulate different arousal thresholds for different response systems, so that a given arousal level might be sufficient to

---

[3]With this concept, level of arousal and critical threshold have been widely used as explanatory principles. In most cases—certainly in most of the human research—level of arousal relative to threshold has been inferred directly from responses without any independent measure of generalized arousal.

activate one response but not another. This refinement protects a de-arousal model against the benign asynchronies of sleep onset. However, the more dramatic asynchronies, such as sleepwalking and sleep talking, would require such large shifts in specific thresholds as to preclude an important role for generalized arousal in response determination.

We now know that mechanisms in the hypothalamus and brain stem participate in the active generation of sleep (see Jones, 1989, and Siegel, 1989, for reviews). An alternative (or an addition) to the de-arousal model would suggest that sleep behaviors result, at least in part, from active induction and modulation by active sleep mechanisms, rather than from a withdrawal of excitatory drive alone. This is abundantly clear in the case of REM sleep, when motoneurons are simultaneously activated and actively inhibited (Chase & Morales, 1989). Although comparable neurophysiological specificity of response modulation has not yet been demonstrated for NREM sleep, it remains a possibility. For example, neurons of the lateral geniculate body (Hirsch, Fourment, & Marc, 1983) and sensorimotor cortex (Pedroarena, Ricciardi, Morales, & Chase, 1993) become more hyperpolarized during NREM sleep than during wakefulness, which could reflect active inhibitory processes rather than simply a withdrawal of excitatory drive. Jacobs, McGinty, and Harper (1973) noted a trend for increased neuronal activity during NREM sleep in structures associated with inhibitory control of behavior, i.e., the amygdala, hippocampus, and medial hypothalamus. It remains to be determined whether NREM sleep behaviors are indeed controlled by active inhibitory mechanisms such as those suggested above, and whether these mechanisms retain some measure of independent action.

Surely, sleep and wakefulness must involve highly coordinated changes in the nervous system; otherwise, sleep and wake behaviors would be intermixed throughout the day. Nevertheless, a relative independence of response modulation mechanisms could account for commonplace asynchronies of sleep onset, whereas occasional failures or innervations of specific modulatory mechanisms could account for the more dramatic asynchronies of sleep. To put it another way, this model proposes that there are separate effector mechanisms that control the different behavioral conditions that, when considered together, constitute "sleep." Although active sleep generators usually stimulate these effector mechanisms in a coordinated manner, in the process of becoming activated (i.e., at sleep onset), the generators do not affect all the effectors or sleep behaviors simultaneously—thus producing the characteristic asynchronies of sleep onset. In more dramatic dissociations of sleep behaviors, a specific modulatory mechanism may not be stimulated or may fail to react altogether. From this perspective, one can think of sleep not only as more or less intense but also as more or less *complete*, depending on the number of response systems effectively modulated.

SUMMARY

The identification of sleep onset requires a definition of sleep. To avoid linguistic confusion, sleep is best defined by the behaviors by which it has long been identified, that is, motor quiescence, reduced response to stimulation, stereotypic posture, reversibility, and, in some cases, subjective impression. Nevertheless, for many purposes, including the identification of sleep onset, the definition of sleep by the physiological correlates of sleep behaviors has advantages that include ease of recording, acquisition of physiological information, differentiation of sleep stages, and monitoring of sleep without disrupting it with behavioral tests. There have been notable successes in finding physiological correlates of sleep-onset behaviors. Nevertheless, there is no hope of defining a specific behavioral or physiological point of sleep onset, except by somewhat arbitrary criteria, because sleep-onset behaviors are not entirely correlated, sleep onset is a gradual process, and there are marked individual differences in sleep-onset patterns. Therefore, the scoring of physiological sleep onset requires judgmental selection from among possible criteria. It is suggested that criteria be selected according to the particular characteristic of sleep that one wishes to emphasize. For example, if the emphasis is on loss of vigilance, then an early sleep indicator, such as slow eye movements, might be selected; if the focus is on functional value, then a later-appearing indicator, such as Stage 2, might be selected.

It is difficult to account for the asynchronies of sleep behaviors by a generalized decrease in neural arousal. It is suggested that active sleep mechanisms may modulate relatively independent sleep behavior systems, and that the asynchronics of sleep may result from differential activation of the modulatory mechanisms.

REFERENCES

Agnew, Jr., H. W., & Webb, W. B. (1972). Measurement of sleep onset by EEG criteria. *American Journal of EEG Technology, 12*, 127–134.

Anliker, J. (1963). Variations in alpha voltage of the electroencephalogram and time perception. *Science, 140*, 1307–1309.

Anliker, J. (1966). Simultaneous changes in visual separation threshold and voltage of cortical alpha rhythm. *Science, 153*, 548–552.

Blake, H., Gerard, R. W., & Kleitman, N. (1939). Factors influencing brain potentials during sleep. *Journal of Neurophysiology, 2*, 48–60.

Chase, M. H., & Morales, F. R. (1989). The control of motoneurons during sleep. In M. H. Kryger, T. Roth, & W. C. Dement (Eds.), *Principles and practice of sleep medicine* (pp. 74–85). Philadelphia: Saunders.

Davis, H., Davis, P. A., Loomis, A. L., Harvey, E. N., & Hobart G. (1937). Changes in human brain potentials during the onset of sleep. *Science, 86*, 448–450.

Everson, C. A., Bergmann, B. M., & Rechtschaffen, A. (1989). Sleep deprivation in the rat: Part 3. Total sleep deprivation. *Sleep, 12*, 13–21.

Foulkes, D., & Vogel, G. (1965). Mental activity at sleep onset. *Journal of Abnormal Psychology, 70*, 231–243.

Hartse, K. M., Eisenhart, S. F., Bergmann, B. M., & Rechtschaffen, A. (1979). Ventral hippocampus spikes during sleep, wakefulness, and arousal in the cat. *Sleep, 1*, 231–246.

Hirsch, J. C., Fourment, A., & Marc, M. E. (1983). Sleep-related variations of membrane potential in the lateral geniculate relay neurons of the cat. *Brain Research, 259*, 308–312.

Jacobs, B. L., McGinty, D. J., & Harper, R. M. (1973). Brain single unit activity during sleep–wakefulness: A review. In M. I. Phillips (Ed.), *Brain unit activity during behavior* (pp. 165–178). Springfield, IL: Thomas.

Jacobson, A., Kales, A., Lehmann, D., & Hoedemaker, F. S. (1964). Muscle tonus in human subjects during sleep and dreaming. *Experimental Neurology, 10,* 418–424.

Jones, B. E. (1989). Basic mechanisms of sleep–wake states. In M. H. Kryger, T. Roth, & W. C. Dement (Eds.), *Principles and practice of sleep medicine* (pp. 121–138). Philadelphia: Saunders.

Kleitman, N. (1963). *Sleep and wakefulness* (rev. ed.). Chicago: University of Chicago Press.

Litchman, J. (1974). *Mentalis EMG in human sleep and wakefulness.* Unpublished doctoral dissertation, University of Chicago.

Makeig, S., & Inlow, M. (1993). Lapses in alertness: coherence of fluctuations in performance and EEG spectrum. *Electroencephalography and Clinical Neurophysiology, 86,* 23–35.

Metz, J., Pivik, R. T., & Rechtschaffen, A. (1975). Phasic facial and extraocular muscle activity during sleep in cats and humans. *Sleep Research, 4,* 35.

Miles, W. (1929). Sleeping with the eyes open. *Scientific American, 140,* 489–492.

Ogilvie, R. D., & Simons, I. (1992). Falling asleep and waking up: A comparison of EEG spectra. In R. J. Broughton & R. D. Ogilvie (Eds.), *Sleep, arousal, and performance* (pp. 73–87). Boston: Birkhauser.

Ogilvie, R. D., Simons, I. A., Kuderian, R. H., MacDonald, T., & Rustenburg, J. (1991). Behavioral, event-related potential, and EEG/FFT changes at sleep onset. *Psychophysiology, 28,* 54–64.

Ogilvie, R. D., & Wilkinson, R. T. (1984). The detection of sleep onset: Behavioral and physiological convergence. *Psychophysiology, 21,* 510–520.

Ogilvie R. D., & Wilkinson, R. T. (1988). Behavioral versus EEG-based monitoring of all-night sleep/wake patterns. *Sleep, 11,* 139–155.

Ogilvie, R. D., Wilkinson, R. T., & Allison, S. (1989). The detection of sleep onset: Behavioral, physiological, and subjective convergence. *Sleep, 12,* 458–474.

Oswald, I. (1959). Experimental studies of rhythm, anxiety, and cerebral vigilance. *Journal of Mental Science, 105,* 269–294.

Pedroarena, C., Ricciardi, L., Morales, F. R., & Chase, M. (1993). An intracellular analysis of pyramidal tract neuron activity during sleep and wakefulness. *Sleep Research, 22,* 450.

Perry, T. J., & Goldwater, B. C. (1987). A passive behavioral measure of sleep onset in high-alpha and low-alpha subjects. *Psychophysiology, 24,* 657–665.

Rechtschaffen, A., & Foulkes, D. (1965). Effect of visual stimuli on dream content. *Perceptual and Motor Skills, 20,* 1149–1169.

Rechtschaffen, A., & Kales, A. (1968). *A manual of standardized terminology, techniques, and scoring system for sleep stages of human subjects.* Los Angeles: Brain Research Institute.

Siegel, J. M. (1989). Brain-stem mechanisms generating REM sleep. In M. H. Kryger, T. Roth, & W. C. Dement (Eds.), *Principles and practice of sleep medicine* (pp. 104–120). Philadelphia: Saunders.

Simon, C. W., & Emmons, W. H. (1956). Responses to material presented during various levels of sleep. *Journal of Experimental Psychology, 51,* 89–97.

Szymusiak, R. S., & McGinty, D. J. (1990). State-dependent neurophysiology of the basal forebrain: Relationship to sleep, arousal, and thermoregulatory function. In M. Mancia & G. Marini (Eds.), *The diencephalon and sleep* (pp. 101–123). New York: Raven Press.

2

Important Underemphasized Aspects of Sleep Onset

Roger Broughton

Given their apparent importance and relative neglect in the literature, four aspects of the sleep-onset process appear to be in need of emphasis. They are the variety of factors involved, the behavioral and cognitive aspects, circasemidian regulation, and phasic events.

FACTORS AFFECTING THE PROBABILITY OF SLEEP ONSET

Our conceptualizations of sleep–wake regulation typically include only two or three factors, yet the number known to influence sleep and its onset is much higher. These may be classed into chronobiological, sleep pressure (homeostatic), constitutional, behavioral and cognitive, environmental, metabolic, symptomatic, and neuropathological.

Chronobiological influences do not include only the circadian domain associated with core body temperature. The important 2/day (circasemidian) component is discussed in a separate section; ultradian 90–120-min "gates" for sleep onset are also documented [Lavie, 1986]). Moreover, it is evident (Broughton, 1989) that intensity of CNS arousal, based on cerebral activation by brain-stem structures, independently exhibits circadian (Edgar, Dement, & Fuller, 1993) and perhaps circa-semidian (Broughton, 1989) endogenous rhythmicities, and that sleep appears possible only during deactivation below a particular threshold.

Sleep pressure (homeostasis) has been said to reflect exclusively or mainly the duration of prior wakefulness. Yet, findings such as those of Bonnet (1985) indicate that continuity of prior sleep is as important for subsequent measures of sleep pressure as is increased prior wakefulness resulting from nocturnal sleep reduction. Moreover, a homeostatic process that responds only to prior wakefulness does not explain strong evidence for selective rebound after deprivation of slow-wave sleep (SWS) or REM sleep.

Constitutional variables are very important. Age has a remarkable effect on probability of onset of sleep, which evolves from the polyphasic sleep in neonates to the common monophasic pattern in adults. There is evidence for large individual variations in sleep need that, at least in part, appear to be genetic or constitutional. Gender is less important but relevant, given the altered sleep patterns in women during the menstrual cycle.

Behavioral–cognitive factors are particularly important in sleep onset. They include degree of desire to fall asleep or to remain awake, motivation and boredom levels, and prior conditioning (learning). This last factor is considered later. Environmental effects on sleep onset are an everyday reality and yet are often ignored. They include levels of ambient temperature, noise and light, and the presence or absence of repetitive hypnogenic stimuli. Metabolic and toxic factors can be important in health and disease. These include the levels and timing of basic metabolic rate, circulating and brain catecholamines, serum cortisol, serum and brain melatonin, and various sleep-facilitating or -inhibiting toxins and drugs. Symptomatic factors affecting sleep onset include presence or absence of pain, stress and anxiety, mood changes (depression or mania), and intensification of hypnagogic events, including simple sensations, hallucinations, and hypnic jerks.

CNS pathology represents an additional potential factor. Lesions in apparent "sleep centers," such as the preoptic hypothalamus (basal fore-brain area), dorso-medial and anterior thalamic nuclei, and midbrain raphé and medullary tractus solitarius areas, have all been documented as leading to insomnia. Similarly, damage to such wake-maintaining areas as the midbrain-pontine-medullary reticular formation, posterior hypothalamus, and mesial thalamic nuclei appear to facilitate sleep onset and lead to hypersomnia.

Even this brief listing indicates that the number of factors potentially affecting sleep onset is great. One of the goals of current research should be to assess their relative importance in influencing sleep-onset probability, sleep structure, and levels of sleepiness or alertness. In any event, efforts to predict sleep onset probability reliably on the basis of only two or three factors appear unlikely to be universally successful.

BEHAVIORAL AND COGNITIVE ASPECTS OF SLEEP ONSET

The behavioral–cognitive aspects of sleep onset have been particularly underemphasized. As sleep is fundamentally a behavioral state, this is regrettable.

Behavioral patterns during sleep onset are in themselves of interest. A recent personal attempt to review the literature on behaviors during sleep episodes in patients with sleep disorders resulted in few useful articles. In the available descriptions for normal subjects, the emphasis was on progressive sleep onsets that are often stereotyped. These may include preliminary exploration of the sleep habitat, rituals, reduced blinking, yawning, adopting a sleeping position, closing the eyes, executing postural shifts for comfort, decreased muscle tone, and slowing of respiration prior to actual sleep onset. Such patterns are typical of reasonably rested individuals.

Yet, under conditions of extreme sleep deprivation in normal subjects, and in patients with excessive daytime sleepiness, sleep onsets may be abrupt with little warning. Episodes may consist of brief "micro-sleeps" (Guilleminault, Billiard, Montplaisir, & Dement, 1975; Oswald, 1962) with rapid transitions into and out of sleep. More prolonged sleep episodes may occur with observable behaviors characteristic of nonrapid eye movement (NREM) or REM sleep (Broughton, 1974), as in narcolepsy. The subject may also enter an apparent dissociated state indicating a "partial sleep onset" expressed as complex behaviors without awareness or later recall. These have been termed *fuguelike states* by Ganado (1958) and *amnesic automatic behaviors* by Guilleminault et al. (1975). Such patterns raise the interesting possibility of the existence of *pathological sleep onsets* considered abnormal by their abruptness, their overwhelmingly irresistible effects, or their partial nature. More detailed behavioral studies of the varieties of sleep onset using, for instance, videotelemetry would be a valuable contribution to knowledge of the field.

Motivation is definitely a major behavioral determinant of sleep onset. Individuals can love or hate going to sleep. Some find sleep a balm; others resist it from fear of sleep-related experiences or risks or consider it a waste of time. Thus, motivation affects sleep-onset latency. Resistance to instructions to fall asleep will falsify the results of the Multiple Sleep Latency Test (MSLT). Similarly, lack of full effort to remain awake will alter the Maintenance of Wakefulness Test. These tests assume full compliance with the instructions, but no measure of compliance is currently part of either.

Motivation to maintain optimal alertness in the presence of marked sleep pressure is not without consequences. The deleterious effects of sustained efforts to suppress sleepiness and sleep have been little documented. These effects include deteriorating performance (fatigability), increasing sleepiness with higher probability of involuntary sleep episodes, and, upon release of such efforts, rebound-heightened sleepiness and, in narcoleptics, even cataplexy (Valley & Broughton, 1981). The long-term health hazards of chronically fighting off diurnal sleep remain to be documented.

Conditioning and learning also affect sleep onset, yet they are little explored. Pavlov (1929) showed that sleep in animals could occur as a conditioned response. More recently, Sterman and collaborators conditioned cats to fall asleep using both classical conditioning to tones before sleep-inducing basal forebrain stimulation (Clemente, Sterman, & Wyrwicka, 1963) and operant conditioning involving food reward (Sterman, 1963; Sterman, & Shouse, 1985). My own laboratories have found that some normal human subjects can fall asleep with very short sleep latencies on MSLT, yet show no subjective, polysomnographic, or performance features suggesting pathological sleepiness: They are typically habitual nappers with a presumed learned facilitation of falling asleep. Similarly, there is marked individual variability in ability to adapt to extreme ultrashort sleep schedules that require a greatly increased number of sleep onsets per 24 hr (Lavie, 1991b).

Conversely, conditioning can suppress sleep onset. Sterman (1963) and Clemente et al. (1963) also conditioned animals to remain awake by pairing tone stimuli with arousing electrical stimulation of the mesial thalamic nuclei. In clinical practice, conditioned insomnias in which environmental stimuli lead to inability to fall asleep have long been recognized. Bootzin (1985) has introduced a "stimulus-controlled therapy" approach with widely confirmed efficacy in such patients.

In short, individual differences exist in sleep-onset ability. These may reflect, in part, genetic constitutional differences; but it seems certain that they can also reflect a learned skill.

CIRCASEMIDIAN (2/DAY) REGULATION OF SLEEP ONSET

A 2/day regulation of sleep onset and sleep probability is typically expressed as one peak in the middle of the night with a second one in the midafternoon evident in a number of variables, paradigms, and conditions (reviewed in Broughton, 1989; Broughton & Mullington, 1992). These include ontogenetic patterns, phylogeny (especially primate), the siesta phenomenon, adult napping in other contexts, performance on tests sensitive to alertness, accidents attributed to sleepiness, sleep latency around the 24 hr in both the entrained state and the constant routine, sleep probability in temporal isolation studies that permit napping, sleep amount during ultrashort sleep schedules, and sleep distribution in certain clinical sleep disorders such as narcolepsy.

The circasemidian regulation is arguably the most powerful chrono-biological regulatory factor after the circadian one.

Equally impressive as the 2/day increases in sleep probability are the interdigitated two periods of low probability that occur typically in the late morning and, more markedly, in the late afternoon and early evening. Even when heightened sleep pressure from prior sleep deprivation exists, subjects seldom fall asleep at these times. These have been called *wake maintenance zones* (Strogatz, 1986) and, less precisely, *forbidden zones for sleep* (Lavie, 1986).

This circasemidian pattern of alternating periods of high and low sleep probabilities is remarkably stable across experimental paradigms. Figure 1 superimposes the following for young healthy adults: sleep latency in a 24-hr version of the MSLT (Richardson, Carskadon, Orav, & Dement, 1982), sleep latency during the constant routine (Carskadon & Dement, 1992), sleep duration in the ultrashort sleep study (7 min for asleep, 13 min for awake; attempt-sleep version) of Lavie (1986), and probability of sleep during temporal isolation with napping permitted (Zulley & Campbell, 1985). These four different paridigms all show an essentially identical major nocturnal peak in sleep propensity at around 0500–0600 hr, a smaller midafternoon peak at 1530–1600 hr, and a powerful evening minimum around 1900–2100 hr.

The only notable differences occur in the morning. The 24-hr curves of entrained sleep latency and the ultrashort sleep amount are essentially superimposable, undoubtedly because sleep amount in the 7-min scheduled naps converts directly to sleep latency. The longer nighttime sleep in temporal isolation, with its consequent shortening and deepening of the morning wake maintenance zone, may be explained by the totally *ad libitum* nature of sleep in this protocol, which leads to prolongation of the major sleep period. However, the earlier minimum of sleep probability in the constant routine data remains less easily explained.

The shape of the sleep propensity curve around the 24 hr can be approximated by averaging all data with the aberrant early morning temporal isolation and constant routine results removed. The resultant

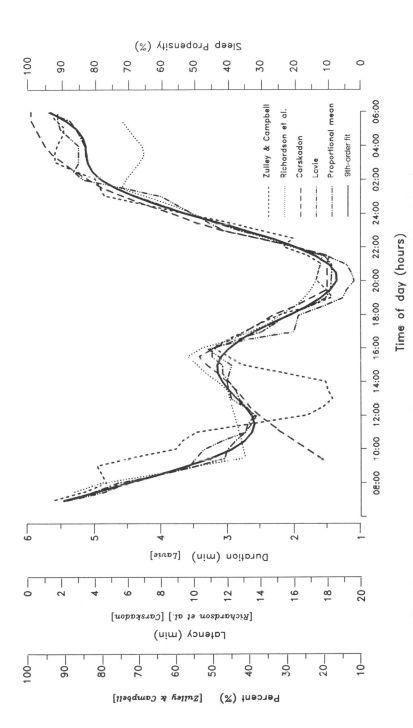

Figure 1

The 24-hr sleep propensity function in young adults. Superimposed are sleep latency (min) in the entrained condition from Richardson et al. (1982) and under a constant routine from Carskadon (unpublished); sleep amount under an ultrashort sleep schedule, attempt sleep version (Lavie, 1986); and sleep probability (%) under temporal isolation with naps permitted (Zulley & Campbell, 1985). All show a virtually identical midafternoon peak, marked early evening trough (wake maintenance zone) and nocturnal peak. The differing morning data for temporal isolation and constant routine were omitted from a proportional mean that was then curve-fitted (continuous line) to describe the function.

curve can then be fitted to derive a descriptive algorithm. To be representative, the curve should explain at least 90% of the variance (Broughton, Campbell, & Dunham, 1993). In Figure 1, this is done using TableCurve (Jandel Scientific, Corte Madre, CA), which compares a large number ($N = 221$) of curve-fitting algorithms with varying assumptions (or none at all).

The best-fit equation involved a ninth-order polynomial regression and explained 99.5% of the variance ($r^2 = .9947$):

$$y = a + bx + cx^2 + dx^3 + ex^4 + fx^5 + gx^6 + hx^7 + ix^8 + jx^9,$$

where $a = 0.994593578$, $b = -0.10960147$, $c = 0.010730631$, $d = -0.00378251$, $e = 0.000676265$, $f = -5.4578e^{-5}$, $g = 2.28901e^{-6}$, $h = -5.2113e^{-8}$, $i = 6.123e^{-10}$, and $j = -2.9133e^{-12}$.

The importance of circasemidian regulation in humans seems to be accepted. It describes a major transitory increase in sleep-onset facilitation during the midday. Under most unmasking circumstances, it is approximately one third as powerful as the circadian variation (Figure 1), and there is evidence that its timing may be altered in certain sleep pathologies (e.g., it is phase advanced in narcolepsy–cataplexy syndrome (Lavie, 1991a; Mullington, Newman, Dunham, & Broughton, 1990; Pollack, Wagner, Moline, & Monk, 1992).

The functional significance of the 2/day phenomenon remains obscure. The following meanings have been suggested: The midday increase may be meant (a) to minimize exposure to the hottest portion of the day, (b) to provide increased flexibility of sleep timing, and (c) to be more efficient in meeting a 24-hr sleep need in two sleep episodes rather than in one.

The mechanism of the circasemidian component has been suggested to be one of the following: a (super)harmonic of the circadian rhythm (Aschoff & Gerkema, 1985; Broughton, 1975), a circa 12-hr rhythm of pressure for SWS (Broughton, 1975), a general evolutionary favoring of fixed-integer ratios (here 2:1) among biological rhythms

(Broughton, 1985), 2/day "gates" of privileged wake-to-sleep transitions (Lavie, 1986), an underlying 2/day rhythm of arousal (Broughton, 1989), and reciprocal inhibition between the two suprachiasmatic nuclei (Pickard & Turek, 1982). Webb (this volume, chapter 4) proposes that it may be explained as a simple combination of homeostatic and circadian processes. This may be so if the circadian process is considered to be one of *arousal* regulated by the suprachiasmatic nuclei as conceptualized by Edgar et al. (1993), rather than by the circadian process-C tested in Borbély, Achermann, Trachsel, and Tobler (1989). The latter model explains poorly both the early morning data and, especially, the evening wake maintenance zone (Broughton & Mullington, 1992). In this context, the nap zone onset would represent the period in time when prior wakefulness has increased sleepiness to a sufficient level to facilitate sleep (process-S), and it is offset the moment in which the circadian arousal process rises sufficiently high to override the sleepiness for several hours.

The importance of the midday increase in sleep propensity is often minimized. This seems to be because, in fully rested individuals, its magnitude is not great. Even when a sleep debt is present, taking naps at this time is optional. Moreover, it is both an everyday experience and a proven biological fact that this transitory period will pass and be followed by one of high alertness. Nevertheless, the robust presence of the phenomenon both in healthy normal subjects and in patients with sleep disorders, and its ontogenetic and phylogenetic persistence, underlie its importance. They also make it mandatory that the mechanisms and functional significance be understood more fully and that the process be incorporated into models predicting sleepiness and probability of sleep onset.

IS SLEEP ONSET A HYPERRESPONSIVE STATE?

In discussing the ongoing tonic features of sleep onset, the transient phasic phenomena have largely been ignored. Indeed, at the Salsamaggiore meeting on phasic events in sleep (Terzano, Halasz, & Declerck, 1991), those at sleep onset were not even considered. Yet, they can be dramatic and may involve motor, sensory, and EEG phenomena, all of which can at times be elicited by external stimuli.

Hypnagogic Massive Jerks

These brief muscular contractions (also called *sleep starts*, *hypnic jerks*, and *predomital myoclonus*) are one of the most impressive phasic phenomena at sleep onset. They involve the entire body or a portion of it in a jerk of greater or lesser intensity. Movement is typically in flexion, then extension. Although usually isolated, the jerks are sometimes repeated. They may awaken the subject, or sleep may continue. At times, hypnagogic jerks are associated with recalled perceptual events, simple *sensory shocks* (discussed later), or interruption of ongoing hypnagogic imagery. They either may be apparently spontaneous or can be provoked by stimuli, whether exteroceptive (Oswald, 1962) or interoceptive, although one reference (McGlade, 1942) quoted by Oswald (1962) referring to an interoceptive trigger clearly involved periodic movements in sleep rather than hypnagogic massive myoclonus.

Hypnagogic massive jerks, when recorded, have nearly always occurred in Stage 1 drowsiness and are usually accompanied by a vertex sharp wave, sometimes followed by an alpha arousal (Oswald, 1959). When multiple superficial EMG leads and full polysomnography have been added (Figure 2), it has been found that the muscles involved show 0.5-s to 1-s duration hypersynchronous potentials (Gastaut & Broughton, 1965; Lugaresi, Cirignotta, Coccagna, & Montagna, 1986) sometimes associated with tachycardia, explosive expiration followed by tachypnea, and an electrodermal response. Prevalence is high: Subjective reports indicate that these jerks are experienced regularly by 10% of individuals, occasionally by 80%, and rarely by 10%. However, as Oswald (1962) pointed out, partner reports are higher.

These events must be differentiated from other forms of myoclonus that may also occur around the time of sleep onset, including the similarly physiologic fragmentary polyclonus of De Lisi and such patho-

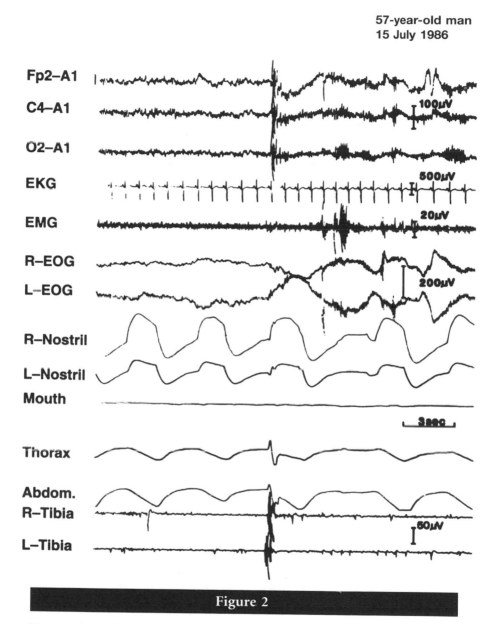

57-year-old man
15 July 1986

Fp2–A1
C4–A1   100μV
O2–A1
EKG   500μV
EMG   20μV
R–EOG
L–EOG   200μV
R–Nostril
L–Nostril
Mouth
    3sec
Thorax
Abdom.
R–Tibia   50μV
L–Tibia

Figure 2

Hypnagogic massive myoclonus. The polysomnogram fragment includes EEG, EKG, submental EMG, oculograms, binasal and mouth airflow, chest and abdominal movement, and bilateral superficial anterior tibialis EMGs. Hypnagogic massive myoclonus occurred in Stage 1 and consisted of a brief hypersynchronous EMG potential seen in the scalp EEG, EOG, and EMG channels associated with sudden expiration and appearance of a diffuse EEG alpha rhythm (arousal).

logical jerks as restless legs, periodic movements in sleep, and epileptic myoclonus. Hypnagogic massive jerks in fact represent a normal phenomenon that is apparently identical to the well-studied startle response (Gogan, 1980; Landis & Hunt, 1939) and its equivalent in the newborn, the Moro reflex. Most investigators of the startle response have considered it to be one of a small group of basic behavioral reflexes that also includes the flexor withdrawal reflex to pain and the orienting response to novel stimuli.

Intensification of hypnagogic massive myoclonus may also occur. Some believe that this may be due to such factors as high caffeine or nicotine consumption, whereas others relate it to nervous personality (Oswald, 1962; Roger, 1931). More important, they may take on medical significance. Accentuation of jerks with recurrent awakening can lead to a form of sleep-onset insomnia first described clinically by Weir Mitchell (1890) and confirmed polygraphically by Broughton (1988). In another medical syndrome, sometimes familial, which combines pathological intensification of startling with loss of its normal habituation upon repeated stimuli (called *startle disease* or the *hyperekplexia syndrome*), spontaneous and stimulus-elicited massive jerks may occur in all sleep stages (Andermann & Andermann, 1986; Gastaut & Broughton, 1972).

Brief Sensory Phenomena

Although much less studied than the phasic motor phenomena, brief *sensory shocks* may also occur at sleep onset (Oswald, 1962). Most common is the sensation of abrupt falling in space, which may be the origin of the expression "falling asleep." Sounds, flashes of light, and other brief simple sensations may occur either in isolation or in association with hypnagogic massive jerks. These events suggest transient activation of sensory as well as of motor mechanisms at sleep onset.

Vertex Sharp Waves

These phasic EEG events often occur during transitional Stage 1 of sleep onset. They are of sufficient amplitude (35–100 μV) to be apparent without averaging in routine EEGs in 30% to 60% of individuals. Vertex sharp waves represent nonspecific evoked responses, although often the eliciting factors are unknown, and they then appear to be "spontaneous." They may occur alone or be repeated in salvos. Yvette Gastaut (1953) and Bancaud, Bloch, & Paillard (1953) contributed detailed topographic studies. The most remarkable feature of these studies is the greatly increased amplitude at sleep onset compared to prior wakefulness. As Niedermeyer (1987, p. 124) said of drowsiness: "Events expressing themselves as evoked potentials, such as the vertex sharp wave, tower over the background activity, whereas the same events have to be extracted by special averaging methods from the electroencephalographic 'noise' of the brain in the waking state."

Our studies using quantitative EEG mapping (Hasan & Broughton, this volume, chapter 13) have shown that the topographic distributions of vertex sharp waves and the sawtooth waves of REM sleep appear identical. The additional fact that vertex sharp waves are a usual accompaniment to both startle responses in wakefulness and hypnagogic massive jerks at sleep onset provides support for the proposal (e.g., Glenn, 1985) that the clusters of phasic activity in REM sleep represent startle patterns that remain partially expressed only because of the normal atonia and paralysis of the REM state. These may be disinhibited clinically in *REM sleep behavior disorder,* during which the motor paralysis is absent and marked generalized (and partial) myoclonus may occur.

The normal intensification of phasic motor, sensory, and EEG phenomena at sleep onset raises several questions. Why should the intensity of the waking startle response be transitorily increased at this time? What are the common and separate neurophysiological mechanisms of these phasic motor, sensory, and EEG events? Does their appearance reflect the actual moment of engagement of mechanisms of sleep onset (or maintenance)? What is the degree of concordance, if any, between the phasic events at sleep onset and those in REM sleep? Above all, why is sleep onset a transitory hyperexcitable state? Does this not help explain the frequent hyperresponsiveness of sleep-deprived individuals?

In closing, I suggest that four of the major challenges concerning sleep onset are to clarify (a) the relative importance, under different conditions, of the numerous factors that can effect sleep onset; (b) the extent and ways in which motivation and learning affect our ability to fall asleep and to resist sleep pressure; (c) the fundamental nature and functional significance of the powerful 2/day circasemidian sleep–wake rhythm; and (d) the apparent transitory hyperexcitable nature of sleep onset and its consequences.

REFERENCES

Andermann, F., & Andermann, E. (1986). Excessive startle syndromes: Startle disease, jumping, and startle epilepsy. In S. Fahn, D. Marsden, & M. Van Woert (Eds.), *Advances in neurology: Vol. 43. Myoclonus* (pp. 321–338). New York: Raven.

Aschoff, J., & Gerkema, M. P. (1985). On diversity and uniformity of ultradian rhythms. In H. Schulz & P. Lavie (Eds.), *Ultradian rhythms in physiology and behavior* (pp. 321–334). Berlin: Springer Verlag.

Bancaud, J., Bloch, V., & Paillard, J. (1953). Contribution EEG à l'étude des potentiels evoqués chez l'homme au niveau de vertex [EEG contribution to the study of evoked potentials in man at the vertex level]. *Revue Neurologique, 89,* 399–418.

Bonnet, M. (1985). The effect of sleep disruption on sleep, performance, and mood. *Sleep, 8,* 11–19.

Bootzin, R. R. (1985). Evaluation of stimulus control instructions, progressive relaxation and sleep hygiene as treatments for insomnia. In W. P. Koella, E. Ruther, & H. Schulz (Eds.), *Sleep '84* (pp. 142–143). Stuttgart, Germany: Fischer.

Borbely, A., Achermann, P., Trachsel, P., & Tobler, I. (1989). Sleep initiation and initial sleep intensity: Interactions of homeostatic and circadian mechanisms. *Journal of Biological Rhythms, 4,* 149–160.

Broughton, R. (1974). Letter to the editor. *Canadian Medical Association Journal, 110,* 1007.

Broughton, R. (1975). Biorhythmic variations in consciousness and psychological functions. *Canadian Journal of Psychology, 16,* 217–230.

Broughton, R. (1985). Three issues concerning ultradian rhythms. In H. Schulz & P. Lavie (Eds.), *Ultradian rhythms in physiology and behavior* (pp. 217–231). Berlin: Springer Verlag.

Broughton, R. (1988). Pathological fragmentary myoclonus, intensified "hypnic jerks" and hypnagogic foot tremor. In W. P. Koella, F. Obal, H. Schulz, & P. Visser (Eds.), *Sleep '86* (pp. 240–243). Stuttgart, Germany: Gustav Fischer.

Broughton, R. (1989). Chronobiological aspects and models of sleep and napping. In D. Dinges & R. Broughton (Eds.), *Sleep and alertness* (pp. 71–98). New York: Raven.

Broughton, R., Campbell, S., & Dunham, W. (1993). Curve fitting of chronobiological data: Some issues and techniques. *Sleep Research, 22*, 395.

Broughton, R., & Mullington, J. (1992). Circadian sleep propensity and the phase-amplitude maintenance model of human sleep/wake regulation. *Journal of Sleep Research, 1*, 93–98.

Carskadon, M. A., & Dement, W. C. (1992). Multiple sleep latency tests during the constant routine. *Sleep, 15*, 396–399.

Clemente, C. D., Sterman, M. B., & Wyrwicka, W. (1963). Inhibitory mechanisms: Conditioning of the basal forebrain induced EEG synchronization and sleep. *Experimental Neurology, 7*, 404–417.

Edgar, D. M., Dement, W. C., & Fuller, C. A. (1993). Effect of SCN lesions on sleep in squirrel monkeys: Evidence for opponent processes in sleep–wake regulation. *Journal of Neuroscience, 13*, 1065–1079.

Ganado, W. (1958). The narcolepsy syndrome. *Neurology, 7*, 197–221.

Gastaut Y. (1953). Les pointes negatives evoquées sur le vertex [Negative points evoked on the vertex]. *Revue Neurologique, 89*, 382–398.

Gastaut, H., & Broughton, R. (1965). A clinical and polygraphic study of episodic phenomena during sleep. *Recent Advances in Biological Psychiatry, 7*, 197–221.

Gastaut, H., & Broughton, R. (1972). *Epileptic seizures.* Springfield, MA: Charles C. Thomas.

Glenn, L. L. (1985). Brainstem and spinal control of lower limb motoneurons with special reference to phasic events and startle reflexes. In D. J. McGinty, R. Drucker-Colin, A. Morrison, & P. L. Parmeggiani (Eds.), *Brain mechanisms of sleep* (pp. 81–96). New York: Raven.

Gogan, P. (1980). The startle response and orienting response in man. *Brain Research, 18*, 117–135.

Guilleminault, C., Billiard, M., Montplaisir, J., & Dement, W. C. (1975). Altered states of conciousness in disorders of daytime sleepiness. *Journal of Neurological Sciences, 26*, 377–393.

Landis, C., & Hunt, W. A. (1939). *The startle pattern.* New York: Farrar & Rinehart.

Lavie, P. (1986). Ultrashort sleep–waking schedule: Part 3. Gates and "forbidden zones" for sleep. *Electroencephalography and Clinical Neurophysiology, 63*, 414–425.

Lavie, P. (1991a). REM cyclicity under ultrashort sleep/wake cycle in narcoleptic patients. *Canadian Journal of Psychology, 45*, 185–193.

Lavie, P. (1991b). The 24-hour sleep propensity function (SPF): Practical and theoretical implications. In T. Monk (Ed.), *Sleep, sleepiness and performance* (pp. 65–96). New York: Wiley.

Lugaresi, E., Cirignotta, F., Coccagna, G., & Montagna, P. (1986). Nocturnal myoclonus and restless legs syndrome. In S. Fahn, D. Marsden, and M. Van Woert (Eds.), *Advances in neurology: Vol. 43. Myoclonus* (pp. 295–307). New York: Raven.

McGlade, H. B. (1942). The relationship between gastric motility, muscular twitching during sleep and dreaming. *American Journal of Digestive Diseases, 9*, 137–140.

Mitchell, S. W. (1890). Some disorders of sleep. *International Journal of Medical Science, 100*, 109–120.

Mullington, J., Newman, J., Dunham, W., & Broughton, R. (1990). Phase timing and duration of naps in narcolepsy–cataplexy. In J. Horne (Ed.), *Sleep '90* (pp. 158–160). Bochum, Germany: Pontenagel.

Niedermeyer, E. (1987). Sleep and EEG. In E. Niedermeyer & F. Lopes da Silva (Eds.), *Electroencephalography* (pp. 93–105). Baltimore: Urban & Schwarzenberg.

Oswald, I. (1959). Sudden body jerks on falling asleep. *Brain, 82*, 92–103.

Oswald, I. (1962). *Sleeping and waking: Physiology and psychology.* Amsterdam: Elsevier.

Pavlov, I. P. (1929). *Conditioned reflexes.* Oxford, England: Oxford University Press.

Pickard, G. E., & Turek, F. W. (1982). Splitting of the circadian rhythms of activity is abolished by unilateral lesions of the suprachiasmatic nuclei. *Science, 215*, 1119–1121.

Pollack, C. P., Wagner, D., Moline, M., & Monk, T. (1992). Cognitive and motor performance of narcoleptic and normal subjects living in temporal isolation. *Sleep, 15*, 202–211.

Richardson, G. S., Carskadon, M. A., Orav, E. J., & Dement, W. C. (1982). Circadian variations of sleep tendency in elderly and young adult subjects. *Sleep, 5*, S82–S94.

Roger, H. (1931). Les secousses nerveuses de l'endormissement [Muscular twitching during sleep]. *Revue de Médecine Française, 12*, 847–852.

Sterman, M. B. (1963). *Basic mechanisms in sleep*. Unpublished doctoral thesis, University of California, Los Angeles.

Sterman, M. B., & Shouse, M. N. (1985). Sleep "centers" in the brain: The preoptic basal forebrain area revisited. In D. J. McGinty, R. Drucker-Colin, A. Morrison, & P. L. Parmeggiani (Eds.), *Brain mechanisms in sleep* (pp. 227–299). New York: Raven.

Strogatz, S. H. (1986). The mathematical structure of the human sleep–wake cycle. *Lecture notes in mathematics, No. 69*. Berlin: Springer-Verlag.

Terzano, M. G., Halasz, P., & Declerck, A. C. (Eds.). (1991). *Phasic events and dynamic organization of sleep*. New York: Raven.

Valley, V., & Broughton, R. (1981). Daytime performance deficits and physiological vigilance in untreated patients with narcolepsy–cataplexy syndrome. *Revue d'EEG et Neurophysiologie Clinique, 11*, 133–139.

Zulley, J., & Campbell, S. (1985). Napping behavior during "spontaneous internal desynchronization." *Human Neurobiology, 4*, 123–126.

3

Immune–Neuroendocrine– Thermal Mechanisms and the Sleep–Wake System

Harvey Moldofsky

Although the physiologic and behavioral correlates to the induction of sleep have been the subject of detailed inquiry for almost four decades, little is known about the questions of why we fall asleep and why we need to sleep or about their corollaries, why we awaken and why we remain awake. The physiologic and behavioral methodologies involve observations of electrophysiologic correlates with changes in performance to characterize the transitions between wakefulness and sleep. Similar methods are used to examine the transitions between states of sleep that are defined as nonrapid eye movement (NREM), or quiet sleep, and rapid eye movement (REM), or dreaming sleep. Such studies in animals and humans have resulted in theoretical models that attempt to account for the timing of such transitions. For example, McCarley and Hobson (1975) proposed a model whereby reciprocal interactions of two chemically defined neuronal groups within the brain result in the oscillations between NREM and REM cycles. Wever (1985, 1987) suggested that the interaction between two oscillators, one cir-

Preparation of this chapter was supported by Medical Research Council of Canada Grant MA-11685.

cadian and one ultradian, simulate the sleep–wake and the NREM–REM cycles. Borbély and colleagues proposed that the timing and duration of sleep are regulated by a two-process model (Achermann & Borbély, 1990; Borbély, 1982; Daan, Beersma, & Borbély, 1984). A homeostatic process, termed *Process S*, increases exponentially during wakefulness and declines exponentially during sleep within the limits set by a circadian process, *Process C*. The time course of Process S relies on measurements of slow wave sleep (SWS) or delta activity of the electroencephalogram (EEG) during sleep episodes over the course of the day. The derived mathematical formulas result in descriptions of the timing of sleep, as well as in the changes of SWS within NREM sleep. However, none of these descriptive theoretical models provides any information on the fundamental mechanisms that underlie the cause and function of the sleeping–waking brain. Recent studies in animals and humans have shown that the coordination of aspects of the immune, neuroendocrine, and temperature rhythms are intimately tied to the sleep–wake brain–behavioral system. In this chapter, I propose to summarize the evidence for the harmonious interrelationship of the circadian pattern of the immune, endocrine, thermal, and sleep–wake systems as important to the cause and function of sleep.

ANIMAL STUDIES

Researchers have shown that specific immunologically active peptides, neuroendocrines, or thermal processes influence the CNS sleep–wake system. However, these endogenous processes do not operate in isolation from one another. There is considerable evidence for a molecular basis for the bidirectional communication between the immune and neuroendocrine systems (Blalock, 1989; Daruna & Morgan, 1990; Dunn, 1989). Not only do aspects of the immune and endocrine systems interact, but various functions of these systems influence or are influenced by the sleeping–waking brain.

The list of specific sleep-promoting immunologically active peptides continues to expand. Initially, Krueger, Pappenheimer, and Karnovsky

(1982) identified a sleep-promoting factor isolated from animals. This substance, Factor S, was shown to be a muramyl peptide (Krueger, Karnovsky, et al., 1984; Pappenheimer, 1983). Subsequently, Factor S was shown to stimulate the production of interleukin-1 (IL-1), an endogenous pyrogenic agent (Krueger, Dinarello, & Chedid, 1983). Initially, it was thought that muramyl peptides were exogenous because they are products of the cell walls of bacteria. However, muramyl peptides also occur endogenously in mammalian tissues and fluids (Krueger, Walter, et al., 1984). Pappenheimer (1983) proposed that muramyl peptide products of bacteria are absorbed through the intestinal wall. The somnolent and pyrogenic effects of muramyl dipeptide that occur through the agency of IL-1 (Krueger, Karnovsky, et al., 1984; Krueger, Walter, et al., 1984; Pappenheimer, 1983) are thought to be mediated by the CNS serotonergic system (Masek & Kadlec, 1983). The link to thermal effects of IL-1 could be disengaged by an antipyretic agent without affecting the sleep-promoting influence of IL-1 (Krueger, Karnovsky, et al., 1984). Nevertheless, no muramyl peptide or product of IL-1 has been found that preserves the somnogenic effect without increasing body temperature (Krueger, Walter, et al., 1984).

Despite the importance of IL-1 to CNS and peripheral functions of the immune system and to the hypothalamic–pituitary axis of the neuroendocrine system (Krueger, 1990), no specific sleep center has been identified with injections of IL-1 into various regions of the third ventricle of the brain stem (Walter, Meyers, & Krueger, 1989). However, cerebrospinal fluid measures of IL-1 are increased during sleep compared to wakefulness in cats (Lue et al., 1988). In addition to IL-1, other sleep-promoting, immunologically active peptides have been uncovered. These include IL-2 (De Sarro, Masuda, Ascioti, Audino, & Nistico, 1990), alpha interferon (De Sarro et al., 1990; Krueger et al., 1987), tumor necrosis factor (Shoham, Davenne, Cady, Dinarello, & Krueger, 1987), prostaglandin D_2 (Ueno, Honda, Inoue, & Hayaishi, 1983), and vasoactive intestinal peptide (Graf & Kastin, 1984; Yehuda, 1986). Another immunologic peptide, prostaglandin E_2, promotes wakefulness in various animals (Hayaishi, 1991). Hayaishi proposed that prostaglandin D_2 and E_2 have a reciprocal influence on the sleep–wake system (Hayaishi, 1991). On the other hand, Krueger, Kapás, Opp, and Obál (1992) were unable to show any significant effect of these two peptides on the EEG sleep–wake physiology of rabbits. Krueger (1990) argued against Hayaishi's specific prostaglandin humoral model for the induction of sleep and wakefulness and proposed that IL-1 is involved in a complex interaction of the various immunologic active peptides and neuroendocrine substances that influence the sleeping–waking brain.

Hormones have been identified that inhibit or promote sleep. Those that inhibit IL-1 and sleep include corticotropin-releasing factor, adrenocorticotropic hormone, alpha melanocyte–stimulating hormone, and glucocorticoids. Those that stimulate IL-1 and promote sleep include insulin, growth hormone (GHRH) releasing factor, growth hormone, somatostatin, and melatonin (Krueger, 1990). The intimate link among IL-1, neurohormones, and sleep is shown by the demonstration that a specific hormone, GHRH, along with IL-1, promotes sleep. Sleep is reduced if the production of GHRH and IL-1 are inhibited by specific antibodies or peptide antagonists (Krueger & Obál, 1993).

Recently, Krueger proposed a neuronal group selection theory of sleep that takes into consideration activation of the brain glial cells that would promote an IL-1 stimulating and IL-1 receptor antagonist system. The net effect would be to produce an oscillatory activation–inactivation cycle that would, in turn, influence local synapses of the CNS. Recruitment of similar neuronal elements would result in the promotion of NREM sleep. Sleep would stabilize the competitive IL-1 agonist–antagonist processes, with the result that wakefulness would emerge. Tissue growth factors, such as GHRH, growth hormone, and insulin-like growth factor, are involved in the neuronal group mechanism. Such an interplay of a neuronal coordinating mechanism with anabolic peptides is proposed to be important in regulating the sleep–wake system and tissue growth and repair (Krueger & Obál, 1993). Furthermore, the promotion of NREM SWS induces brain and body cooling, which results in lower energy use, reduced cerebral metabolism, protection of the brain against elevated temperatures of wakeful-ness, and facilitation of immune defense processes. This thermoregu-latory influence of sleep is organized in the medial preoptic region of the anterior hypothalamus and basal forebrain neuronal network (McGinty & Szymusiak, 1990). The increased production of IL-1 with sleep may contribute to the thermoregulatory processes. Possibly, tem-perature-sensitive regions of the hypothalamus are stimulated so that body temperature would begin to rise during the latter part of noctur-nal sleep, when REM sleep is more evident and cortisol production increases.

The sleep–immune–neuroendocrine–thermal system is especially prominent when homeostatic influences are challenged, such as by in-fection. Toth and Krueger (1989) showed that the pyrogenic and som-nogenic effects of microbial challenge depend on the type of infectious organism and the route of its administration in the animal. For ex-ample, *E. coli*, administered intravenously to rabbits, produced a more rapid increase in SWS than when the animals were inoculated with *S. aureus* (Toth & Krueger, 1989). These authors also showed that the induction of pasteurellosis in rabbits by intranasal administration fa-cilitated a later and longer somnogenic and pyrogenic effect than when this pathogen was given by intravenous injection (Toth & Krueger, 1990).

The homeostatic influence of sleep on these infectious challenges to the organism is shown to occur in animals that have been sleep deprived. Brown, Pang, Husband, and King (1989) showed that sleep-deprived mice that were administered influenza virus, after they had been immunized previously with the virus, had the virus particles in their lungs. On the other hand, those mice that were not deprived of sleep did not have any evidence of the virus in their lungs. These au-thors showed that rats challenged with sheep red blood cells following eight hours of sleep deprivation showed reduced antibody responses three days later. However, IL-1 and muramyl dipeptide prevented this decreased antibody response (Brown, Price, King, & Husband, 1989). Toth and Krueger (1990) showed that the duration and amount of SWS produced by an infectious organism influenced the survival from infection in animals. Animals that had reduced SWS and high levels of plasma cortisone showed a much higher mortality than those that had increased SWS and low cortisone levels. In parallel with these studies is the important observation that rats died when they were deprived of sleep for an average of 21 days. Over that time, the rats showed a hypermetabolic state, skin lesions, hypoalbuminemia, and loss of body weight. Just prior to death, core temperature declined and there was impaired heat production (Rechtschaffen, Bergmann, Everson, Kushida, & Gilliland, 1989). Until recently, the etiology of the death of these prolonged sleep-deprived animals was unknown. Everson (1993) showed that such animals harbored opportunistic microbes, but had no febrile response. These animal studies show not only the interplay between the CNS sleep–wake system and the immune–neuroendocrine–thermal system, but also that organ functions are safeguarded against disease and death by these CNS regulatory operations.

HUMAN STUDIES

Clinical research studies have shown circadian variations in the cellular immune system. Eosinophils, mononuclear cells, lymphocytes, and T and B cells were found to increase between 2400 hr and 0200 hr (Bertouch, Roberts-Thompson, & Bradley, 1983; Haus, Lakatua, Swoyer, & Sackett-Lundeen, 1983; Pownall, 1984; Ross, Pollak, Akman, & Bachur, 1980). One study did not show circadian variations in polymorphonuclear phagocytosis (Bongrand, Bouvent, Bartolin, Tatossian, & Bruguerolle, 1988). The major difficulties in interpreting these studies are as follows: They rely on infrequent blood sampling over 24 hr (as few as four and often no more than six samples per day); statistical extrapolations are based on the questionable assumption of a diurnal cosinor function; and there are few or no overnight samples and no references to sleep physiology.

By analyzing immune functions and hormones from serial, repeated blood samples while monitoring diurnal sleep–wake physiology, aspects of cytokines, peripheral cellular immune functions, and neuroendocrines were shown to be linked to sleep and wakefulness in humans. Plasma IL-1 and IL-2 activities were found to be related to the sleep–wake cycle and not to the external clock time. Maximal plasma IL-1 activity occurred at sleep onset and was greater during SWS than during daytime waking, wakefulness after bedtime lights out, and Stages 1 and 2 sleep (Moldofsky, Lue, Eisen, Keystone, & Gorczynski, 1986). Covelli et al. (1992) confirmed and extended these initial findings. They observed that the nocturnal rise of plasma IL-1β occurred during undisturbed sleep. On the other hand, plasma IL-1β was not detected in two subjects whose sleep was disturbed. Plasma beta-endorphin was inversely related to IL-1β. These authors suggested that stressful situations that would disturb sleep might result in a negative feedback influence of the corticotropin-releasing hormone on IL-1β. In a study of 12 men (Gudewill et al., 1992), measures of plasma IL-1β and IL-6 were not detected in four subjects from 1900 hr to 0700 hr. In the others, IL-1 and IL-6 exceeded the detection limit of the assays more frequently during nocturnal sleep than during the wakefulness period before sleep. No temporal association of these cytokines was found with stages of sleep. Furthermore, the plasma tumor necrosis factor-α (TNF-α) was distributed randomly throughout the night and was not specifically associated with sleep.

Although IL-1 appears to be related to sleep, the type and sensitivity of the assay, the presence of unknown and known inhibitors (e.g., IL-1β receptor antagonist), feedback mechanisms involving the hypothalamic–pituitary–neuroendocrine axis, and sleep disturbances remain to be clarified. Whereas IL-6 was shown to be related to sleep in humans, this cytokine was not shown to promote sleep in rabbits (Opp, Obál, & Krueger, 1989). Similarly, whereas TNF-α was somnogenic in these animals, plasma levels of TNF-α (Shoham et al., 1987) did not vary with wakefulness and sleep in humans (Gudewill et al., 1992). Additional studies are required in various mammalian species to determine the specificity of CNS infusions of various cytokines for sleep promotion or association of plasma measures of IL-1 and other cytokines to sleep–wake behavior.

Thus far, all the human studies have focused on the natural occurrence of changes in cytokines and peripheral immune measures with the normal daytime wake and nocturnal sleep physiology. Because these nocturnal effects could not be distinguished from diurnal chronobiologic influences, Shahal et al. (1994) examined the diurnal influence of two-hour naps scheduled at six-hour intervals beginning at midnight. They showed that irrespective of time of day, plasma IL-1 tended to be higher in Stage 4 SWS than in wakefulness. However, plasma IL-1 levels may not be specifically linked to sleep behavior. In subjects who remained awake for 40 hr, the predisposition to nocturnal sleepiness may have been influenced by increased plasma IL-1 activity during the night of deprived sleep, when plasma IL-1 was compared to baseline nocturnal sleep and resumed sleep on the third night (Moldofsky, Lue, Davidson, & Gorczynski, 1989).

Aspects of peripheral cellular immune functions vary with sleep and wakefulness. In our initial study of young men, B-cell lymphocyte responsiveness, assessed with the in vitro pokeweed mitogen (PWM) assay, showed greater activity during nocturnal sleep. Natural killer (NK) cell activity declined precipitously following sleep onset and reached its lowest levels during Stage 4 SWS (Moldofsky et al., 1986). The reason for the diminished activity is unknown. There may be reduction in NK cell function with sleep. Another possibility is that many NK cells may disappear from the peripheral circulation, to be distributed in the tissues to perform immune surveillance and lysis of pathogenic cells. A similar sleep-related decline in NK functional activity was observed in healthy young women. However, the timing of the decline was related to plasma progesterone. With low plasma progesterone, the nocturnal pattern of decline of NK activity was similar to that of the young men. During the phase of the menstrual cycle in which the plasma progesterone was elevated, Stage 4 SWS was delayed and reduced, as were the NK activities (Moldofsky, Lue, Shahal, Jiang, & Gorczynski, 1991).

The association of these cellular functions with sleep was assessed further in studies of the influence of nocturnal sleep deprivation and of napping at various times during the day. Early clinical studies showed that peripheral immune functions were altered following sleep deprivation. Seventy-two hours of sleep deprivation resulted in reduced phagocytosis by polymorphonuclear granulocytes, increased interferon production by lymphocytes, and increased plasma cortisol (Palmblad et al., 1976). Forty-eight hours of wakefulness were followed by reduced phytohaemagglutinin (PHA) mitogen response (Palmblad, Petrini, Wasserman, & Åkerstedt, 1979). However, these studies were flawed by their reliance on single morning blood samples and by the emotional distress of the experimental procedure.

Our study of the effects of 40 hr of wakefulness showed not only increased plasma IL-1 and IL-2 functions during the night of wakefulness but also dramatic changes in cellular immune functions. The nocturnal rise of PWM response that occurred during the normal baseline 24-hr wake–sleep cycle was delayed by sleep deprivation. The diurnal PHA mitogen response showed no change with sleep loss. The activity of NK cells did not decline during nocturnal wakefulness, as it had during baseline sleep. The NK activity remained reduced throughout the night of resumed sleep. These changes in peripheral immune functions were unrelated to changes in the circadian pattern of cortisol, thus indicating that the changes did not occur as the result of possible physiological stress from the procedures that were used in the study (Moldofsky, Lue, Davidson, & Gorczynski, 1989).

In our 64-hr study of the effects of prolonged wakefulness, there was disruption of the normal undisturbed diurnal pattern of PWM and NK cell activities. Furthermore, two of the five subjects who participated in the study experienced upper respiratory infections, and one subject encountered asthmatic symptoms for the first time within the week that followed the study (Moldofsky, Lue, Davidson, Jephthah-Ochola, et al., 1989). These studies showed that sleep deprivation does alter the diurnal pattern of cellular and humoral immune functions. Although the observations were anecdotal, sleep deprivation may predispose some vulnerable people to infectious illness. This notion is consistent with the animal experimental studies.

By displacing sleep to two-hour naps at six-hour time intervals starting at 2400 hr and concluding after the 1800-hr nap, NK activity was found to be associated with sleep (Shahal, Lue, Jiang, MacLean, & Moldofsky, 1992). That is, whenever the subjects slept, there was a coincident decline in NK activity. NK activity was least during Stage-4 sleep versus wakefulness. Although rectal temperature and plasma cortisol showed the typical reduction during the night and early morning rise, both the temperature and plasma cortisol were reduced during the naps compared to wakefulness. Plasma IL-1 activity was higher during Stage 4 sleep versus wakefulness. There were no specific sleep-related changes with plasma IL-1 receptor antagonist and IL-2 or responses to PHA and PWM. This study demonstrates that aspects of cellular (NK cells) and humoral (IL-1) activity are related to sleep rather than to diurnal influences. Plasma cortisol and temperature showed both diurnal and sleep-related effects.

SUMMARY AND CONCLUSIONS

The data from both animal and human studies show that certain cytokines (e.g., IL-1) and aspects of peripheral immune cellular functions (e.g., NK cell activities), together with neuroendocrine and thermal functions, are intimately connected to the circadian sleep–wake system. Sleep deprivation not only perturbs these brain and peripheral functions but may also predispose subjects to disease. The harmonious interrelationship of the sleeping–waking brain with the immune–neuroendocrine and thermal mechanisms are shown to be important for the cause and function of sleep.

REFERENCES

Achermann, P., & Borbély, A. A. (1990). Simulation of human sleep: Ultradian dynamics of electroencephalographic slow-wave activity. *Journal of Biological Rhythms, 5,* 141–157.

Bertouch, J. V., Roberts-Thompson, P., & Bradley, J. (1983). Diurnal variation of lymphocyte subsets identified by monoclonal antibodies. *British Medical Journal, 286,* 1171–1172.

Blalock, J. E. (1989). A molecular basis for bidirectional communication between the immune and neuroendocrine systems. *Physiological Reviews, 69,* 1–32.

Bongrand, P., Bouvent, G., Bartolin, R., Tatossian, J., & Bruguerolle, B. (1988). Are there circadian variations in polymorphonuclear phagocytosis in men? *Chronobiology International, 5,* 81–83.

Borbély, A.A. (1982). A two-process model of sleep regulation. *Human Neurobiology, 1,* 195–204.

Brown, R., Pang, G., Husband, A. J., & King, M. G. (1989). Suppression of immunity to influenza virus infection in the respiratory tract following sleep deprivation. *Regulatory Immunology, 2,* 321–325.

Brown, R., Price, R. J., King, M. G., & Husband, A. J. (1989). Interleukin-1β and muramyl dipeptide can prevent decreased antibody response associated with sleep deprivation. *Brain Behavior and Immunity, 3,* 320–330.

Covelli, V., Massari, F., Fallarca, C., Munno, I., Jirrilo, F., Savastano, S., Tommaselli, A., & Lombardi, G. (1992). Interleukin-1 beta and beta endorphin circadian rhythms are inversely relaxed in normal and stress-altered sleep. *International Journal of Neuroscience, 63,* 299–305.

Daan, S., Beersma, D. G. M., & Borbély, A. A. (1984). Timing of human sleep: Recovery process gated by a circadian pacemaker. *American Journal of Physiology, 246,* R161–R183.

Daruna, J. H., & Morgan, J. E. (1990). Psychosocial effects on immune function: Neuroendocrine pathways. *Psychosomatics, 31,* 4–12.

De Sarro, G. B., Masuda, Y., Ascioti, C., Audino, M. G., & Nistico, G. (1990). Behavioral and E CoG spectrum changes induced by intracerebral infusion of interferons and interleukin-2 in rats are antagonized by naloxone. *Neuropharmacology, 29,* 167–179.

Dunn, A. J. (1989). Psychoneuroimmunology for the psychoneuroendocrinologist: A review of animal studies of nervous system–immune system interactions. *Psychoneuroendocrinology, 14,* 251–274.

Everson, C. A. (1993). Sustained sleep deprivation impairs host defense. *American Journal of Physiology, 265,* R1148–R1154.

Graf, M. V., & Kastin, A. J. (1984). Delta-sleep-inducing peptide (DSIP): A review. *Neuroscience Biobehavior Review, 8,* 83–93.

Gudewill, S., Pollmächer, T., Vedder, H., Schreiber, W., Fassbender, K., & Holsboer, F. (1992). Nocturnal plasma levels of cytokines in healthy men. *European Archives of Psychiatry and Clinical Neuroscience, 242,* 53–56.

Haus, E., Lakatua, D. J., Swoyer, J., & Sackett-Lundeen, L. (1983). Chronobiology in haematology and immunology. *American Journal of Anatomy, 168,* 467–517.

Hayaishi, O. (1991). Molecular mechanisms of sleep–wake regulation: Roles of prostaglandins D_2 and E_2. *FASEB Journal, 5,* 2575–2581.

Krueger, J. M. (1990). Somnogenic activity of immune response modifiers. *TIPS, 11,* 122–126.

Krueger, J. M., Dinarello, C. A., & Chedid, L. (1983). Promotion of slow wave sleep (SWS) by a purified interleukin-1 (IL-1) preparation. *Federation Proceedings, 42,* 356.

Krueger, J. M., Dinarello, C. A., Shoham, S., Davenne, D., Walter, J., & Kubillus, S. (1987). Interferon α-2 enhances slow wave sleep in rabbits. *International Journal of Immunopharmacology, 9,* 23–30.

Krueger, J. M., Kapás, L., Opp, M.R., & Obál, F. (1992). Prostaglandin E_2 and D_2 have little effect on rabbit sleep. *Physiology Behavior, 51,* 481–485.

Krueger, J. M., Karnovsky, M. L., Martin, S. A., Pappenheimer, J. R., Walter, J., & Biemann, K. (1984). Peptidoglycans as promoters of slow wave sleep: Part 2. Somnogenic and pyrogenic activities of some naturally occurring muramyl peptides: Correlations with mass spectrometric structure determination. *Journal of Biological Chemistry, 259,* 12659–12662.

Krueger, J. M., & Obál, F. (1993). A neuronal group theory of sleep function. *Journal of Sleep Research, 2,* 63–69.

Krueger, J. M., Pappenheimer, J. R., & Karnovsky, M. L. (1982). The composition of sleep-promoting factor isolated from human urine. *Journal of Biological Chemistry, 259,* 1664–1669.

Krueger, J. M., Walter, J., Karnovsky, M. L., Chedid, L., Choay, J. P., Lefrancier, P., & Lederer, E. (1984). Muramyl peptides: Variation of somnogenic activity with structure. *Journal of Experimental Medicine, 159,* 68–76.

Lue, F. A., Bail, M., Jephthah-Ochola, J., Carayanniotis, K., Gorczynski, R. M., &

Moldofsky, H. (1988). Sleep and cerebrospinal fluid interleukin-1 like activity in the cat. *International Journal of Neuroscience, 42*, 179–183.

Masek, K., & Kadlec, O. (1983). Sleep factor, muramyl peptides, and the serotoninergic system. *Lancet, 2*, 1277.

McCarley, R. W., & Hobson, J. A. (1975). Neuronal excitability modulation over the sleep–wake cycle: A structural and mathematical model. *Science, 189*, 58–60.

McGinty, D., & Szymusiak, R. (1990). Keeping cool: A hypothesis about the mechanisms and functions of slow wave sleep. *Trends in Neuroscience, 13*, 480–487.

Moldofsky, H., Lue, F. A., Davidson, J. R., & Gorczynski, R. (1989). Effects of sleep deprivation on human immune functions. *FASEB Journal, 3*, 1972–1977.

Moldofsky, H., Lue, F. A., Davidson, J. R., Jephthah-Ochola, J., Carayanniotis, K., & Gorczynski, R. (1989). The effect of 64 hours of wakefulness on immune functions and plasma cortisol in humans. In J. Horne (Ed.), *Sleep '88* (pp. 185–187). New York: Gustav Fischer Verlag.

Moldofsky, H., Lue, F. A., Eisen, J., Keystone, E. C., & Gorczynski, R. M. (1986). The relationship of interleukin-1 and immune function to sleep in humans. *Psychosomatic Medicine, 48*, 309–318.

Moldofsky, H., Lue, F., Shahal, B., Jiang, C. G., & Gorczynski, R. M. (1991). Circadian immune functions and the menstrual cycle in healthy women. *Sleep Research, 20A*, 552.

Opp, M., Obál, F., Jr., & Krueger, J. M. (1989). Corticotropin-releasing factor attenuates interleukin-1-induced sleep and fever in rabbits. *American Journal of Physiology, 257*, R528–R535.

Palmblad, J., Cantell, K., Strander, H., Froberg, J., Karlsson, C. G., Levi, L., Granstom, M., & Unger, P. (1976). Stressor exposure and immunological response in man: Interferon producing capacity and phagocytosis. *Journal of Psychosomatic Research, 20*, 193–199.

Palmblad, J., Petrini, B., Wasserman, J., & Åkerstedt, T. (1979). Lymphocyte and granulocyte reactions during sleep deprivation. *Psychosomatic Medicine, 41*, 273–278.

Pappenheimer, J. R. (1983). Induction of sleep by muramyl peptides. *Journal of Physiology, 335*, 1–11.

Pownall, R. (1984). Biological rhythms in cell-mediated immunity: Their relevance in rheumatology. *British Journal of Clinical Practitioners, 33*(Suppl.), 20–23.

Rechtschaffen, A. W. S., Bergmann, B. M., Everson, C. A., Kushida, C. A., & Gilliland, M. A. (1989). Sleep deprivation in the rat: Integration and discussion of the findings. *Sleep, 12*, 68–87.

Ross, D., Pollak, A., Akman, S. A., & Bachur, N. R. (1980). Diurnal variation of circulating human myoloid progenitor cells. *Experimental Hematology, 8*, 954–960.

Shahal, B., Jiang, C. G., Lue, F. A., MacLean, A. W., Gorczynski, R. M., & Moldofsky, H. (1994). *Immune functions in sleep and wakefulness during naps.* Manuscript submitted for publication.

Shahal, B., Lue, F. A., Jiang, C. G., MacLean, A., & Moldofsky, H. (1992). Circadian and sleep–wake related changes in immune functions. *Journal of Sleep Research, 1*(Suppl.), 210.

Shoham, S., Davenne, D., Cady, A. B., Dinarello, C. A., & Krueger, J. M. (1987). Recombinant tumor necrosis factor and interleukin-1 enhance slow wave sleep. *American Journal of Physiology, 253*, R142–R149.

Toth, L. A., & Krueger, J. M. (1989). Effects of microbial challenge on sleep in rabbits. *FASEB Journal, 3*, 2062–2066.

Toth, L. A., & Krueger, J. M. (1990). Somnogenic, pyrogenic thematologic effects of experimental pasteurellosis in rabbits. *American Journal of Physiology, 258*, R536–R542.

Ueno, R., Honda, K., Inoue, S., & Hayaishi, O. (1983). Prostaglandin D_2, a cerebral sleep-inducing substance in rats. *Proceedings of the National Academy of Science, 80*, 1735–1737.

Walter, J. S., Meyers, P., & Krueger, J. M. (1989). Microinjection of interleukin-1 into brain: Separation of sleep and fever response. *Physiologic Behavior, 45*, 169–176.

Wever, R. A. (1985). Modes of interaction between ultradian and circadian rhythms: Towards a mathematical model of sleep. *Experimental Brain Research* (Suppl.), 309–317.

Wever, R. A. (1987). Mathematical models of circadian one- and multioscillator systems. In G. A. Carpenter (Ed.), *Lectures on mathematics in the life sciences. Some mathematical questions in biology: Circadian rhythms* (pp. 205–265). Providence, RI: American Mathematical Society.

Yehuda, S. (1986). *DSIP—Physiological, pharmacological and immunological effects.* New York: Academy of Sciences.

PART TWO

Predictive Models

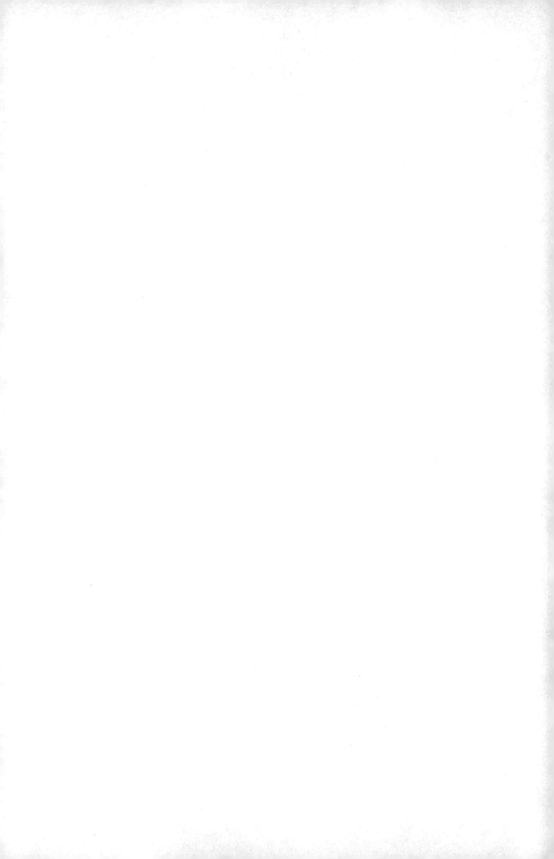

4

Prediction of Sleep Onset

Wilse B. Webb

Aristotle informed us that we may have wisdom about a phenomenon in four ways: formal, material, efficient, and final. Thus, we may know about a tree by its formal characteristics (shape, leaves, etc.), its material characteristics (physical and cellular structures, etc.), its efficient characteristics (seed, soil, water, sunlight, time, etc.), and its purposes or final causes (fruit, shade, etc.). In other chapters of this volume, the reader will learn a great deal about the formal and material aspects of sleep onset. In this chapter, I have focused on the efficient causes of sleep onset, that is, on the determinants of sleep onset.

THE PREDICTION OF SLEEP ONSET

In science, efficient causes are established as predictor variables. In an earlier article, I proposed a three-factor behavioral model of sleep in an attempt to develop a predictive model of sleep (Webb, 1988). This was an extension of the Borbély-Daan two-factor model (Daan, Beersma, & Borbély, 1984), which is based on sleep demand and circadian variables. My extended three-factor model proposed that sleep responses were predictable from three primary variables: sleep demand, circadian timing, and behavioral facilitation or inhibition. In this chapter, I specify this model relative to the prediction of a major parameter of sleep and the topic that is the focus of this book: sleep onset.

As noted later, the major determining variables are modulated by four additional variables: age, individual differences, variations in the neurophysiological system, and species. In my initial considerations of sleep demand, circadian tendencies, and behavioral determinants, these modulators are "controlled" by considering averaged data drawn from human young adults with "clean" central nervous systems.

The three primary variables are defined by objectively observable measures. Sleep demand increases as a function of time of wakefulness prior to sleep onset and decreases as a function of sleep following sleep onset. The circadian timing variable is defined by the sidereal time at which sleep onset is measured and the sleep process that ensues. The behavioral component is defined by the behavioral activities engaged in at the time of sleep onset and within ensuing sleep. The dependent variable, sleep onset, is defined by electroencephalogram (EEG) measures.

I will consider the primary variables separately in turn by holding two of the variables constant, varying one of the variables, and determining its relationship to sleep-onset latencies.

SLEEP DEMAND AND SLEEP ONSET

In young adult human sleep, the relationship between sleep-onset latencies and prior wakefulness appears to be a simple exponential function. Figure 1 shows data drawn from laboratory-measured sleep onsets at 11 p.m. (behavioral and circadian variables held constant) as a function of prior wakefulness amounts (Webb & Agnew, 1971). The likelihood that this is *the* functional relationship for sleep demand and sleep-onset latency is bolstered by the fact that these data were drawn

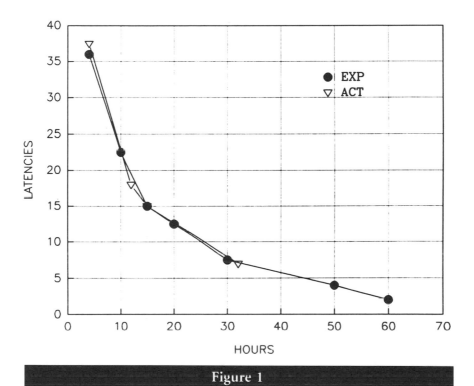

Figure 1

Sleep latencies (min) and prior wakefulness. NOTE: EXP = exponential curve values, ACT = obtained experimental values. Modified from Webb and Agnew (1971).

from three independent studies and that the simple exponential relationship is a form that nature seems to favor for many biological functions.

Because this is a simple asymptotic function, more formally the sleep demand (relative to sleep onset) can be defined mathematically as

$$\text{sleep demand} = M - M\, e^{i\,\text{TP}},$$

where M is the maximum sleep demand level, e is the exponential function, i is a simple logarithmic function, and TP is the time of prior wakefulness.

CIRCADIAN TENDENCIES AND SLEEP ONSET

The initial Borbély-Daan model proposed that the circadian tendencies acted on sleep onset by determining the sleep–waking thresholds. Sleep onset was determined by an interaction between the circadian tendency and a rising Process S (sleep demand) and a decreasing demand associated with sleep. The form of the circadian tendency (Process C) was a skewed sinusoid rising from awakening to a peak during the day and beginning to fall to a nadir in the midsleep period.

Since the early 1980s, there has been a plethora of proposed circadian models. In a recent review by Borbély and Achermann (1992), six circadian-rhythm, three interactive, and 11 "miscellaneous" models are noted. A special issue of *Journal of Sleep Research* (1992) includes 15 additional research papers on concepts and models relative to sleep regulation. A survey of these models revealed no precise tests of predictions of sleep onset in young adults; therefore, I have turned to the empirical data.

There is a set of data on the relationship between sleep-onset latencies and circadian tendencies. The requirements of such data would be measures of sleep-onset latencies where prior wakefulness and the behavioral sets were held constant and the times of sleep onset varied across the 24 hr. Other-than-24-hr sleep–wake regimes (alternate or varied day schedules) provide such data.

Table 1 presents six studies from which it was possible to derive sleep-onset data across a 24-hr period. This table cites the study, the time interval of prior wakefulness, the sleep period, the number of days for which the schedules were maintained, and the number of subjects in each study. Table 2 cites the hourly schedules of these studies. Latencies were reported in only one of the experiments (Webb & Agnew, 1975). However, all of the experiments reported on the stages of sleep within the circadian intervals of sleep time, and graphs of these data, were presented.[1]

---

[1]The specific sources of data from which onset latencies were estimated were as follows: Weitzman et al. (1976, Figure 1, p. 1021); Carskadon and Dement (1975, Figure 2, p. 129); Moses et al. (1975, Figure 1, p. 629, less the first measure); Webb and Agnew (1975, Figure 2, p. 639); Lavie (1986, Figure 1 and Figure 2, p. 418).

Table 1

Alternate Schedule Experiments

	W	S	S/24	D	N
Weitzman et al. (1976)	120	60	8	10	7
Carskadon & Dement (1975)	60	30	8	5.3	10
Moses et al. (1975)	160	60	6.5	1.7	10
Webb & Agnew (1975)	360	180	8	6	4
Lavie (1986), Exp I & II	13	7	8.4	1	12

NOTE: W = wake interval (min), S = sleep interval (min), S/24 = sleep available per 24 hr, D = duration (days), and N = number of subjects.

The data, except Webb and Agnew's, presented total sleep stage times per interval. Latencies were derived by subtracting total sleep time (sum of sleep stages) from the total interval time available. Thus, in the Lavie experiments, latencies were derived by subtracting total sleep time per testing period from seven minutes. Two-hour averages of the six data points for the two experiments constitute each data point. As may be seen in Table 1, the Weitzman et al., Carskadon and Dement, and Webb and Agnew experiments repeated these schedules over a number of days, and the data points are averaged across these days in

Table 2

Circadian Schedules of Alternate Experiments

Weitzman et al. (1976)	12M...3A...6A...9A....etc.
Carskadon & Dement (1975)	12M...1:30A...3A...4:30A...etc.
Moses et al. (1975)	8:17 A...11:49A...3:28P...etc.
Webb & Agnew (1975)	2A...11A...8P...5A...2P...etc.
Lavie (1986)	7:20P...7:40P...8P...etc. and
	7:20A...7:40A...8A...etc.

the studies. The Moses et al. and Lavie experiments are a series of single data points.

Several limitations of the data should be noted. First, this method would result in the inclusion of some awake time after sleep onset. However, because all of the intervals (except Webb and Agnew's) were short, these are likely to be limited. Second, in the short sleep intervals of the Lavie and the Carskadon and Dement experiments (7 and 30 min, respectively), there were intervals in which sleep did not occur. During these intervals, sleep latencies are underestimated. Finally, sleep-demand levels are not completely controlled. As sleep schedules are modified "away" from the 8-hr asleep/16-hr awake schedule, sleep becomes increasingly less efficient (Webb & Agnew, 1975), and less sleep occurs per 24 hr. As a consequence, in these shorter sleep–wake schedules, a sleep "debt" accrues as the schedule is extended. However, the data of both Weitzman et al. (1976) and Lavie (1986) provide evidence that this factor may shorten the latencies but the general circadian effect is maintained.

On the positive side, these data points are drawn from a substantial number of subjects and from repeated measures. For example, the Weitzman et al. data, at any given time interval, say 3 p.m. to 4 p.m., are the average of 100 measures (10 subjects over 10 days). Whereas the Lavie data points were obtained only once across a 24-hr period, the data presented here are the 2-hr averages of three within-hour measures of 13 subjects, or 78 measures at each data point. The lowest number of measures per interval is that drawn from Moses et al. because the intervals were not repeated. However, each of these data points is the average of 10 subjects.

Figures 2 and 3 present the data from these latency estimates. Figure 2 displays the latencies as a function of time of day of the Weitzman et al., Carskadon and Dement, and Webb and Agnew experiments, and Figure 3 displays these data for the Lavie and Moses et al. experiments. Each set of data begins with the shortest latency period and ends with this initial latency replotted. The scale of values of each experiment is given on the abscissa of each figure. Each of these sets of data has a

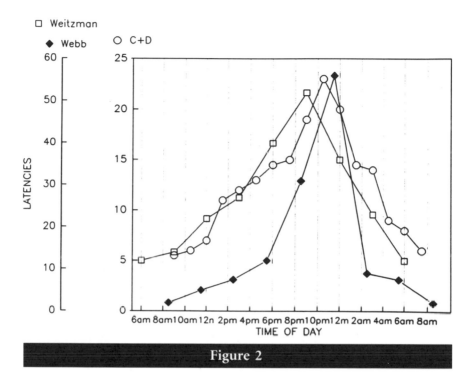

Figure 2

Sleep latencies (min) and time of day. Data derived from Weitzman et al. (1976), Carskadon and Dement (1975), and Webb and Agnew (1975). Scale of Weitzman et al. and Webb and Agnew = 0–60 min; scale of Carskadon and Dement = 0–25 min.

common form, rising from a low point in the early morning hours to a peak in the evening hours, with a steeper return slope to the early morning hours.

Although the daytime rises in latencies display different forms, the nighttime descending slopes are remarkably similar. Figure 4 displays these latencies taken from the highest to the lowest latency from the five experiments. A linear slope from 10 p.m. to 6 a.m. (method of averages) provides an excellent fit for these data. A linear fit can also be applied to the rising slope. However, the standard error of estimate is much higher.

Assuming that the young adults of these experiments had a normal sleep–wake pattern with sleep set between approximately 11 p.m. and

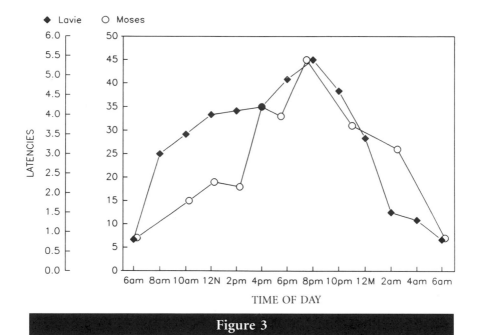

Figure 3

Sleep latencies (min) and time of day. Data derived from Lavie (1986) and Moses et al. (1975). Scale of Lavie = 0 to 6 min; scale of Moses et al. = 0 to 50 min.

7 a.m., the data indicate that, other variables being controlled, sleep-onset latencies begin to rise linearly before sleep termination, for about 16 hr to approximately 10 p.m. From this point, they fall linearly for a period of 8 hr.

A remarkable affirmation of this circadian tendency can be found in temperature data, which is an alternative index of circadian biological tendencies. Figure 5, adapted from Monk and Embrie (1981), displays oral temperature measures obtained at 2-hr intervals from six shift workers over a one-month period on rapidly rotating 12-hr shifts (7 a.m. to 7 p.m.). These are "grand mean averages" formed by averaging the rhythms of the six individuals and are based on either three or four night-shift and day-shift sessions for each subject. These temperature

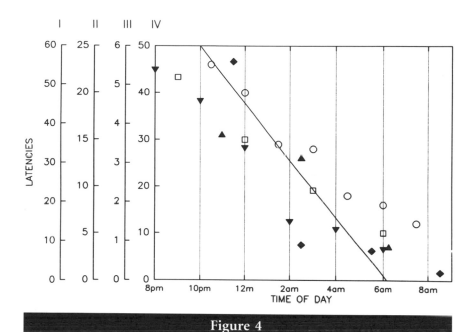

Figure 4

Sleep latencies from highest evening to lowest morning values. Data from Figures 2 and 3. Scale I = Weitzman et al. and Webb and Agnew; Scale II = Carskadon and Dement; Scale III = Lavie; Scale IV = Moses et al.

measures rise in an essentially linear fashion from 6 a.m. and fall in a linear fashion from 8 p.m. They differ from the latencies data by only a slightly earlier (8 p.m. vs. 10 p.m.) peak.

BEHAVIORAL DETERMINANTS OF SLEEP ONSET

In my original formulation of behavioral determinants, I proposed that behavioral determinants might be facilitative or inhibitory. I now propose that behavioral determinants operate simply as an inhibitory variable. In regard to sleep onset, for a given sleep-onset tendency determined by sleep demand and circadian tendencies, sleep onset may be inhibited by behavioral responses. Thus, with muscularly relaxed and

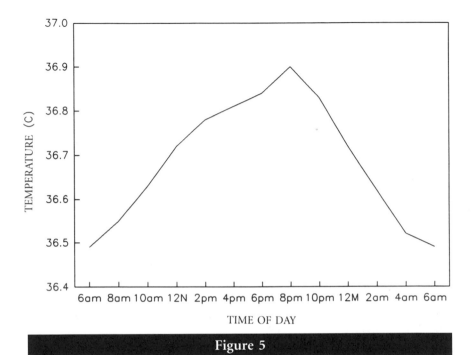

Figure 5

Temperature and time of day on a rotating shift schedule. Data derived from Monk and Embrie (1981).

nonthinking behavior as a baseline, behavioral responses that modify this condition will inhibit sleep onset. More formally, the inhibition of sleep onset latencies will be increased by behavioral responses that lead to muscular tension, cognitive activity, or both.

The difficulty posed by such a broad definition lies in the selection of particular behaviors and in the task of dimensionalizing them. A few selected dimensions of behavior variables relative to sleep latencies illustrate the intuitive force of the role of behavioral variables and the experimental problems that would be posed by exploring these determinants. It is reasonable to argue that the following changes in behavior will systematically increase sleep-onset latencies at a set period of sidereal time after equal periods of prior wakefulness:

- supine–sitting–erect–walking
- passive responding–goal directed responding–escape/avoidant responding
- silence–random noise–relevant information–danger signals
- darkness–undifferentiated light–low information–high information
- nonpain–pain

Although it is apparent that sleep onset is affected by conscious and unconscious behavioral responses and that the therapeutic control of sleep onset focuses on relaxation of muscular and control of cognitive activities, systematic studies of these relationships are rare. A few exemplary studies can be cited to illustrate their complexities. A recent study by Nau (1992) illustrates a thin line of studies attempting to clarify the complex cognitive–physiological aspects of relaxation training begun by Borkovec, Kaloupek, and Slama (1975). Nau found a significant and superior differential effect on sleep-onset latencies of attentional focusing compared with muscular relaxation. The effects of instructional sets were explored sporadically because Hartse, Roth, and Zorick (1982) reported a significant difference on using the directive "try to fall asleep" as opposed to the directive "try to stay awake" using the repeated daytime measures of the Multiple Sleep Latency Test after a normal night's sleep. This effect was not present after a night of sleep deprivation. Lavie (1986) used two sets of accepting versus resisting sleep in his controlled, short-regime studies. He found no significant differences between sets. Alexander, Blagrove, and Horne (1991), however, reported a significant effect on latencies of sleep-deprived subjects using a maintenance of wakefulness test when financial incentives were added.

Unfortunately, as a predictor variable, behavioral responding cannot be indexed simply by a single, unidimensional variable such as the passage of time or time of day. Each instance must be characterized as an obvious, necessary, and, on occasion, sufficient variable. However, this variable is definable only in an ad hoc and contextual manner.

INTERACTIONS OF SLEEP DEMAND, CIRCADIAN TENDENCIES, AND BEHAVIORAL ACTIVITIES

In my original formulation, I had sleep demand and circadian effects interacting multiplicatively (sleep demand $\times$ circadian tendencies), with an addition or subtraction contributed by behavioral responding. My review of the sleep-onset literature dictates modifications of this formulation.

In considering the interaction between sleep demand and circadian tendencies relative to sleep onset, the data indicate that an increasing sleep tendency is generated by sleep demand as a simple exponential function. This rising tendency interacts with circadian sleep tendencies, rising for approximately 16 hr across the daytime hours (circa 6 a.m. to 10 p.m.) and falling across approximately 8 nighttime hours (circa 10 p.m. to 6 a.m.).

These interactions, generally, have long been apparent in performance and subjective measurements during extended sleep deprivation. The data clearly demonstrate that the sleep deprivation effects on these measures increase with time of prior wakefulness (sleep demand). It is also apparent that these are not linearly increasing effects but are effects that are systematically related to sidereal time of measurement (circadian). Unfortunately, such data can be related to sleep-onset latencies only inferentially.

There is, however, an extensive set of data available on sleep demand and circadian tendency interactions. I refer to the data obtained in the exploration of the Multiple Sleep Latency Test (MSLT) measurements. In this paradigm, measurements of sleep onset are obtained at intervals across sidereal time. Because sleep time is sharply restricted in each test interval, each testing occurs with increased amounts of prior wakefulness. Moreover, behavioral responses are held constant.

Figure 6 presents three selected sets of representative data from the MSLT paradigm, which extends across a 24-hr period from 8 a.m. to 8 a.m. Data from Clodore, Benoit, Forêt, & Bouard (1990) are latency measures from 10 a.m. through 8 p.m. The Sugerman & Walsh (1989)

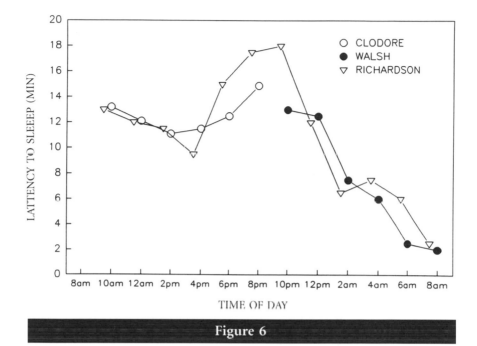

Figure 6

Multiple sleep latencies across 24 hr. Data derived from Clodore et al. (1990); Richardson et al. (1982); and Sugerman & Walsh (1989).

obtained latencies from 10 p.m. to 8 a.m. Richardson, Carskadon, Orav, & Dement (1982) measured latencies for 24 hr from 9:30 a.m. to 9:30 a.m. These data display relatively high latencies in the morning hours, a bowed effect across the day with a low point in the early afternoon, and rising latencies in the evening hours. These latencies then fall rapidly to a low point in the early morning.

Considering the data from the perspective of an interaction between sleep demand and circadian tendencies across the 24-hr period, Figure 7 plots a hypothetical exponential effect of prior wakefulness and linear circadian effects across a 24-hr period based on our earlier considerations. This figure plots wakefulness tendencies of these variables: decreasing wakefulness as a function of sleep demand and an increasing and then decreasing wakefulness associated with circadian tendencies.

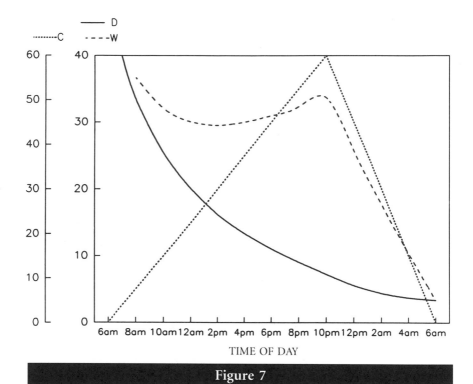

Figure 7

Hypothetical wakefulness tendencies of sleep demand and circadian variables and their interaction. NOTE: C = circadian tendencies (scale = 0 to 40); D = sleep demand tendencies (scale = 0 to 60); W = summed interaction (scale = 0 to 60).

The assumptions of the figure are simple and few. There is an exponential sleep demand effect beginning at awakening (7 a.m.). A maximum wakefulness tendency of 60 min is assumed at awakening as a result of no sleep demand. A wakefulness tendency of 5 min is assumed after 24 hr. This, of course, would return to 60 min if sleep occurred during the night. A linear circadian arousal effect of two thirds the strength of the sleep demand effect is assumed to start before awakening at 6 a.m., with a peak at 10 p.m. and returning to 0 at 6 a.m.

These summed wakefulness tendencies resulting from the demand and circadian tendencies interact and form a wakefulness tendency reflected in latencies of sleep onset. These are plotted as "W" (using the demand scale) in Figure 7. It is apparent that they are similar to the latencies displayed empirically in Figure 6: high latencies in the morning, a bowed effect across the day with a minimum at 2 p.m., and a sharp decrease during the evening hours.

These data and hypothetical assumptions indicate that, within the 24-hr period, sleep onset may be predicted from a simple summative interaction between the sleep demand and circadian tendencies with behavioral responding held constant.

Although the results are beyond the scope of my consideration of sleep onset, I cannot resist pointing out that this two-factor interaction between sleep demand and circadian tendencies has provocative implications for several independently developed concepts and empirical sleep phenomena as follows.

Napping

Strong arguments have been put forth suggesting that napping provides evidence that sleep is an endogenous circasemidian or biphasic system (cf. Broughton & Mullington, 1992). The bowed MSLT effect is used in support of this type of theorizing. The present two-factor interactive model would derive this afternoon-sleep propensity as a relatively weak tendency resulting from offsetting demand and circadian tendencies. This position reflects the less than robust presence of napping in adults and the apparent ease of override by behavioral and cultural variables (Webb & Dinges, 1992).

Sleep Gates or Forbidden Zones

There is considerable evidence that, paradoxically, sleep propensity is reduced in the early evening hours (cf. Lavie, 1986). According to the two-factor interaction, this is a simple expression of the continuously rising, circadian lower sleep tendencies at this time with a relative stable sleep demand tendency. The midafternoon, secondary gate may simply reflect the interaction with increasing sleep demand that results in the particular experimental design.

Sleep Lag

In attempting to model performance and subjective data, Folkard and Åkerstedt (1992) proposed the addition, to sleep demand and circadian tendencies, of a waking-up component lasting for several hours after awakening tendencies. This addition was used to account for lowered morning performance measures. The assumption of near-maximum circadian sleep tendencies in the early morning hours makes this added component unnecessary.

Only general statements can be made about the interaction of behavioral responding with the sleep demand and circadian variables. Within the boundary of 24 hr, sleep onset can be readily delayed or eliminated by behavioral responding. However, this capacity, even within this boundary, is bounded by time. Greater behavioral arousal is required in the later part of the 24-hr period as a dual function of a high sleep demand and lowered, offsetting circadian tendencies (Figure 7).

With extended sleep deprivation, there are predictable relations between behavioral responding and sleep onset. With increasing prior wakefulness, sleep demand increases, and increased behavioral responding is required to delay sleep onset. At some hypothetical point, wakefulness cannot be maintained. However, this is a wavelike function reflecting circadian tendencies, with more or less behavioral responding being required, depending on the sidereal time within the 24-hr cycle.

THE MODULATORS

To this point, I have focused on averaged data drawn from young human adults. In my original model, I noted that there were four primary modulator variables relative to the three primary determinants: age, neurophysiological variations, individual differences, and species. Each of these, although not changing the determinative role of the three primary variables, requires modifications in its parameters. Such changes permit the extension of the model to allow predictions across age, varied neurophysiological conditions, species, and individual subjects. Brief reminders are given here about these modulators relative to sleep onset.

Age

The most systematic laboratory data on sleep onset at bedtime and on age (Williams, Karacan, & Hursh, 1974) indicate a limited effect on sleep onset until the sixth decade. The sleep latencies of older subjects, in these data and in other studies of older persons, show a significant increase in both sleep-onset latencies and their standard deviation. These changes are generally attributed to changes in the circadian system. Sleep-onset measures obtained from MSLTs show distinct and provocative age-related changes in both amplitude (e.g., longer latencies in adolescents) and circadian tendencies.

Neurophysiological Variables

Neurophysiological variables modify the sleep response. They include such variables as drugs and neurophysiological anomalies, such as narcolepsy and sleep apnea. Pharmacological studies have documented a wide range of effects on sleep-onset latencies, and MSLTs, with demonstrated effects, have been widely applied to various clinical conditions.

Individual Differences

There are certainly stable, individual, longer or shorter latencies brought about by acquired and persisting state tendencies. These are evident in persistent insomnias. However, among normal, healthy adults, *trait* individual differences do not appear to be primary determinants of latencies. Night-to-night correlations of sleep latencies in such subjects are quite low (cf. Webb & Agnew, 1971). In short, within-subject onset-latency traits appear to have limited force.

Species Differences

Observations of sleep onsets across species reveal a wide range of differences in intervals of prior wakefulness and the placement of sleep onsets within circadian periods. Furthermore, the behavioral determinants of sleep vary widely across species relative to such determinants as predator–prey role and foraging needs. The prediction of sleep onset in any particular species requires a specification of the sleep demand, circadian, and behavioral parameters of that species.

SUMMARY AND CONCLUSIONS

I have stated that, in young adult humans, there are three efficient causes of sleep onset: sleep demand, circadian tendencies, and behavioral responding at sleep onset. These variables are indexed by observable and measurable antecedents: prior wakefulness, sidereal time, and behaviors at the time of sleep onset. The experimental evidence indicates that, with two of these variables held constant, remarkably accurate predictions of sleep onset are possible. This is particularly true for the easily indexed variables of sleep demand and circadian tendencies. Experimental data also indicate that, under conditions of interaction of these variables (e.g., sleep deprivation and MSLT measurements), the three variables yield predictive results. The use of four modulator variables (age, species, neurophysiological variables, and individual differences) permits the extension of these predictor variables to a broad range of phenomena. Because prediction is a powerful criterion for a theoretical position with regard to sleep latencies, the three-factor model proposed shows promise.

In an Aristotelian sense of efficient causality, one can conclude that sleep onset may be sufficiently attributed to three causal variables: sleep demand (defined by prior wakefulness), circadian tendencies (defined by sidereal time), and behavioral responding (defined by sleep-antagonistic responding). In the current hegemony of science, explanation reduces to prediction, control, or both. Even within this exalted context, our explanation of sleep onset is approaching a satisfactory state.

Whereas behavioral responding, particularly with regard to control, remains a major challenge, our ability to predict the probability or strength of a sleep onset is remarkably advanced.

REFERENCES

Alexander, C., Blagrove, M., & Horne J. (1991). Subject motivation and the Multiple Sleep Latency Test. *Sleep Research*, *20*, 403.

Borbély, A., & Achermann, P. (1992). Concepts and models of sleep regulation: An overview. *Journal of Sleep Research*, *1*, 63–79.

Borkovec, T. D., Kaloupek, D. G., & Slama, K. (1975). The facilitative effect of muscle-tension release in relaxation treatment of sleep disturbance. *Behavior Therapy*, *6*, 301–309.

Broughton, R., & Mullington, J. (1992). Circasemidian sleep propensity and the phase–amplitude maintenance model of human sleep/wake regulation. *Journal of Sleep Research*, *1*, 93–98.

Carskadon, M., & Dement, W. (1975). Sleep studies on a 90 minute day. *Electro encephalography and Clinical Neurophysiology*, *39*, 145–155.

Clodore, M., Benoit, O., Forêt, J., & Bouard G. (1990). The Multiple Sleep Latency Test: Individual variability and time of day effect in normal young adults. *Sleep*, *13*, 385–394.

Daan, S., Beersma, D., & Borbély, A. (1984). Timing of human sleep: Recovery process gated by a circadian pacemaker. *American Journal of Physiology*, *246*, R161–R178.

Folkard, S., & Åkerstedt, T. (1992). A three-process model of the regulation of alertness–sleepiness. In R. J. Broughton & R. D. Ogilvie (Eds.), *Sleep, arousal and performance* (pp. 11–26). Cambridge, MA: Birkhauser Boston.

Hartse, K., Roth, T., & Zorick, F. (1982). Daytime sleepiness and daytime wakefulness: The effect of instruction. *Sleep*, *5*, S107–S118.

Journal of Sleep Research. (1992). Concepts and models of sleep regulation [Special issue].

Lavie, P. (1986). Ultrashort sleep–waking schedule: Part 3. Gates and "forbidden zones" for sleep. *Electroencephalography and Clinical Neurophysiology*, *63*, 414–425.

Monk, T., & Embrie, D. (1981). A field study of circadian rhythms in actual and interpolated performance. In A. Reinberg, M. Vieux, & P. Andlauer (Eds.),

Night and shift work: Biological and social aspects (pp. 473–480). New York: Pergamon.

Moses, J., Hord, D., Lubin, A., Johnson, L., & Naitoh, P. (1975). Dynamics of nap sleep during a 40 hour period. *Electroencephalography and Clinical Neurophysiology, 39,* 627–633.

Nau, S. (1992). Sleep tendency during relaxation training. *Sleep Research, 21,* 108.

Richardson, G., Carskadon, M., Orav, E., & Dement, W. (1982). Circadian variation of sleep tendency in elderly and young adult subjects. *Sleep, 5,* S82–S94.

Sugerman, J., & Walsh, J. (1989). Physiological sleep tendency and ability to maintain alertness at night. *Sleep, 12,* 106–112.

Webb, W. (1988). An objective behavioral model of sleep. *Sleep, 11,* 488–496.

Webb, W., & Agnew, H. (1971). Sleep latencies in human subjects: Age, prior wakefulness, and reliability. *Psychonomic Science, 24,* 253–254.

Webb, W., & Agnew, H. (1975). Sleep efficiency for sleep–wake cycles of varied length. *Psychophysiology, 12,* 637–641.

Webb, W., & Dinges, D. (1992). Cultural perspectives on napping and the siesta. In D. Dinges & R. Broughton (Eds.), *Sleep and alertness* (pp. 247–266). New York: Raven.

Weitzman, E., Nogeire, C., Perlow, M., Fukushima, D., Sassin, J., Macgregor, P., Gallagher, T., & Hellman, L. (1976). Effects of a prolonged 3-hour sleep–wake cycle on sleep stages, plasma cortisol, growth hormones and body temperature. *Journal of Clinical Endocrinological Metabolism, 38,* 1018–1030.

Williams, R., Karacan, I., & Hursh, C. (1974). *Electroencephalography (EEG) of human sleep: Clinical applications.* New York: Wiley.

5

Prediction of Intentional and Unintentional Sleep Onset

Torbjorn Åkerstedt and Simon Folkard

Sleep onset may be either intentional, that is, initiating a conventional sleep episode, or unintentional, initiating a sleep intrusion into an ongoing waking activity. The latter constitutes an obvious problem if the waking activity involves work or some other purposeful activity. However, the intentional sleep onset is also of major importance if it fails to occur. Electroencephalogram (EEG) studies conducted during actual work have demonstrated that 25% of process operators fall asleep during work and sleep for 5 to 30 min without being aware that sleep has occurred (Torsvall, Åkerstedt, Gillander, & Knutsson, 1989). Similar results have been demonstrated for train drivers and truck drivers, although these groups lack full-fledged sleep and rather present a picture of a continuous series of short sleep onsets while fighting sleep (Kecklun & Åkerstedt, 1993; Torsvall & Åkerstedt, 1987). Observations such as these have led us to develop a quantitative model of alertness regulation.

The purpose of this chapter is to describe some of our recent work to improve the model in terms of its ability to predict the timing of unintentional sleep onset during work and to predict the latency of intentional sleep. The chapter also discusses the development of a rating scale coupled to EEG changes and sleepiness behavior.

THE THREE-PROCESS MODEL OF ALERTNESS

The inspiration for the development of the alertness model was the "two-process model of sleep regulation," which had shown that sleep length and slow wave activity could be described by a combination of homeostatic and circadian influences (Borbély, 1982). This model was based on the amount of EEG slow wave activity during sleep, but it seemed likely that a similar approach could be used to model and predict alertness variations.

To construct the model, we used published data from experiments with life on a 22-hr day (Folkard, Hume, Minors, Waterhouse, & Watson, 1985), sleep deprivation (Folkard & Åkerstedt, 1991; Fröberg, 1977; Fröberg, Karlsson, Levi, & Lidberg, 1975), and other studies. It should be emphasized that these studies are completely independent of those used for the Borbély model and use a completely different parameter: subjective sleepiness. We found that subjective sleepiness (or alertness) was, indeed, predictable using three processes : S, C, and W. Space does not permit a discussion of the derivation of the model, but the reader is referred to Folkard and Åkerstedt (1991). Here, we will describe the main traits of the model.

Process *C* represents sleepiness because of circadian influences and has the general sinusoidal form indicated in Figure 1 and Table 1. Our attempts to model empirical data suggest that the phase estimate may have to be delayed by up to four hours in students, shift workers, or other groups in whom evening-type preferences dominate.

Process *S* is an exponential function of the time since awakening. Maximum alertness is reached upon awakening, although alertness initially falls rapidly and then levels out and gradually approaches an asymptote. The rate of decrease of the exponential function corresponds to 3.5% of the previous value per hour. At sleep onset, process *S* is reversed and called *S'*, and recovery occurs as an exponential function

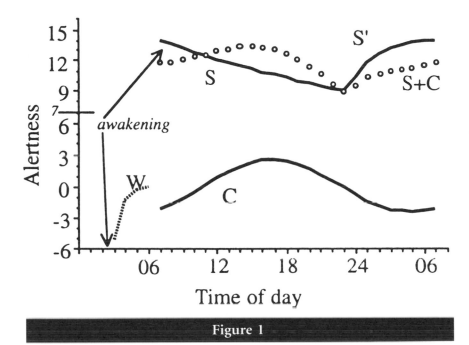

Figure 1

Parameters of the three-process model of alertness regulation. S = homeostatic component during waking; S' = homeostatic component during sleep; C = circadian component; W = wake-up component; $S + C$ = the alertness prediction (excluding W); and 7 = level of risk.

that initially increases at a very rapid rate but subsequently levels off toward an upper asymptote. The rate of increase of the exponential function is 28.7% per hour (i.e., much steeper than the decay during the day). It is of interest to note that the exponential functions arrived at are very similar to those demonstrated by Borbély (1982).

The final component is the wakeup process W, or sleep inertia, after forced awakenings. This function is also exponential but with an even steeper initial decrease: 62.7% per hour (i.e., already, after the first hour, most of the inertia has dissipated). W is subtracted from the $S + C$ level. Spontaneous awakenings constitute a special problem because the exact time of awakening is often not available and because the time between the first formal awakening and the time of final rising

Table 1

Mathematical Functions of the Model of Alertness Regulation

$C = M \cos (t\partial - p)\pi/12$ or $C = 2.5 \cos (t - 16.8)\pi/12$.

$S = (S_a - L)e - 0.0353t + L$ or $S = (14 - 2.4)e - 0.0353t + 2.4$.

$S' = U - (U - S_r)e - 0.381t$ or $S' = 14.3 - (14.3 - 7.96)e - 0.381t$.

$W = 5.72e - 1.51t$.

$A = C + S$ (or S') $- W$.

$S' + C' = U$.

NOTE: M = amplitude (in arbitrary units on a scale from 1 to 21); p = acrophase (in decimal hours); $t\partial$ = time of day (in decimal hours); S_a = value of S at awakening; L = lower asymptote; t = time since awakening (in functions S and W) or time since going to bed (in function S'); S_r = S value at retiring; and U = upper asymptote.

might be considerable. Tentatively, we assume that such a process might take approximately 1 hr.

The estimated alertness (or sleepiness) is then expressed as the arithmetic sum of the three functions above ($S + C$, in Figure 1). It should be emphasized that the homeostatic function involves not only prior time awake but also the amount of prior sleep. It also recognizes that recuperation is more rapid in the initial hours of sleep and that loss of alertness is more rapid during the initial hours of wakefulness. Furthermore, the recuperative process (S') increases in speed with increasing sleep loss, and the loss of alertness is less rapid if initial alertness is low. Incidentally, the S' function has been demonstrated to predict slow wave activity (Åkerstedt, Gillberg, & Folkard, 1992) and total sleep length (Åkerstedt & Folkard, 1994).

PREDICTION OF INVOLUNTARY SLEEP

Using the three-process model, we have found it possible to predict with high accuracy the variation of subjective sleepiness under conditions of sleep deprivation and various experimental or naturally occurring alternations of sleep–wake behavior (Folkard & Åkerstedt, 1991).

In these validation studies, we also found that Level 7 of predicted alertness corresponded to a point at which slow eye movements (SEMs) started to occur during waking polysomnography under conditions of 5 min of open eyes. This has been taken to indicate a level of sleep-onset risk. It is admittedly arbitrary but contains considerable face validity.

To continue the validation work, we tried to predict the alpha-power density (APD), after spectral analysis of the Cz Pz derivation, in two field studies with ambulatory EEG recordings (Åkerstedt & Folkard, in press). The first APD derives from 15 truck drivers during a night drive (Kecklun & Åkerstedt, 1993). On the whole, APD rises as predicted alertness falls (Figure 2). The right part of the figure illustrates the close relation between the APD and predicted alertness. Baseline levels (100%) coincide with predicted levels of 10 and above and characterized daytime driving (not in Figure 1). This means that the relationship between predicted alertness and alpha (and theta) intrusions is in effect curvilinear because daytime values (not in the figure) oscil-

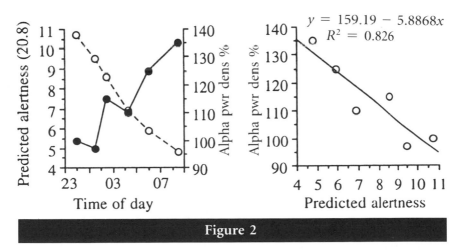

Figure 2

Left: Mean APD and predicted alertness plotted against time of day for truck drivers working at night. Right: Mean APD plotted against predicted alertness for the same group. 100% = baseline (daytime values); N = 15 subjects at each point.

late closely around 100% (the point of inflection appears around the level of 7–8). This is very close to the earlier observation that SEM (as well as alpha and theta intrusions) are completely absent for high-to-medium levels of alertness (14–9) but start to appear around 7, together with perceptions of fighting sleep (Folkard & Åkerstedt, 1991).

A similar analysis was conducted with 15 train drivers during night work (Torsvall & Åkerstedt, 1987). Here, the covariation between predicted alertness and APD during the night drive was even higher than for the truck drivers ($R^2 = 0.94$, with $y = 515 - 44x$, where $y =$ alpha % of baseline and $x =$ predicted alertness). Again, daytime driving was associated with an absence of alpha or theta activity beyond baseline and with high-to-medium levels of predicted alertness. Thus, the true relationship is curvilinear between predicted alertness and sleep intrusions into the waking EEG, and the first increase above baseline occurs around Level 7–8 of predicted alertness.

To test further the prediction of the model, we used a 64-hr sleep deprivation study (Gillberg & Åkerstedt, 1981) in which EEG measures were obtained in connection with performance tests. The study involved 12 male subjects living on a semiconstant routine. The latter included isolation from environmental time cues and a three-hourly control of activity and intake of food and fluid. In each 3-hr module, ratings of sleepiness were carried out and a 32-min monotonous vigilance test was used.

Figure 3 shows the time elapsed before the first miss because of sleep (scored visually), plotted against time together with predicted alertness from the model (the acrophase was set to 2048 hr). The data in the left panel show a very pronounced fall across time awake, together with a superimposition of a circadian pattern. The right panel shows that the amount of variance accounted for by the model prediction is considerable. The number of minutes without a miss increases by 2.5 for each level of the scale (above the intercept). Performance without misses appears to require a level of 13, whereas a rapid onset (i.e., less than 10 min) of misses occurs around 3. No obvious "critical

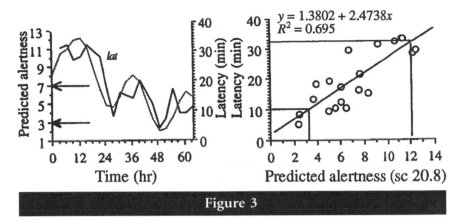

Figure 3

Left: Mean latency to first miss caused by sleep and predicted alertness, plotted against time awake across 64 hr in three-hour intervals ($N = 12$). Right: Latency to miss plotted against predicted alertness.

point" appears to exist in these data, but the probability of missing due to sleep is linearly related to predicted alertness.

Taken together, the data suggest that the alertness model may be used to define levels of critical sleepiness, but that the outcome will be influenced by the activity of the subject and by the environmental setting. At Level 3 and below, occurrences of sleep seem highly likely almost regardless of the situation. Between Levels 3 and 7, the probability of sleep intrusions is high, at least for average sedentary activity. Between Levels 7 and 10, the risk of sleep intrusions is reduced but is definitely present for monotonous situations. Above Level 10, sleep is unlikely unless the situation is highly conducive to it.

PREDICTION OF RATED UNINTENTIONAL SLEEP

Self-rated sleepiness is frequently a necessary substitute for EEG measures of sleepiness, and high levels of objective sleepiness appear to reflect episodes of sleep onset, although immediately aborted (Åkerstedt & Gillberg, 1990). Most rating scales for this purpose make use of the visual analogue approach—a 100-mm line between the verbal descriptors "very alert" and "very sleepy" on which the subjects are asked to mark their level of sleepiness. This approach has useful psychometric properties, but it is a relative scale. Different subjects use it differently depending on their frame of reference.

To circumvent the problem of relativity, we have developed an absolute nine-point rating scale with verbal anchors. The steps are 1 = very alert; 3 = alert; 5 = neither alert nor sleepy; 7 = sleepy, but no effort required to keep awake; and 9 = very sleepy, fighting sleep, an effort to keep awake (Åkerstedt & Gillberg, 1990). This Karolinska Scale of Sleepiness (KSS) is closely related to the visual analogue scale of alertness and to changes in the EEG/electrooculogram (EOG). Both APD and slow eye movements during a control situation with five minutes of open eyes increase in a curvilinear way as a function of KSS sleepiness rating. No EEG/EOG changes occur until the individual starts to rate him- or herself as "sleepy" (Level 7). At Level 9, which denotes "very sleepy, fighting sleep, an effort to keep awake," alpha activity and slow eye movements are largely continuous.

The three-process model of sleepiness is derived from data obtained with various types of rating scales for sleepiness–alertness, all predating the KSS scale. Because this scale is based on perceptions of transients of sleep onset (fighting sleep), it is of interest to use it to validate further the predictions of the three-process model of alertness.

Figure 4 contains data from a laboratory study of irregular sleep with two-hourly self-ratings of sleepiness (Åkerstedt & Gillberg, 1986b). The covariation between KSS and predicted sleepiness is quite high ($R^2 = 0.64$), and the function was KSS $= 10.3 - 0.5x$, where $x =$ predicted sleepiness. Incidentally, much of the residual variance appears to be due to a 12-hr ultradian rhythm. The regression function yields approximately the following pairs of data: high subjective sleepiness (Level 9—fighting sleep, an effort to keep awake) coincides with a predicted alertness level of 3. A KSS value of 7 (sleepy but not fighting sleep) corresponds to a predicted alertness of 7. Intermediate KSS sleepiness (Level 5) corresponds to a predicted alertness of 10–11,

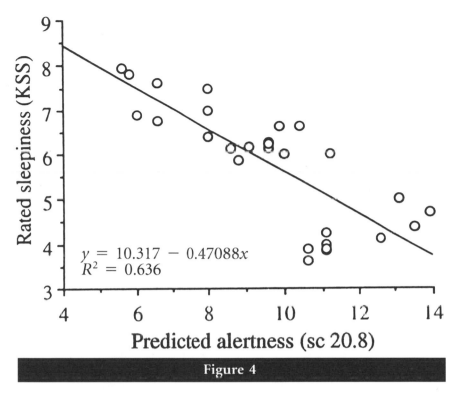

$$y = 10.317 - 0.47088x$$
$$R^2 = 0.636$$

Figure 4

Mean sleepiness (KSS) at different points of irregular sleep experiment plotted against predicted alertness ($N = 8$).

whereas a KSS level of 3 (alert) corresponds to a predicted alertness of about 14.

Figure 5 shows mean rated sleepiness (KSS) plotted against predicted sleepiness (acrophase set to 2048 hr) for 50 air crew on intercontinental flights (Stockholm–Los Angeles) and for 15 three-shift workers (operators in a nuclear power plant) on the night shift (unpublished data). Both groups rose at about 0700 hr and did not nap. The shift workers reported from their second night shift. Both groups show alertness during the daytime with increasing sleepiness toward the morning, reaching a maximum of 7.5 on the KSS scale, that is, just above "sleepy but not fighting sleep." This corresponded to 4–5 of

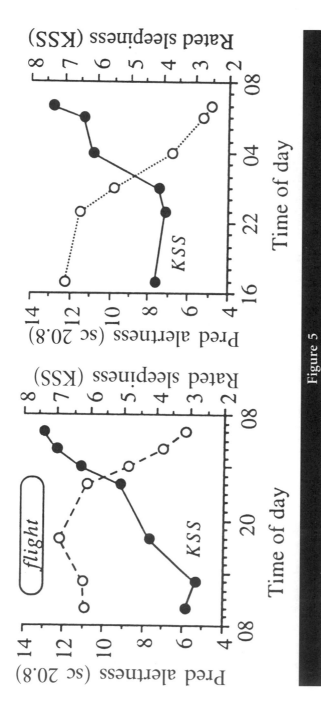

Figure 5

Predicted and rated (mean) alertness for air crew during day of westward flight and for three-shift workers during day with the second night shift.

predicted alertness. It is very similar to what would be predicted from the regression function from Figure 5. The regression function for the shift workers was KSS $= 9 - 0.4x$ ($R^2 = 0.91$) and for air crew KSS $= 11.6 - 0.7x$ ($R^2 = 0.76$), where $x =$ predicted alertness. It is interesting to note that the rated sleepiness in the morning is exceptionally low, probably reflecting the stress of preflight preparation and the initial burst of activity during the first hours after takeoff. On the whole, then, the three-process model also predicts subjective alertness with high accuracy.

PREDICTING SLEEP ONSET OF INTENDED SLEEP

Onset of an intended sleep episode is a different issue from that of unintended sleep, but it should also be possible to predict this phenomenon from the three-process model of alertness. For this purpose, we obtained sleep latency data from two laboratory studies conducted under semiconstant conditions (Åkerstedt & Gillberg, 1981; Åkerstedt & Gillberg, 1986a). One involved sleep episodes displaced from a baseline bedtime at 2300 to 0300 hr, 0700 hr, 1100 hr, 1500 hr, 1900 hr, and 2300 hr, respectively. The other involved four conditions, all with a sleep episode scheduled to 1100 hr, but preceded either by no prior night sleep or by sleep between 2300 hr and 0700 hr, 0300 hr and 0700 hr, or 0500 hr and 0700 hr. Both studies contained considerable influence on alertness by circadian and homeostatic factors.

The group mean values of sleep latency for the different conditions were then combined into one set of data and regressed on the alertness prediction from the model, given the particular conditions of retiring and rising. The analysis was repeated with different acrophase estimates (1648 to 2148 hr) and with both linear and exponential regression to find the optimum fit (Åkerstedt & Folkard, 1994). Figure 6 shows that a very high multiple correlation was reached for an exponential fit with the acrophase set at 2048 hr. As a rule, linear fits provided a slightly poorer fit, whereas the effect of acrophase was considerable; the poorest fit ($R^2 = 0.49$) was obtained for the acrophase set at 1648 hr.

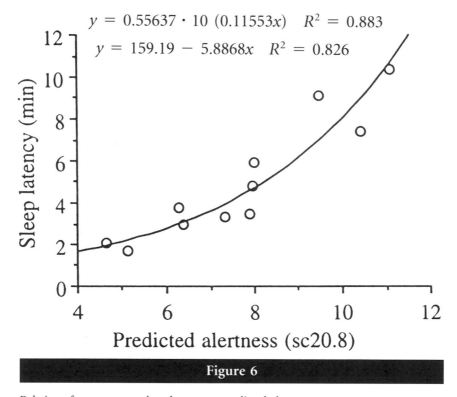

$$y = 0.55637 \cdot 10\ (0.11553x) \quad R^2 = 0.883$$
$$y = 159.19 - 5.8868x \quad R^2 = 0.826$$

Figure 6

Relation of group mean sleep latency to predicted alertness.

The resulting optimum function indicates that, at the lowest level of the model alertness, sleep latency amounts to 0.5 min. This is, of course, reasonable because it is the lowest possible measurable sleep latency, and one that occurs at the circadian trough with long prior waking. As predicted, as alertness rises, so does sleep latency. At normal levels of model alertness (10–12), sleep latency is around 10 min. At very high levels of predicted alertness (13–17), the sleep latency exceeds 20 min, and the marginal increase becomes very steep. Presumably, sleep latencies here become so long that sleep attempts are easily aborted. These levels may occur only for evening sleep episodes preceded by very short periods of prior waking. These may occur after a long afternoon nap or in connection with very irregular sleep patterns.

The prediction of sleep latency has not been systematically validated yet. We have, however, applied the prediction to several field studies with ambulatory polysomnography of sleep (in the subject's home). In a study of three-shift work, we obtained data from 25 workers on rotating three shifts (Åkerstedt, Kecklun, & Knutsson, 1991). Twenty-four-hour polysomnography was carried out during the second 24-hr period on each of the morning (0600–1400 hr), afternoon (1400–2200 hr), and night (2200–0600 hr) shifts. All subjects slept in their own bedrooms and at their spontaneously determined bedtime. The model used an acrophase of 2048 hr, and its prediction came reasonably close to the obtained values. Thus, before the morning shift, we predicted 11 min versus the obtained 13 min. After the morning shift, the values were 11 versus 8 min; and after the evening shift, they were 9 versus 5 min.

CONCLUSION

The data presented here suggest that unintentional as well as intentional sleep onset may be predicted from a simple model based on circadian and homeostatic regulation of sleep. Both are determined by circadian phase, prior time awake, and length of prior sleep. This knowledge makes it possible to predict, with considerable accuracy, the sleep–wake consequences at altered sleep–wake patterns. One direct practical application would be the evaluation of work schedules with regard to sleepiness, accident risk, and sleep disturbances.

REFERENCES

Åkerstedt, T., & Folkard, S. (1994). *Prediction of sleep length from Process C and S of the three process model of alertness regulation.* Manuscript submitted for publication.

Åkerstedt, T., & Folkard, S. (in press). Validation of Process S and C of the three-process model of alertness regulation, and the construction of an alertness nomogram. *Sleep.*

Åkerstedt, T., & Gillberg, M. (1981). The circadian variation of experimentally displaced sleep. *Sleep, 4,* 159–169.

Åkerstedt, T., & Gillberg, M. (1986a). A dose-response study of sleep loss and spontaneous sleep termination. *Psychophysiology, 23,* 293–297.

Åkerstedt, T., & Gillberg, M. (1986b). Sleep duration and the power spectral density of the EEG. *Electroencephalography and Clinical Neurophysiology, 64,* 119–122.

Åkerstedt, T., & Gillberg, M. (1990). Subjective and objective sleepiness in the active individual. *International Journal of Neuroscience, 52,* 29–37.

Åkerstedt, T., Gillberg, M., & Folkard, S. (1992). Slow wave activity and prior sleep/wakefulness on an irregular schedule. *Journal of Sleep Research, 2,* 118–121.

Åkerstedt, T., Kecklun, G., & Knutsson, A. (1991). Spectral analysis of sleep electroencephalography in rotating three-shift work. *Scandinavian Journal of Work Environment and Health, 17,* 330–336.

Borbély, A. (1982). Sleep regulation: Circadian rhythm and homeostasis. In D. Ganten & D. Pfaff (Eds.), *Sleep: Clinical and experimental aspects* (pp. 83–104). Berlin: Springer Verlag.

Folkard, S., & Åkerstedt, T. (1991). A three-process model of the regulation of alertness and sleepiness. In R. Broughton & R. Ogilvie (Eds.), *Sleep, arousal and performance: Problems and promises* (pp. 11–26). Cambridge, MA: Birkhauser Boston.

Folkard, S., Hume, K. I., Minors, D. S., Waterhouse, J. M., & Watson, F. L. (1985). Independence of the circadian rhythm in alertness from the sleep/wake cycle. *Nature, 313,* 678–679.

Fröberg, J. E. (1977). Twenty-four hour patterns in human performance, subjective and physiological variables and differences between morning and evening active subjects. *Biological Psychology, 5,* 119–134.

Fröberg, J., Karlsson, C. G., Levi, L., & Lidberg, L. (1975). Circadian variations of catecholamine excretion, shooting range performance and self-ratings of fatigue during sleep deprivation. *Biological Psychology, 2,* 175–188.

Gillberg, M., & Åkerstedt, T. (1981). Possible measures of "sleepiness" for the evaluation of disturbed and displaced sleep. In A. Reinberg, N. Vieux, & P. Andlauer (Eds.), *Night and shift work: Biological and social aspects* (pp. 155–160). Oxford: Pergamon Press.

Kecklun, G., & Åkerstedt, T. (1993). Sleepiness in long distance truck driving: an ambulatory EEG study of night driving. *Ergonomics, 36,* 1007–1017.

Torsvall, L., & Åkerstedt, T. (1987). Sleepiness on the job: Continuously measured EEG changes in train drivers. *Electroencephalography and Clinical Neurophysiology, 66,* 502–511.

Torsvall, L., Åkerstedt, T., Gillander, K., and Knutsson, A. (1989). Sleep on the night shift: 24 hr EEG monitoring of spontaneous sleep–wake behavior. *Psychophysiology, 26,* 352–358.

6

Entrained Phase of the Circadian Pacemaker Serves to Stabilize Alertness and Performance Throughout the Habitual Waking Day

Charles A. Czeisler, Derk-Jan Dijk, and Jeanne F. Duffy

The endogenous circadian pacemaker, located in the suprachiasmatic nucleus of the hypothalamus, is considered to be a major determinant of variations in subjective alertness and cognitive performance. Early evidence supportive of a clock mechanism underlying variations in alertness and performance was derived from long-term sleep deprivation experiments. In these experiments, alertness and performance exhibited rhythmic variations with a period close to 24 hr, superimposed on a steady deterioration of alertness and performance attributable to sleep loss (Åkerstedt & Fröberg, 1977; Fröberg, Karlsson, Levi, & Lidberg, 1975). The notion that alertness and performance are determined by the interaction of these two processes, that is, a circadian and a sleep–wake-dependent process, is widespread and

This project was supported in part by USPHS NIH awards NIA-R01-AG06072, NIA-P01-AG09975, NIMH-R01-MH45130 and GCRC-M01-RR02635; and the Swiss National Science Foundation Grant 31.32574.91.
    We thank the following individuals: J. M. Ronda and M. P. Johnson for data analysis; R. A. Sanchez, A. E. Ward, T. L. Shanahan, E. B. Martin, Jr., and D. W. Rimmer for supervising the studies; L. DiFabio for editorial assistance; the technicians for data collection; and the subject volunteers for their participation in the studies.

has been formalized in mathematical models (Åkerstedt & Folkard, 1990; Daan, Beersma, & Borbély, 1984; Folkard & Åkerstedt, 1989). The circadian contribution to variations in alertness and performance is generated by the light-sensitive circadian pacemaker that also drives the circadian rhythms of core body temperature, plasma cortisol, and plasma melatonin; in fact, scheduled light exposure shifts the rhythms of all of these variables by an equivalent amount (Czeisler, Johnson, et al., 1990; Czeisler et al., 1989; Shanahan & Czeisler, 1991). Despite the consensus on the significance of both a circadian and a sleep–wake-dependent process in the regulation of alertness and performance, attempts to quantify the contribution of both these processes to observed rhythms in alertness and cognitive performance have been scarce, and few adequate protocols to separate the circadian and sleep–wake-dependent processes have been developed (Folkard & Åkerstedt, 1989; Monk, 1987).

This chapter gives an overview of the current understanding of how the output of the circadian pacemaker interacts with the sleep–wake-dependent oscillatory process to generate the daily time course of alertness and cognitive performance under normal entrained conditions, under free-running conditions, among night workers, and during desynchronization of the sleep–wake and circadian systems, such as is seen in blind individuals.

TIME COURSE OF ALERTNESS DURING A CONSTANT ROUTINE

During our habitual waking day and during sleep deprivation, the circadian phase and the amount of prior wakefulness change simultaneously. In addition, alertness and performance are affected by caffeine intake, meals, exercise, variation in light intensity, and other exogenous factors. To document the time course of alertness and subjective performance in the absence of the confounding influences of such exogenous factors, we investigated these variables in a constant routine protocol (Czeisler et al., 1985; Mills, Minors, & Waterhouse, 1978) in 24 subjects.

Whereas previous authors have stressed variations in the daily time course of alertness, including the presence of 12-hr oscillatory components (Broughton, 1975, 1989; Brunner et al., 1992), we draw attention to the remarkable stability of alertness during the habitual day (Figure 1). After an initial rise in alertness shortly after awakening (called *sleep inertia* [Åkerstedt & Folkard, 1990]), alertness remains stable throughout the period that coincides with the habitual waking day. A sudden drop in alertness occurs close to habitual bedtime, and a minimum of alertness is reached shortly after the minimum of the endogenous rhythm of core body temperature (see Johnson et al., 1992, for further discussion). Thereafter, an upswing in alertness occurs at the beginning of the second day of the constant routine (CR). The data indicate that, in the absence of knowledge of clock time, the simultaneous variation in prior wakefulness and in circadian phase results in stable levels of alertness and performance during the habitual waking day.

THE FORCED DESYNCHRONY PROTOCOL

Separation of circadian and wake-dependent aspects of alertness and performance cannot be achieved by sleep deprivation experiments, or by classical free-running studies, or by those in which the sleep–wake cycle becomes desynchronized from the output of the circadian pacemaker because, in those experiments, the circadian phase and the duration of prior wakefulness either vary simultaneously or are not controlled (Czeisler, Weitzman, Moore-Ede, Zimmerman, & Knauer, 1980). The forced desynchrony protocol (Czeisler, Allan, & Kronauer, 1990) allows for a separation of these two processes. In this protocol, subjects live in a laboratory free of time cues for approximately one month, during which time they follow a 28-hr rest–activity cycle of which one third is spent in bed in darkness. After three baseline days, the initial endogenous circadian phase is assessed in a 40-hr CR. At the end of

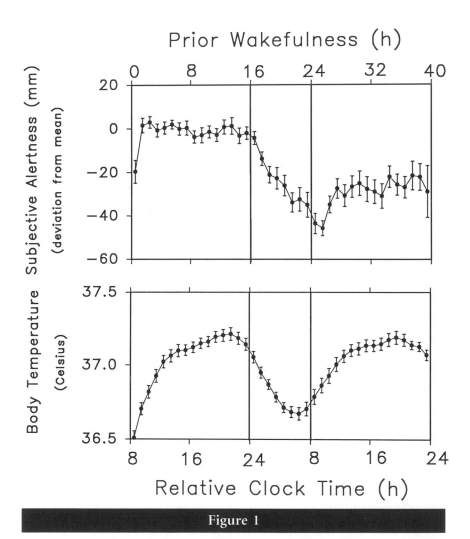

Figure 1

Time course of subjective alertness (upper panel) and core body temperature (lower panel) during a constant routine in 24 subjects. Data were averaged at 1-hr intervals. Alertness data for each subject are expressed as deviation from the entrained mean. Vertical bars represent ± 1 SEM. All data are plotted relative to habitual wake time, which was assigned a reference value of 8 a.m. (Adapted from Dijk, Duffy, & Czeisler, 1992.)

the forced desynchrony protocol, endogenous circadian phase is again assessed in a CR. To ensure that the endogenous circadian pacemaker is free running with a stable period, light intensity during the wake episodes is kept at very low levels, ca. 15 lux (Klerman, Dijk, Czeisler, & Kronauer, 1992). As shown in Figure 2, under these conditions, the sleep–wake cycle and its associated light–dark cycle can be scheduled at a period ($T = 28$ hr) that is outside the range of entrainment of the endogenous circadian pacemaker. Under such conditions, the circadian pacemaker, as reflected by the endogenous component of the body temperature cycle, continues to oscillate at a stable, near-24-hr period (Figure 2a and 2b). As a consequence, scheduled sleep and wake episodes cover virtually all phases of the endogenous circadian cycle, whereas the variation in sleep duration preceding wake episodes is minimized by instructing the subjects to stay in bed and in darkness, for 9 hr and 20 min of every 28-hr day. Similarly, the duration of wakefulness preceding sleep episodes is controlled, since subjects are scheduled to be awake for 18 hr and 40 min of every 28-hr day. Thus, sleep deprivation does not affect the evaluation of alertness and cognitive performance. During the scheduled waking episode, alertness is assessed approximately every 20 min, and calculation performance tests are given hourly.[1]

SEPARATION OF CIRCADIAN AND SLEEP–WAKE-DEPENDENT ASPECTS OF ALERTNESS AND PERFORMANCE

The contribution of the two processes to alertness and performance were separated by folding the data at either the endogenous circadian period (τ) or the period of the rest–activity cycle (T). Tau was assessed by nonparametric spectral analysis of the core body temperature data (Czeisler, 1978) obtained during the forced desynchrony part of the

---

[1]Details on subject selection and on the alertness and performance measures may be found in the original publications (Johnson, et al., 1992; Klerman, Dijk, Czeisler, & Kronauer, 1992).

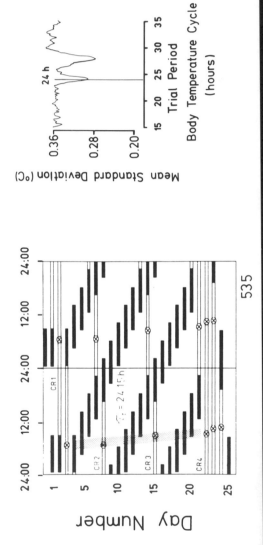

Figure 2

Forced desynchrony protocol. Left panel: Double raster plot of the protocol of subject 535. The rest–activity pattern is double-plotted in a raster format with successive days plotted next to and beneath each other. Solid bars represent scheduled bedrest episodes, open bars represent the constant routine protocol, and the encircled X represents the minimum of the core body temperature rhythm assessed during each CR. After two baseline nights and a 40-hr CR, the subject underwent fifteen 28-hr days (corresponding to 18 calendar days). This was followed by a 69-hr CR and a recovery sleep episode. Right panel: Nonparametric spectral analysis of core body temperature data collected during forced desynchrony protocol. Results indicate an endogenous component with an intrinsic period of 24.15 hr, as well as an endogenous component corresponding to the imposed period of the 28.0-hr rest–activity schedule.

protocol and also by the change in phase of the minimum of the core body temperature rhythm fitted with a dual-harmonic regression model (Brown & Czeisler, 1992) between the initial and final CR. The estimates of both methods are in good agreement with each other and with assessments of τ derived from plasma melatonin data (Shanahan & Czeisler, 1991). Assuming that the pacemaker oscillates with a stable period under these conditions, a circadian phase can be assigned to every minute of the protocol and thus to every alertness and performance measurement. Similarly, each value can be referenced to the duration of prior wakefulness at which it was collected. When averaged across circadian phases, a robust circadian oscillation in both subjective alertness and cognitive performance can be extracted from the data (Figure 3, left panels). Perhaps more surprising is the equivalent strength of the contribution of prior wakefulness to the level of alertness within the normal range of the duration of the daily waking episode. Even when the sleep–wake/dark–light cycle is scheduled to a period of 20 hr, reducing the length of the "daily" waking episode to 13 hr and 20 min, the striking impact of prior waking on alertness during the scheduled day can be extracted from these data (Figure 4, right panel). Alertness is significantly lower at the end of an episode of waking as short as 13.3 hr.

This wake-dependent deterioration of alertness cannot be seen under entrained conditions because the circadian contribution to alertness counteracts the wake-dependent decline in the latter half of the day. Likewise, the sleep-dependent restoration of alertness is not observed under entrained conditions because the timing of awakening coincides with the circadian trough of alertness, and alertness shortly after awakening is further suppressed by sleep inertia. However, data collected under conditions of forced desynchrony may be used to analyze how the two processes interact by *holding prior waking constant* and averaging the data train at selected durations of prior waking. In Figure 5a, the circadian modulation of alertness is illustrated as a function of the duration of prior wakefulness; whereas in Figure 5b, the circadian modulation of cognitive performance is illustrated as a function of the du-

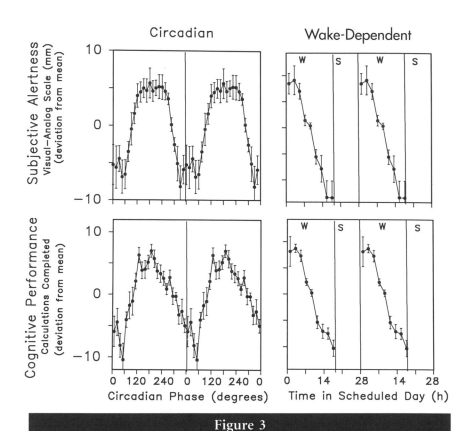

Figure 3

Circadian and wake-dependent variation of subjective alertness (upper panel; 8 subjects, total number of observations—6,142) and cognitive performance (lower panel; 9 subjects, total number of observations—2,277) as assessed in the forced desynchrony protocol ($T = 28$ hr). Data are expressed as a deviation from each subject's mean value during the forced desynchrony protocol. Data from each subject were first averaged per bin, and then the bin values were averaged across subjects. Vertical bars indicate ± 1 SEM. Left panels: Circadian component; data were averaged by phase of the endogenous component of the core body temperature rhythm, derived from the intrinsic period (τ_t) of each subject, with the minimum of the educed waveform of the core temperature rhythm assigned a reference value of 0 degrees. Right panels: Wake-dependent component; data were averaged with reference to the rest–activity cycle, at the imposed period of 28 hr (T). W = the scheduled 18.67-hr waking episode; S = the scheduled 9.33-hr rest episode. (Reanalysis of data from Dijk, Duffy, & Czeisler, 1992, and Johnson et al., 1992.)

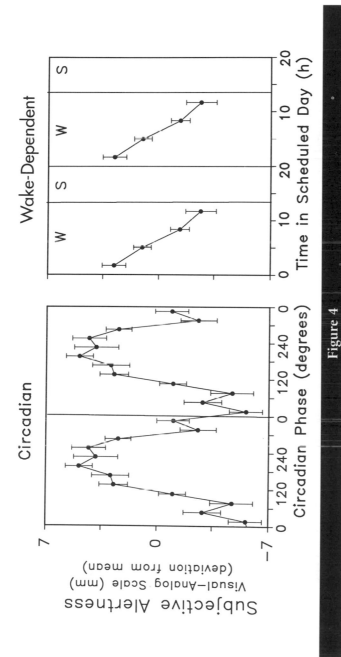

Figure 4

Circadian and wake-dependent variation of subjective alertness in subject 1111, scheduled to a 20-hr day. Data are expressed as the deviation from the subject's overall mean alertness level during the period of forced desynchrony (mean alertness value = 70.8). Data were averaged per bin, and vertical bars indicate ±1 SEM. Left panel: Data were averaged at the intrinsic period of the subject, with the minimum of the educed waveform of the core temperature rhythm assigned a reference value of 0 degrees. Right panel: Data were folded at the forced period of the rest–activity cycle (T = 20 hr). W = scheduled 13.33-hr waking episode; S = scheduled 6.67-hr rest episode.

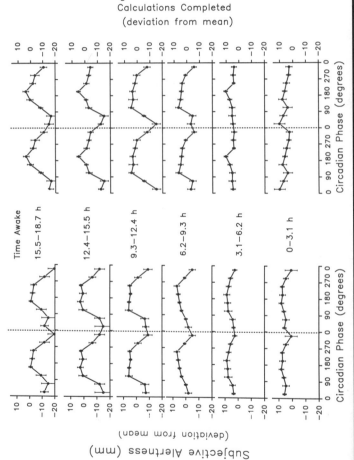

Cognitive Performance
Calculations Completed
(deviation from mean)

Subjective Alertness (mm)
(deviation from mean)

Time Awake

15.5–18.7 h

12.4–15.5 h

9.3–12.4 h

6.2–9.3 h

3.1–6.2 h

0–3.1 h

Circadian Phase (degrees)

Figure 5

Circadian modulation of alertness and cognitive performance for different durations of prior wakefulness from 9 young subjects on the forced desynchrony protocol ($T = 28$ hr). Definitions as in Figure 3. (Reanalysis of data from Dijk, Duffy, & Czeisler, 1992, and Johnson et al., 1992.)

ration of prior wakefulness. The data show that little circadian modulation of alertness or performance can be observed during the first 3 hr of the waking day. By contrast, the influence of the circadian pacemaker on alertness and performance becomes more pronounced when subjects have been awake for at least 6 hr. Once they have been awake for 16 hr, both alertness and performance are impaired at an adverse circadian phase. The maximum circadian facilitation of alertness and performance occurs at the circadian phase that, under entrained conditions, would coincide with the middle or later part of the habitual waking day.

Similarly, alertness data collected under forced desynchrony conditions can be used to analyze the interaction between the wake-dependent deterioration of alertness and circadian phase by *holding circadian phase constant* and averaging the data with regard to the length of prior waking (Figure 6). The results indicate that the effect of prior waking on alertness is most pronounced only around the minimum of the endogenous circadian rhythm of core body temperature.

Although these analysis techniques are useful for separating the effects of circadian phase from those of prior waking on alertness, they do not correspond with actual observations because neither temporal dimension (i.e., circadian phase or length of prior waking) can progress in time while the other is held constant. Figure 7, therefore, illustrates the dynamic interaction of the length of prior waking and circadian phase during the course of waking days commencing at different circadian phases. The data were averaged to correspond with particularly relevant circadian phases of waking. Panel A illustrates the typical time course of alertness, derived from data collected in the forced desynchrony protocol, expected to correspond to entrained conditions in which subjects awaken 0–3 hr after the fitted minimum of their endogenous circadian temperature cycle. Levels of alertness begin to drop only after ~16 hr of waking, corresponding to the time of habitual bedtime, presuming ~8 hr of sleep per day. Panel B illustrates the typical time course of alertness, derived from the data collected in the forced desynchrony protocol, expected to correspond to free-running

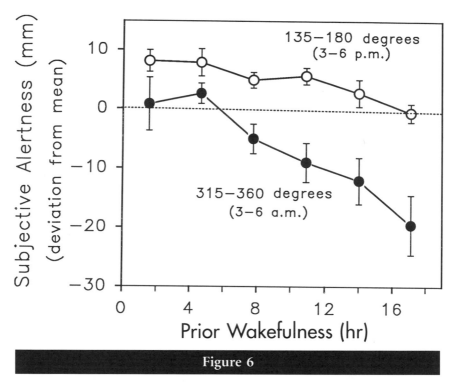

Figure 6

Effect of variations in prior wakefulness on subjective alertness at two different circadian phases (135–180 degrees and 315–360 degrees). Definitions as in Figure 3. (Reanalysis of data from Dijk, Duffy, & Czeisler, 1992, and Johnson et al., 1992.)

conditions during synchrony between the sleep–wake and body temperature cycles. Under those conditions, young normal subjects typically elect to go to sleep near the minimum of the endogenous component of the circadian temperature cycle and wake 7–9 hr later (Czeisler, 1978; Wever, 1973; Zulley, Wever, & Aschoff, 1981). Note that levels of alertness begin to drop 3–4 hr before the average time at which bedtime is selected under these conditions (~16½ hr after wake time). Panel C illustrates the typical time course of alertness, derived from the data collected in the forced desynchrony protocol, expected to correspond to that experienced by a permanent night-shift worker

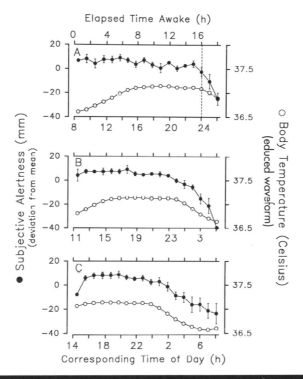

Figure 7

Time course of alertness (filled circles) and core body temperature (open circles) for wake episodes starting at three circadian phases. Data are derived from forced desynchrony studies shown in Figure 3. Panel A: Wake episodes beginning at 0–45 degrees, typical of entrained conditions (corresponding to wake times of 6–9 a.m.). Panel B: Wake episodes beginning at 45–90 degrees, typical of synchronized free-run conditions when subjects normally choose to go to bed near their temperature minimum and awaken 7–9 hr later. Panel C: Wake episodes beginning at 90–135 degrees, corresponding to the times at which a night-shift worker who sleeps from 9 a.m. to 2 p.m. would be awake. (Reanalysis of data from Dijk, Duffy, & Czeisler, 1992, and Johnson et al., 1992.)

sleeping between 0900 and 1400 hr each day and attempting to remain awake and alert while at work between 2400 and 0800 hr. Because the circadian pacemaker typically fails to adjust to such attempted inversions of the sleep–wake schedule (Czeisler, Allan, et al., 1990; Roden, Koller, Pirich, Vierhapper, & Walhauser, 1993), both the circadian and wake-dependent components of alertness are in phase with each other throughout the waking day. Thus, in the permanent night-shift worker, both components contribute to high alertness during the first half of the waking day, and both components lead to a deterioration of alertness during the working night.

RELATION TO THE CIRCADIAN REGULATION OF SLEEP

Current models of the regulation of sleep have stressed that sleep propensity and sleep structure are determined by the interaction of the circadian pacemaker and of a sleep–wake-dependent process (Borbély 1982; Borbély, Achermann, Trachsel, & Tobler, 1989; Borbély & Achermann, 1992; Daan, Beersma, & Borbély, 1984). The contributions of sleep–wake-dependent and circadian processes to sleep structure and sleep propensity have been assessed in the forced desynchrony protocol (Dijk & Czeisler, 1991, 1992, 1993, 1994). We have found that the circadian drive for wakefulness is greatest near the end of the habitual waking day, whereas the circadian drive for sleep is strongest near the end of the habitual sleep episode. By contrast, the sleep-dependent or homeostatic drive for sleep is greatest at the beginning of the sleep episode, and the propensity for wakefulness increases progressively throughout the sleep episode (Dijk & Czeisler, 1994). We conclude from these data that a consolidated bout of sleep can be achieved best when sleep is initiated just after the maximum of the circadian drive for wakefulness ($\sim$90 degrees before the endogenous circadian temperature minimum). Additional support for this notion may be found in the sleep data from blind subjects whose circadian pacemaker is not synchronized to the 24-hr day and who nonetheless adhere to a 24-hr sleep–wake schedule (Klein et al., 1993; Sack, Lewy, Blood, Keith, &

Nakagawa, 1992). These blind people experience a chronic state of forced desynchrony between their sleep–wake and circadian cycles. They suffer from recurring sleep disturbances with a period that is related directly to the circadian period (Folkard, Arendt, Aldhous, & Kennett, 1990; Klein et al., 1993; Nakagawa, Sack, & Lewy, 1992).

An analysis of three months of polygraphically recorded sleep in a blind subject suffering for more than three decades from a recurring sleep disturbance that recurred cyclically every three months, may be used to illustrate the circadian contribution to sleep propensity (Figure 8). The endogenous circadian rhythms of core body temperature and plasma cortisol were free running with a period of 24.27 hr. During this time, the subject was living on a 24-hr schedule; therefore, his sleep occurred at virtually all circadian phases. Sleep was most disturbed near the crest of the body temperature cycle and least disturbed near the temperature nadir. The propensity to initiate sleep, as estimated by the latency to sleep onset, is plotted as a function of circadian phase at the time of lights out. Shortest sleep latencies were observed at the trough of the endogenous circadian rhythm of core body temperature, whereas longest latencies were present several hours after the crest of the temperature cycle.

If the duration of prior wakefulness were not a factor, entrained subjects would choose to go to sleep at the time of the greatest circadian propensity to initiate sleep, which occurs approximately 1 to 2 hr before their habitual wake time. Ironically, the low point of the circadian sleep propensity rhythm occurs just before the habitual bedtime. This paradoxical phase relationship between the sleep propensity rhythm and the timing of the habitual sleep–wake cycle had been previously observed in ultradian day studies, including 0.3-hr, 1.5-hr, and 3-hr day studies (Carskadon & Dement, 1975, 1980; Lavie, 1986; Nakagawa et al., 1992; Webb & Agnew, 1975; Weitzman et al., 1974). In each of these studies, the circadian nadir of sleep efficiency occurred in the late evening, near the subjects' habitual bedtimes, whereas the circadian peak in sleep efficiency occurred near the subjects' habitual wake times. Such findings perplexed observers at the time. Given the present data, however, it is

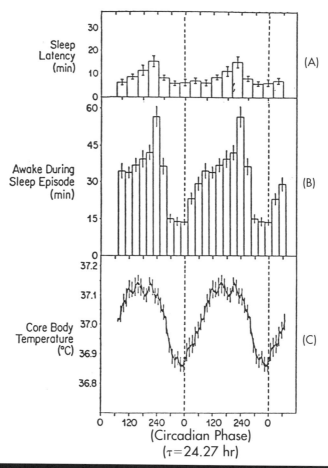

Figure 8

Sleep latency and amount of wakefulness within scheduled sleep episodes as a function of circadian phase in a blind man. Data were collected during a three-month study in which the subject's cortisol and core body temperature rhythms were free running with an intrinsic period of 24.27 hr, despite adhering to a 24-hr rest–activity schedule. Sleep data from each night of the study were assigned a circadian phase derived from the educed waveform of the core temperature rhythm (Panel C). Latency to sleep onset (Panel A) and minutes of wakefulness per hour of sleep (Panel B) were found to vary with the phase of the core temperature and cortisol rhythms. Vertical bars represent ±1 SEM. (Modified from Klein et al., 1993.)

apparent that the ultradian day protocols quench the influence of the wake-dependent increase in sleep tendency and unmask the circadian rhythm of sleep propensity. This is consistent with the view expressed by Webb in the present volume (chapter 4). Similarly, the daily variation in Multiple Sleep Latency Test (MSLT) results, with the reliable midday increase in sleep tendency, may reflect the interaction of these two processes. The long sleep latencies observed on MSLTs in the first third of the waking day in entrained subjects may reflect primarily the short duration of prior waking at those test times; by contrast, the long sleep latencies observed in the evening hours may reflect primarily the circadian peak in alertness occurring at those test times. Shorter sleep latencies recorded in the midafternoon may occur because neither system promotes wakefulness at that time (Borbély et al., 1989).

FUNCTIONAL CONSIDERATIONS

In summary, under normal entrained conditions, the circadian minimum of alertness and performance and the circadian minimum of wake propensity occur near the habitual wake time, whereas the maximum of the circadian rhythms of these variables occur near the end of the habitual day. Although these findings might seem, at first glance, difficult to understand, they may provide insight into how the output of the circadian pacemaker interacts with other regulatory processes in the CNS to generate stable levels of alertness and performance during the habitual waking episode, and into how these same interactions might generate a consolidated sleep episode. By providing a signal that counteracts the wake-dependent increase in fatigue and sleep propensity during the habitual waking day, the circadian system allows for stable levels of alertness through the wake episode and facilitates the consolidation of the wake episode (Figure 9). Likewise, the increase in sleep propensity toward the early morning, when we have already been asleep for several hours, serves to consolidate sleep. By providing a signal that counteracts sleep–wake-dependent changes in sleep–wake tendency, the

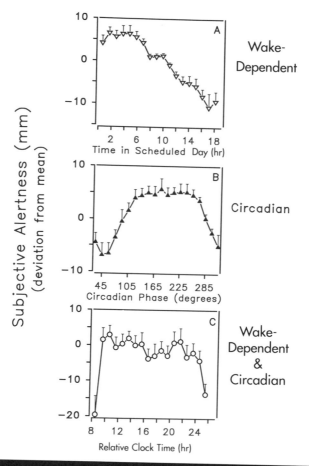

Figure 9

Components of subjective alertness. Panels A and B were derived from data collected in the forced desynchrony protocol. Data for each subject are expressed as a deviation from the individual mean score during the forced desynchrony segment ($N = 7$). Panel A: Variation of subjective alertness in relation to length of the scheduled wake episode. Data were averaged at the forced period of the rest–activity cycle (28 hr). Panel B: Circadian variation of alertness during the fraction of the circadian cycle that coincides with the wake episode and the first few hours of the sleep episode during entrainment (8 a.m.–3 p.m.). Data were folded at the observed period (τ_r) of the core body temperature rhythm, with the minimum of the educed waveform assigned a reference value of 0 degrees. Panel C: Time course of alertness during an 18-hr episode of wakefulness on a constant routine immediately following release from entrainment ($n = 24$ subjects). Data are plotted with regard to habitual wake time, which was assigned a reference value of 8 a.m. (Reanalysis of data from Dijk, Duffy, & Czeisler, 1992, and Johnson et al., 1992.)

circadian pacemaker is ideally positioned to facilitate the consolidation of sleep and waking, a phenomenon that is uncommon in other mammals.

Taken together, these data indicate that the seemingly paradoxical phase relation between the sleep–wake cycle and the endogenous circadian rhythm of alertness and sleep propensity serves to maintain constant high levels of alertness and performance and low levels of sleepiness throughout the waking day. This phase relationship further assures that sleep remains consolidated until the end of the nightly sleep episode despite the sleep-dependent increase of wake propensity. The contribution of endogenous and exogenous factors to the establishment of this phase relationship between the sleep–wake cycle and the endogenous circadian pacemaker remains to be established.

REFERENCES

Åkerstedt, T., & Folkard, S. (1990). A model of human sleepiness. In J. Horne (Ed.), *Sleep '90* (pp. 310–340). Bochum, Germany: Pontenagel Press.

Åkerstedt, T., & Fröberg, J. E. (1977). Psychophysiological circadian rhythms in women during 72 h of sleep deprivation. *Waking Sleeping, 1,* 387–394.

Borbély, A. A. (1982). A two-process model of sleep regulation. *Human Neurobiology, 1,* 195–204.

Borbély, A. A., & Achermann, P. (1992). Concepts and models of sleep regulation: An overview. *Journal of Sleep Research, 1,* 63–79.

Borbély, A. A., Achermann, P., Trachsel, L., & Tobler, I. (1989). Sleep initiation and initial sleep intensity: Interaction of homeostatic and circadian mechanisms. *Journal of Biological Rhythms, 4,* 149–160.

Broughton, R. J. (1975). Biorhythmic variations in consciousness and psychological functions. *Canadian Psychological Review, 16,* 217–230.

Broughton, R. J. (1989). Chronobiological aspects and models of sleep and napping. In D. F. Dinges & R. J. Broughton (Eds.), *Sleep and alertness: Chronobiological, behavioral, and medical aspects of napping* (pp. 71–98). New York: Raven Press.

Brown, E. N., & Czeisler, C. A. (1992). The statistical analysis of circadian phase and amplitude in constant routine core temperature data. *Journal of Biological Rhythms, 7*, 177–202.

Brunner, D. P., Wirz-Justice, A., Kräuchi, K., Graw, P., Haug, H. J., & Leonhardt, G. (1992). Is there an endogenous mid-afternoon dip of subjective alertness? *Journal of Sleep Research* (Suppl. 1), 33.

Carskadon, M. A., & Dement, W. C. (1975). Sleep studies on a 90-min day. *Electroencephalography and Clinical Neurophysiology, 39*, 145–155.

Carskadon, M. A., & Dement, W. C. (1980). Distribution of REM sleep on a 90-minute sleep–wake schedule. *Sleep, 2*, 309–317.

Czeisler, C. A. (1978). *Internal organization of temperature, sleep–wake, and neuroendocrine rhythms monitored in an environment free of time cues.* Unpublished doctoral dissertation, Stanford University, California.

Czeisler, C. A., Allan, J. S., & Kronauer, R. E. (1990). A method for assaying the effects of therapeutic agents on the period of the endogenous circadian pacemaker in man. In J. Montplaisir & R. Godbout (Eds.), *Sleep and biological rhythms: Basic mechanisms and applications to psychiatry* (pp. 87–98). New York: Oxford University Press.

Czeisler, C. A., Brown, E. N., Ronda, J. M., Kronauer, R. E., Richardson, G. S., & Freitag, W.O. (1985). A clinical method to assess the endogenous circadian phase (ECP) of the deep circadian oscillator in man. *Sleep Research, 14*, 295.

Czeisler, C. A., Johnson, M. P., Duffy, J. F., Brown, E. N., Ronda, J. M., & Kronauer, R. E. (1990). Exposure to bright light and darkness to treat physiologic maladaptation to night work. *New England Journal of Medicine, 322*, 1253–1259.

Czeisler, C. A., Kronauer, R. E., Allan, J. S., Duffy, J. F., Jewett, M. E., Brown, E. N., & Ronda, J. M. (1989). Bright light induction of strong (Type 0) resetting of the human circadian pacemaker. *Science, 244*, 1328–1333.

Czeisler, C. A., Weitzman, E. D., Moore-Ede, M. C., Zimmerman, J. C., & Knauer, R. S. (1980). Human sleep: Its duration and organization depend on its circadian phase. *Science, 210*, 1264–1267.

Daan, S., Beersma, D. G. M., & Borbély, A. A. (1984). Timing of human sleep: Recovery process gated by a circadian pacemaker. *American Journal of Physiology, 246*, R161–R178.

Dijk, D. J., & Czeisler, C. A. (1991). A quantitative assessment of the circadian influence on sleep propensity and sleep structure by forced desynchrony of the sleep–wake cycle and core-body-temperature rhythm [Abstract]. *Sleep Research, 20A*, 531.

Dijk, D. J., & Czeisler, C. A. (1992). The consolidation of human sleep is codetermined by the output of the endogenous circadian pacemaker and a sleep-dependent process [Abstract]. *Proceedings of the 3rd Meeting of the Society for Research on Biological Rhythms*, 69.

Dijk, D. J., & Czeisler, C. A. (1993). Sleep-dependent disinhibition of REM sleep in humans [Abstract]. *Sleep Research, 22*, 400.

Dijk, D. J., & Czeisler, C. A. (1994). Paradoxical timing of the circadian rhythm of sleep propensity serves to consolidate sleep and wakefulness in humans. *Neuroscience Letters, 166*, 63–68.

Dijk, D. J., Duffy, J. F., & Czeisler, C. A. (1992). Circadian and sleep/wake dependent aspects of subjective alertness and cognitive performance. *Journal of Sleep Research, 1*, 112–117.

Folkard, S., & Åkerstedt, T. (1989). Towards the prediction of alertness on abnormal sleep/wake schedules. In A. Coblentz (Ed.), *Vigilance and performance in automated systems* (pp. 287 296). Norwell, MA: Kluwer Academic.

Folkard, S., Arendt, J., Aldhous, M., & Kennett, H. (1990). Melatonin stabilises sleep onset time in a blind man without entrainment of cortisol or temperature rhythms. *Neuroscience Letter, 113*, 193–198. Fröberg, J. E., Karlsson, C. G., Levi, L. & Lidberg, L. (1975). Circadian rhythms of catecholamine excretion, shooting range performance and self-ratings of fatigue during sleep deprivation. *Biological Psychology, 2*, 175–188.

Johnson, M. P., Duffy, J. F., Dijk, D. J., Ronda, J. M., Dyal, C. M., & Czeisler, C.A. (1992). Short-term memory, alertness and performance: A reappraisal of their relationship to body temperature. *Journal of Sleep Research, 1*, 24–29.

Klein, T., Martens, H., Dijk, D. J., Kronauer, R. E., Seely, E. W., & Czeisler, C.A. (1993). Chronic non-24-hour circadian rhythm sleep disorder in a blind man with a regular 24-h sleep–wake schedule. *Sleep, 16*, 333–343.

Klerman, E. B., Dijk, D. J., Czeisler, C. A., & Kronauer, R. E. (1992). Simulations using self-selected light–dark cycles from "free-running" protocols in humans result in an apparent tau significantly longer than the intrinsic tau [Abstract]. *Proceedings of the 3rd Meeting of the Society for Research on Biological Rhythms*, 78.

Lavie, P. (1986). Ultrashort sleep–waking schedule: Part 3. Gates and "forbidden zones" for sleep. *Electroencephalography and Clinical Neurophysiology, 63,* 414–425.

Mills, J. N., Minors, D. S., & Waterhouse, J. M. (1978). Adaptation to abrupt time shifts of the oscillator[s] controlling human circadian mechanisms. *Journal of Physiology, 285,* 455–470.

Monk, T. H. (1987). Subjective ratings of sleepiness—The underlying circadian mechanisms. *Sleep, 10,* 343–353.

Nakagawa, H., Sack, R. L., & Lewy, A. J. (1992). Sleep propensity free-runs with the temperature, melatonin, and cortisol rhythms in a totally blind person. *Sleep, 15,* 330–336.

Roden, M., Koller, M., Pirich, K., Vierhapper, H., & Walhauser, F. (1993). *American Journal of Physiology, 34,* R261–R267.

Sack, R. L., Lewy, A. J., Blood, M. L., Keith, L. D., & Nakagawa, H. (1992). Circadian rhythm abnormalities in totally blind people: Incidence and clinical significance. *Journal of Clinical Endocrinology and Metabolism, 75,* 127–134.

Shanahan, T. L., & Czeisler, C. A. (1991). Intrinsic period of the endogenous circadian rhythm of plasma melatonin is consistent with that of core body temperature during forced desynchrony in a 21-year-old man [Abstract]. *Sleep Research, 20A,* 557.

Webb, W., & Agnew, H. (1975). Sleep efficiency for sleep–wake cycles of varied length. *Psychophysiology, 12,* 637–641.

Weitzman, E. D., Nogeire, C., Perlow, M., Fukushima, D., Sassin, J., McGregor, P., Gallagher, T. F., & Hellman, L. (1974). Effects of a prolonged 3-hour sleep–wake cycle on sleep stages, plasma cortisol, growth hormone, and body temperature in man. *Journal of Clinical Endocrinology and Metabolism, 38,* 1018–1030.

Wever, R. (1973). Internal phase-angle differences in human circadian rhythms: Causes for changes and problems of determinations. *International Journal of Chronobiology, 1,* 371–390.

Zulley, J., Wever, R., & Aschoff, J. (1981). The dependence of onset and duration of sleep on the circadian rhythm of rectal temperature. *Pfluegers Archives, 391,* 314–318.

PART THREE

Behavioral, Physiological, and Cognitive Changes

7

Vigilance Decrement and Sleepiness

Nancy Barone Kribbs and David Dinges

The natural investigation of sleep onset requires patience and little interference with the potential sleeper because healthy individuals seldom experience a transition from full, conscious wakefulness to sleep more than a few relatively unpredictable times in every 24-hr period (Carskadon & Dement, 1989). As those who have experienced and studied insomnia are well aware, sleep onset cannot be forced or persuaded when it is not timely or when it is aggravated by internal or external factors (e.g., noise or persistent worries [Hauri, 1989; Roehrs, Zorick, & Roth, 1989]). The study of sleep onset can be facilitated by inducing sleepiness with a sleep deprivation paradigm that will increase the occurrence of sleep onsets. Pathological sleepiness resulting from obstructive sleep apnea can also be used opportunistically as a means of studying sleepiness closely (Kribbs et al., 1993). The frequent dis-

Preparation of this chapter was supported in part by National Institute of Mental Health Grant MH 44193, NASA Grant NCC-2-599, National Institutes of Health (NIH) Grant SCOR HL 42236, NIH Clinical Research Center Grant RR00040, and the Institute for Experimental Psychiatry Research Foundation.

We are grateful to Kelly A. Gillen, John N. Henry, Geoffrey E. Ott, and John W. Powell for their assistance in the research.

ruptions of sleep caused by apneic airway obstruction result in sleepiness and, therefore, more frequent sleep onsets. In fact, experimental sleep disruption alone, in the absence of a loss of total sleep time (including Stage 1 sleep), has also been demonstrated to result in sleepiness (Bonnet, 1986; Stepanski, Lamphere, Roehrs, Zorick, & Roth, 1987).

The study of sleepiness itself is, in effect, also the study of sleep onset or of the processes leading to sleep onset. The physiological sleep system and the brain's need for sleep are so powerful that, by imposing wakefulness or sleep disruption, one is able to study sleepiness and sleep onset with great frequency and throughout the 24-hr period in which sleep is normally not likely or not easily obtained. Thus, during sleep deprivation, sleep onsets occur frequently and often uncontrollably. Therefore, sleepiness can be conceptualized as brain state lability, the hallmark of which is an increased probability of transition from wakefulness to sleep onset (Dinges, 1989, 1990).

Sleep deprivation, sleep disruption, and pathological sleepiness not only increase the frequency of sleep onsets but also enhance the *rate* of sleep onset. We propose that this accelerated rate of sleep onset is the product of a facilitatory interaction between the sleep system and the environment of the person, and that this interaction can result in performance in which the performer is *functionally asleep* (i.e., that there is, in effect, a diminished functioning as the transition to sleep onset increases). This chapter illustrates this concept by drawing upon examples of the effects of sleepiness, caused by sleep loss and sleep apnea, on psychomotor vigilance performance.

FUNCTIONAL SLEEP ONSET

The concept of functional sleep onset is, by definition, performance based. Thus, from a behavioral perspective, we posit that a sleepy individual who can no longer respond, or respond appropriately, to a stimulus is, in effect, functionally asleep. Although we used electrophysiological measures of sleep onset to determine the basis of performance changes, they were not essential criteria for our concept of functional sleep onset.

CONTEXTUAL DEPENDENCE

A common misconception that has persisted in the sleep literature is that easy tasks, such as those related to simple reaction time, are not readily impaired by one night of sleep deprivation, whereas complex, longer duration, and more difficult cognitive tasks and decision-making capability do suffer (Dinges & Kribbs, 1991). Certainly, longer duration tasks can reveal the effects of sleep loss, but there is also ample experimental evidence to dispute the claim that performance, including vigilance performance, is affected *only* when the test is prolonged to the range of 30 to 60 min. If the signal rate is high and the response modality appropriately sensitive, repetitive tasks of 10-min duration will expose the limits of performance capability in sleepy subjects (Dinges, 1992).

We now know, as will be demonstrated, that performance decrements resulting from sleep deprivation can be observed in simple and relatively short tasks if changes across time are analyzed (Dinges & Powell, 1988). The performance of boring and monotonous tasks, even if of short duration, during which shifts in attention are detrimental to performance, traps the brain into a repetitive, rhythmic cycle, thereby providing an environment that is conducive to sleep, despite the performer's desire to stay awake. This kind of task is very difficult to perform well when combined with sleep deprivation *if* the goal is to remain alert. It is no coincidence that a common folk remedy for sleeplessness is to "count sheep" in the mind's eye. What could be more simple, monotonous, and repetitive yet still require constant observation? Therefore, the degree to which performance is impaired depends very much on the environment in which it occurs. That is, there is a "contextual dependence" that results from the brain's interaction with, and reliance on, the environmental context for stimulation.[1] That is why it is usually far easier to remain awake late at night while at a party than it is to remain awake while driving home from the party.

THE PSYCHOMOTOR VIGILANCE TASK

In studying impairment from sleep loss and pathological sleepiness, we used a performance domain that is highly sensitive to sleepiness, yet has little of the practice effects and other confounds that can often make neuropsychological probes difficult to interpret (Dinges & Kribbs, 1991). This performance, referred to as the *psychomotor vigilance task* (PVT), requires sustained attention, rapid response to a stimulus, and data analyses that reflect the many ways in which the brain can be impaired by sleep loss. Broadly, these analyses yield at least six performance parameters: lapses, false responses, optimum response shifts, slowing, lapse duration, and vigilance decrement functions (i.e., time-on-task decrements; Dinges & Powell, 1985). We refer to the latter as a *fatigability function* (Dinges et al., in press).

The PVT takes 10 min to complete and was administered in our studies once every 2 hr during wakefulness. A reaction time stimulus consists of the digits "000" appearing in the color red in a LED window on the device and increasing in milliseconds until the response button is pushed. The resulting number at the button press is the reaction time in milliseconds. The subject's task is to press the button as soon as the stimulus appears, making an effort to keep response times as short as possible throughout the task, but not to press before the stimulus appears. There is a variable 1–10-sec interstimulus interval. The data are then downloaded digitally to a computer for processing. Although similar simple reaction time tasks have been used in experimentally induced sleep deprivation studies in normal subjects (Dinges, Orne, Whitehouse, & Orne, 1987; Glenville, Broughton, Wing, & Wilkinson,

---

[1]This theory has been articulated at some length (Dinges, 1989).

1978; Lisper & Kjellberg, 1972), we also used them to gather extensive data in apneic patients before and after treatment with nasal continuous positive airway pressure (CPAP; Kribbs et al., 1993) and in transoceanic flight crews (Dinges, Graeber, Connell, Rosekind, & Powell, 1990; Rosekind et al., 1993). In addition, dependent variables were extracted from these task data beyond those used by other investigators (see Dinges & Powell, 1985, 1988, 1989).

TIME-ON-TASK DECREMENT

One calculation that we used is the time-on-task or vigilance decrement function. If results *across* time are analyzed, even for a task as brief as the 10-min PVT, decrements in performance are observed. As is demonstrated in Figure 1, grand means of four daily tests on 14 untreated apneic subjects (PRE-TX) show a steeper slope in the response speed regression line with time on task and a lower y-intercept (mean response speed), relative to performance after treatment (POST-TX) with nasal CPAP. (The reaction times were reciprocally transformed to normalize the data, thus decreasing the influence of performance lapses on the mean.) The performance regression line of the apneic subjects following treatment improved but, interestingly, not to the levels found in rested young adults (see Kribbs et al., 1993, for further discussion). This suggests that apneic patients are not yet fully recovered after 30 days of treatment. However, caution must be taken in such an interpretation of the findings because of age differences between the patient group and the young adult group.

Vigilance decrement may be observed as evidence of fatigue (because of inadequate waking rest) even in well-motivated subjects with adequate sleep. This decrement manifests itself as a shallow decline in the time-on-task slope. When the subject is sleep-deprived, it appears to be impossible to sustain attention enough to maintain peak performance across the entire duration of a high-signal-load task such as the PVT. Sleep loss *accelerates* the degradation process (i.e., increases the

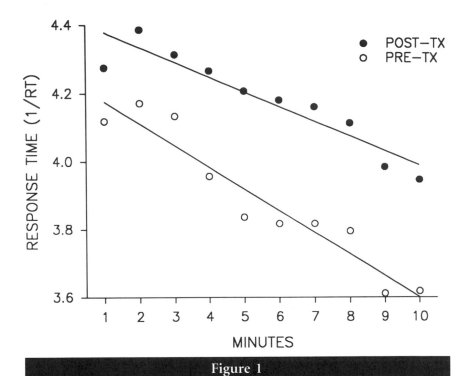

Figure 1

Least-squares regression lines fitted to grand mean reciprocal reaction times (in min) for each minute of the 10-min PVT administered in four daily testing sessions per subject, to 14 obstructive sleep apnea patients before (PRE-TX; $R = .96$, slope $= .064$) and after (POST-TX; $R = .94$, slope $= .043$) treatment with nasal CPAP. The overall PRE-TX mean reciprocal reaction time, collapsing across minutes, of 3.9 ($SD = 0.52$) was significantly lower than the POST-TX mean of 4.2 ($SD = 0.56$) ($t = 3.16$, $p < .05$).

negative slope). This is why analysis of the overall mean response often does not truly reflect the entire impairment process and, in fact, may sometimes obscure actual performance impairment.

VARIABILITY OF PERFORMANCE

In addition to performance degradation over time, an investigation of the variability in performance with time on task provides further valuable information about performing while sleepy and during sleep onset. One parameter that reflects performance variability is the number of reaction time performance *lapses* that occur during a trial. Lapses, generally defined as reaction times that are greater than twice the baseline average, have historical significance in sleep-deprivation research (Dinges & Kribbs, 1991). Usually, the lapses within a test period are counted, and the numbers are compared for different conditions. Lapses are generally infrequent unless the sleep deprivation is prolonged. A count of the number of lapses provides a gross estimate of the level of impairment but fails to extract systematic changes in lapsing with time on task.

If the lapses are observed over time, one obtains a better picture of the acceleration of impairment, reflective of fatigability. Figure 2 shows an increase in lapses across time on task for sleep-deprived normal subjects. As is evident in the figure, as sleep deprivation increases in time, an increase in the mean number of lapses occurs each minute across the 10-min task. Consequently, the effect of sleep deprivation beyond 24 hr is not clearly apparent until the final 5 min of the 10-min task (relative to the first 5 min). After two nights without sleep, lapses increase conspicuously from the third to the tenth minute. If one sets a criterion of 2 or more lapses in 1 minute of PVT performance as indicative of being functionally asleep (a *very* liberal criterion), then by the third minute of performance, the subjects would be functionally asleep following 48–64 hr of deprivation. If the criterion is no more than 1 lapse per minute (a liberal criterion), then sleep loss of 24–36 hr would reveal functional sleep by the eighth minute of PVT time. Obviously, even more rigorous standards will yield discrimination in the first few minutes on the PVT. Figure 3 shows similar data for patients with sleep apnea before and after treatment with CPAP. In both Figures 2 and 3, the relatively nonsleepy conditions show a shallower slope and smaller mean, as is the case for mean response speed (Figure 1).

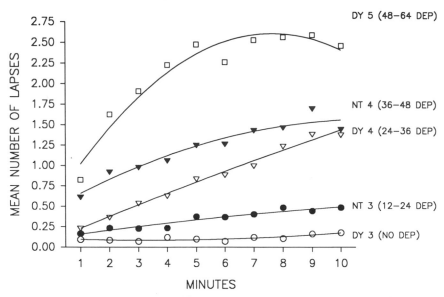

Figure 2

Quadratic (second-order polynomial) regression lines fitted to grand mean number of lapses (i.e., reaction times > 500 msec) for each minute of the 10-min PVT in 20 healthy young adults. Testing was conducted in six daily/nightly sessions when the subjects were alert during the day (DY 3, no deprivation; $M = .11$ lapse, $SD = .04$), during the night after 12 to 24 hr of sleep deprivation (NT 3; $M = .34$ lapse, $SD = .12$), during the day after 24 to 36 hr of sleep deprivation (DY 4; $M = .85$ lapse, $SD = .41$), during the night after 36 to 48 hr of sleep deprivation (NT 4; $M = 1.22$ lapses, $SD = .32$), and during the day after 48 to 64 hr of sleep deprivation (DY 5; $M = 2.15$ lapses, $SD = .56$).

PROBING THE BRAIN'S ATTENTIONAL CAPACITY

Kjellberg (1977a, 1977b, 1977c) proposed that one way in which the environment and physiological sleepiness interact is through the fundamental central nervous system (CNS) process of habituation (Dinges & Kribbs, 1990). Although there are a number of reasons why we are not certain that habituation is the specific physiological mechanism underlying PVT vigilance decrement functions in sleepy subjects (e.g.,

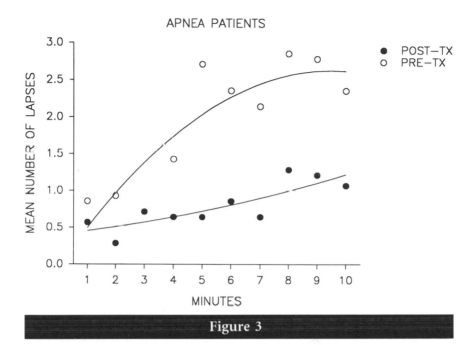

Figure 3

Quadratic (second-order polynomial) regression lines fitted to grand mean number of lapses (i.e., reaction times > 500 msec) for each minute of the 10-min PVT in 14 obstructive sleep apnea patients. Testing was conducted in four daily sessions before (PRE-TX) and after (POST-TX) treatment with nasal CPAP. The overall mean number of lapses, collapsing across minutes, was significantly higher for PRE-TX (19.36, $SD = 27.71$) compared to POST-TX (7.64, $SD = 13.37$) ($t = 2.25$, $p < .05$).

Figure 1), we posit that sleepiness can moderate the ability of the brain to respond to environmental stimuli, especially to those that are monotonous and repetitive. We believe that this acceleration of performance deterioration with time on task is reflective of a shortening of sleep-onset latency in which the brain is "driven" to sleep (Dinges, 1989; Dinges & Kribbs, 1990). In other words, a monotonous or repetitive task that measures performance over time acts as a CNS probe, revealing the brain's sleep tendency, and because it also reveals performance failures, it reflects the fundamental ability (or inability) to remain attentive.

It is our experience that time-on-task decrements in sleepy persons are to be seen most likely in tasks that demand a high attentional capacity (e.g., high or sustained signal load), like the PVT. The accelerated decrements with time on task are indicative of escalating failures of attention.

The observed pattern of attentional shifts, demonstrated by decrements with time on task, is hypothesized to be a reflection of underlying neurophysiological events within the CNS. Electrophysiologic measures during time on task show promise as indicators of direct CNS involvement in reaction time capability and time-on-task decrements. Average event-related brain potentials (ERPs) can be used for the simultaneous evaluation of brain electroencephalographic activity during performance tasks sensitive to sleepiness (see Harsh, chapter 18; Ogilvie, Battye, & Simons, chapter 16; and Salisbury, chapter 17, in this volume for further information.) Responses in the 50–400-ms range, known as slow cognitive potentials, have been measured during reaction-time tasks. For example, the P300 waveform has been widely studied. This evoked potential component appears at about 300 ms following the occurrence of a rare target stimulus, to which the subject has been instructed to attend. The rare stimulus appears infrequently against a background of frequently occurring standard stimuli, in a procedure also known as an *oddball* paradigm. To elicit a P300, the subject must actively attend to stimuli and maintain some level of consciousness. Decreases in the amplitude and latency of this waveform component have been linked to the processes of sleep onset (Campbell, Bell, & Bastien, 1992; Harsh, chapter 18, this volume). Other studies have demonstrated a P300 amplitude decline across testing time, attributed to a habituation process (see Wesensten, Badia, & Harsh, 1990, for an example and review.)

The N100 response that peaks at 80–100 ms following stimulus presentation, occurring both when subjects are instructed to ignore or attend to the stimulus, is also a potential ERP indicator of sleepiness and sleep onset mechanisms in the CNS. Previous research has shown this waveform to be sensitive to state, in that its amplitude decreases with sleep onset and depth of sleep (Campbell et al., 1992). Our own preliminary work has shown a decrease in the N100 component over a 10-min period of time, as would be anticipated by habituation.

Therefore, in future studies, it may be possible, with an appropriate CNS probe presentation rate, to analyze the data further and to show a general decline not only in performance over time but also in the pattern of attention as it shifts and oscillates.

CONCLUSION

We have presented behavioral evidence indicating that accelerated time-on-task performance decrements, especially in attention-based tasks, can reflect sleepiness and lead to functional sleep onsets with severe impairment; that is, high sleep pressure from sleep loss results in a rapid deterioration of performance over brief periods of test time. The reaction time lapse findings also point to the importance of studying the variability of performance with sleepiness. For example, a sleepy driver may undergo many descents toward sleep (lapses) within one excursion and demonstrate wild fluctuations in driving capability, without actually achieving EEG sleep or being involved in an accident. Investigation of these frequent functional sleep onsets, and the mechanisms by which they occur, should be one of our research goals if we wish to understand fully the relationship between sleepiness and performance capability.

REFERENCES

Bonnet, M. H. (1986). Performance and sleepiness as a function of frequency and placement of sleep disruption. *Psychophysiology, 23*, 263–271.

Campbell, K., Bell, I., & Bastien, C. (1992). Evoked potential measures of information processing during natural sleep. In R. J. Broughton & R. D. Ogilvie (Eds.), *Sleep, Arousal, and Performance* (pp. 88–116). Boston: Birkhauser.

Carskadon, M. A., & Dement, W. C. (1989). Normal human sleep: an overview. In M. H. Kryger, T. Roth, & W. C. Dement (Eds.), *Principles and practice of sleep medicine* (pp. 3–13). Philadelphia: W. B. Saunders.

Dinges, D. F. (1989). The nature of sleepiness: causes, contexts, and consequences. In A. J. Stunkard & A. Baum (Eds.), *Eating, Sleeping, and Sex* (pp. 147–179). Hillsdale, NJ: Erlbaum.

Dinges, D. F. (1990). Are you awake? Cognitive performance and reverie during the hypnopompic state. In R. Bootzin, J. Kihlstrom, & D. Schacter (Eds.), *Sleep and cognition* (pp. 159–175). Washington, DC: American Psychological Association.

Dinges, D. F. (1992). Probing the limits of functional capability: The effects of sleep loss on short-duration tasks. In R. J. Broughton & R. D. Ogilvie (Eds.), *Sleep, Arousal, and Performance* (pp. 177–188). Boston: Birkhauser.

Dinges, D. F., Gillen, K., Powell, J., Carlin, M., Ott, G., Orne, E. C., & Orne, M. (in press). Discriminating sleepiness by fatigability on a psychomotor vigilance task. *Sleep Research, 23.*

Dinges, D. F., Graeber, R. C., Connell, L. J., Rosekind, M. R., & Powell, J. W. (1990). Fatigue-related reaction time performance in long-haul flight crews. *Sleep Research, 19,* 117.

Dinges, D. F., & Kribbs, N. B. (1990). Comparison of the effects of alcohol and sleepiness on simple reaction time performance: enhanced habituation as a common process. *Alcohol, Drugs and Driving, 5/6,* 329–339.

Dinges, D. F., & Kribbs, N. B. (1991). Performing while sleepy: Effects of experimentally induced sleepiness. In T. H. Monk (Ed.), *Sleep, Sleepiness, and Performance* (pp. 97–128). New York: Wiley.

Dinges, D. F., Orne, M. T., Whitehouse, W. G., & Orne, E. C. (1987). Temporal placement of a nap for alertness: contributions of circadian phase and prior wakefulness. *Sleep, 10,* 313–329.

Dinges, D. F., & Powell, J. W. (1985). Microcomputer analyses of performance on a portable, simple visual RT task during sustained operations. *Behavioral Research Methods, Instruments & Computers, 17,* 652–655.

Dinges, D. F., & Powell, J. W. (1988). Sleepiness is more than lapsing. *Sleep Research, 17,* 84.

Dinges, D. F., & Powell, J. W. (1989). Sleepiness impairs optimum response capability; It's time to move beyond the lapse hypothesis. *Sleep Research, 18,* 366.

Glenville, M., Broughton, R., Wing, A. M., & Wilkinson, R. T. (1978). Effects of sleep deprivation on short duration performance compared to the Wilkinson auditory vigilance task. *Sleep*, *1*, 169–176.

Hauri, P. (1989). Primary insomnia. In M. H. Kryger, T. Roth, & W. C. Dement (Eds.), *Principles and practice of sleep medicine* (pp. 442–447). Philadelphia: W. B. Saunders.

Kjellberg, A. (1977a). Sleep deprivation and some aspects of performance: I. Problems of arousal changes. *Waking and Sleeping*, *1*, 139–143.

Kjellberg, A. (1977b). Sleep deprivation and some aspects of performance: II. Lapses and other attentional effects. *Waking and Sleeping*, *1*, 145–148.

Kjellberg, A. (1977c). Sleep deprivation and some aspects of performance: III. Motivation, comment and conclusions. *Waking and Sleeping*, *1*, 149–153.

Kribbs, N. B., Pack, A. I., Kline, L. R., Getsy, J. E., Schuett, J. S., Henry, J. N., & Dinges, D. F. (1993). The effects of one night without nasal CPAP treatment on sleep and sleepiness in patients with obstructive sleep apnea. *American Review of Respiratory Disease*, *147*, 1162–1168.

Lisper, H.-O., & Kjellberg, A. (1972). Effects of 24-hour sleep deprivation on rate of decrement in a 10-minute auditory reaction time task. *Journal of Experimental Psychology*, *96*, 287–290.

Roehrs, T., Zorick, F., & Roth, T. (1989). Transient insomnia and insomnias associated with circadian rhythm disorders. In M. H. Kryger, T. Roth, & W. C. Dement (Eds.), *Principles and Practice of sleep medicine* (pp. 433–441). Philadelphia: W. B. Saunders.

Rosekind, M. R., Graeber, R. C., Dinges, D. F., Connell, L. J., Rountree, M., Spinweber, C. L., & Gillen, K. A. (1993). Crew factors in flight operations : IX. Effects of cockpit rest on crew performance and alertness in long-haul operations. In *NASA Technical Memorandum Report N. 103884* (pp. 10–252). Moffett Field, CA: NASA.

Stepanski, E., Lamphere, J., Roehrs, T., Zorick, F., & Roth, T. (1987). Experimental sleep fragmentation in normal subjects. *International Journal of Neuroscience*, *33*, 207–214.

Wesensten, N. J., Badia, P., & Harsh, J. (1990). Time of day, repeated testing, and interblock interval: Effects on P300 amplitude. *Physiology and Behavior*, *47*, 653–658.

8

Impact of the Level of Physiological Arousal on Estimates of Sleep Latency

Michael H. Bonnet and Donna A. Arand

S tudies have reported that insomniacs misperceive how long it takes them to fall asleep and underestimate their total sleep time compared with normally scored EEG values (Moore, 1981). By contrast, normal sleepers can generally estimate their sleep latency accurately (Moore, 1981). For example, data from seven studies of insomniacs indicated that the insomniacs overestimated their sleep latencies by about 36 min, whereas normal sleepers (NSs) overestimated their sleep latencies by about 0.5 min (Moore, 1981). These differences are commonly explained as an insomnia problem related to increased cognitive or physiological activity at sleep onset (Frankel, Buchbinder, Coursey, & Snyder, 1973; Monroe, 1967) or as an inability to differentiate sleep from waking (Downey & Bonnet, 1992). However, the differences could also be the result of a simple mathematical phenomenon. Because insomniacs have much longer objective sleep latencies, one would expect the error around those larger numbers to be larger as well. Therefore, simple mathematics might predict that small overestimates of short latencies might grow to larger overestimates of long latencies independently of an individual's status as an insomniac or NS. One means of "correcting" for this potential error might be to express the subjective and objective sleep latencies as a ratio. If a linear increase in overestimation as a function of latency length existed, the subjective-to-objective ratio would be similar in insomniacs and in NSs. Examination of the ratio data reveals that insomniacs still have larger ratios than NSs. (Therefore, they still overestimate.) However, a nonlinear increase in overestimation may exist as a function of sleep latency.

A recent examination of the relationship between arousal levels and the production of insomnia (Bonnet & Arand, 1992) revealed that EEG-defined insomniacs have an increased 24-hr metabolic rate compared with age-, sex-, and weight-matched NSs (Bonnet, McNulty, & Arand, 1993). In a different design, it was found that the chronic administration of 400 mg of caffeine (t.i.d.) to NSs increased their metabolic rate and produced many of the symptoms commonly reported by insomniacs (Bonnet & Arand, 1992). These findings have led to the hypothesis that the degree of accuracy seen in sleep-latency estimates may be related to the arousal level at the time of sleep onset. The alternative hypothesis is simply that the degree of overestimation is a nonlinear mathematical function of the actual objective sleep latency.

There are many ways to vary arousal levels at sleep onset. In general, manipulations such as sleep deprivation or the use of benzodiazepines will decrease the level of arousal and are hypothesized to decrease the subjective-to-objective ratio of sleep latencies. Conversely, administration of caffeine, which increases arousal levels, should also increase the latency ratio. A series of experiments to test these hypotheses is presented in Table 1. Although these experiments were performed for other reasons, they provide data to test the current hypotheses. The studies to be presented include observations from single subjects and trend data. It is important that the presentation be evaluated as a whole (i.e., as a combination of several discrete observations or a meta-analysis) rather than as a series of unrelated observations. Estimated data for short and long intervals from NSs and insomniacs will also be presented as a control for the effects of length of interval estimated.

Table 1

Tests of the Relationship Between Arousal Level and Estimates of Subjective and Objective Sleep Latency

Ratio of subjective to objective sleep latencies should be decreased when arousal level is decreased by

- administration of benzodiazepines
- sleep deprivation

Ratio of subjective to objective sleep latencies should be increased when arousal level is increased by

- administration of caffeine
- sleep during the daytime (circadian arousal)

AROUSAL LEVEL DECREASES

Administration of Benzodiazepines

In one study (Bonnet, 1991), triazolam (0.125 mg) or a placebo was given to independent groups of 12 normal, young adult male sleepers before 2-hr or 4-hr naps. In other groups, 0.25 or 0.50 mg of triazolam was given before 8-hr naps. The subjective-to-objective sleep latency ratios for the various groups and doses are plotted in Figure 1, which shows that the difference in subjective/objective ratios between the drug and each matched placebo group grows as a function of triazolam dose, with the largest difference between placebo and triazolam estimates found at the .5-mg dose. All four increasing triazolam doses compared with those of placebo indicate lower ratios with medication and lower ratios as medication dose increases. Overall, the subjective-to-objective sleep latency ratios were significantly lower after triazolam compared with placebo ($F(1,47) = 4.16$, $p < .05$).

In another benzodiazepine study (Bonnet, Kramer, & Roth, 1981), one of three doses of diazepam or a placebo was given 30 min before the beginning of a normal night of sleep. A dose response decrease in

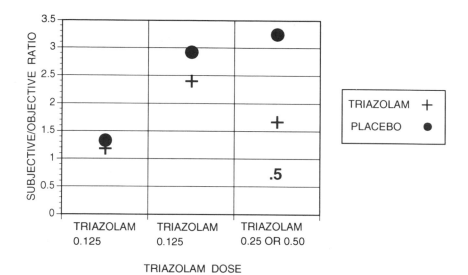

Figure 1

A comparison of subjective-to-objective sleep latency values for groups of young adults given either 0.125 mg of triazolam or matched placebo at two times or 0.25, 0.50 mg of triazolam or placebo at another time.

the subjective-to-objective ratio occurs in these data as well (as plotted by the regression line), although the differences are not so apparent as in the triazolam study (see Figure 2) because of the increased subjective/objective ratio in the 0.50-mg condition.

Sleep Deprivation

Subjective-to-objective sleep latency ratios were calculated in 104 normal, young adult male subjects (Ss) from baseline nights and the recovery night after a 64-hr period during which groups of Ss were allowed 0, 2, 4, or 8 hr of sleep (Bonnet, 1991). As would be expected, the median latency ratio was decreased on the recovery night compared with baseline at all four levels of sleep deprivation (see Figure 3). More impressive is that the difference in the subjective/objective ratio from the matched baseline for each group increased as a direct function of

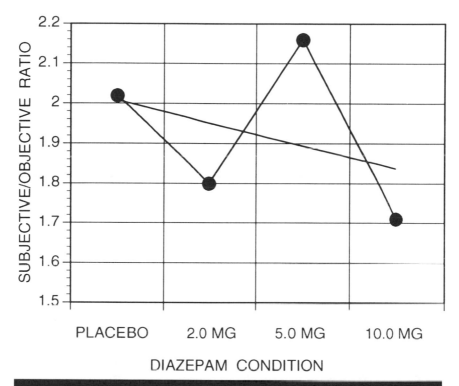

A comparison of subjective-to-objective sleep latency values for groups of young adults given matched placebo or 2, 5, or 10 mg of diazepam prior to bedtime. The line through the middle of the figure is the linear regression line.

the amount of sleep lost during the 64-hr period. The differences in sleep latency ratios from baseline to recovery sleep, therefore, also show a dose response relationship very similar to that seen in the triazolam study cited earlier. The difference in sleep latency ratios from baseline was significantly less for groups receiving no sleep or 2 hr of sleep during the sleep deprivation.

In a different type of study, a patient with documented psycho-physiological insomnia was partially sleep deprived (*sleep restriction therapy*) for seven nights. Figure 4 presents a graphic representation of

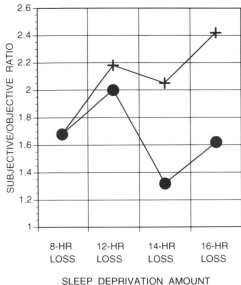

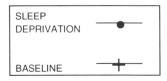

Figure 3

A comparison of subjective-to-objective sleep latency values for groups of young adults on baseline and on recovery after deprivation of a total of 0, 2, 4, or 8 hr of sleep over a 64-hr period (corresponding to 16, 14, 12, or 8 hr of lost sleep).

the subjective-to-objective sleep latency ratios for this patient. It is noteworthy that the ratios decline toward 1 ("correct" estimates) early during the partial sleep deprivation and that the ratios actually dropped below the 1 level on some nights. The first nonrestricted recovery night was night R1. The result of this was a "good" night of sleep. However, the insomnia returned on the next night, and R2 was accompanied by the expected increase in subjective-to-objective sleep latency ratio. This case illustrates that it is perhaps not one's status as an insomniac or NS that accounts for characteristic overestimation of sleep-onset latency. Clearly, the level of arousal, as indexed here by degree of sleep deprivation, seems to play a role in the degree of misperception of how long it takes to fall asleep. In these four studies, in which the level of arousal was decreased by benzodiazepines or sleep deprivation, subjec-

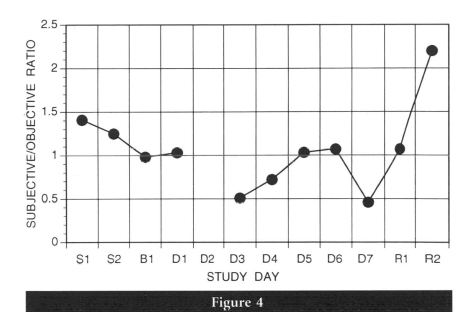

Figure 4

A comparison of subjective-to-objective sleep latency values for one psychophysiological insomniac undergoing screening (S), baseline (B), sleep restriction (D), and recovery (R).

tive-to-objective sleep latency ratios were decreased in comparison with placebo or baseline conditions in 11 of 12 comparisons, and effects appeared to be dose related. Because the effects were common to medication and sleep deprivation conditions, the latency ratings cannot be specific to memory or to other effects of benzodiazepines.

AROUSAL LEVEL INCREASES

Administration of Caffeine

In an experiment by Bonnet and Arand (1992), caffeine (400 mg t.i.d.) or a placebo was administered to normal, young adult male Ss for seven days. Figure 5 shows that the caffeine resulted in an increase in the subjective-to-objective ratio, whereas the ratio did not change in Ss

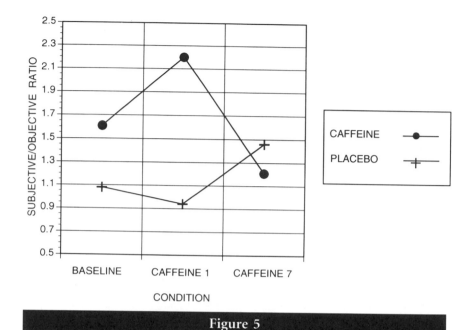

Figure 5

A comparison of subjective-to-objective sleep latency values for young adults given placebo or caffeine (400 mg t.i.d.) for one week.

receiving the placebo. Furthermore, the ratio returned to baseline levels by the seventh night of caffeine administration. This return to baseline in sleep latency ratio reflects the finding that tolerance to the metabolic effect of caffeine had developed by the seventh night, and that the metabolic rate was no longer significantly elevated by caffeine.

Circadian Effects

The well-known circadian physiological arousal curve implies that there should be a tendency to have greater subjective-to-objective sleep latency ratios as a function of the time of day when the sleep period begins. In a nap study by Bonnet (1991), sleep onsets occurred at 1200, 1600, 1800, and 2300 hr following a normal night of sleep in independent groups of normal young adults. Figure 6 shows the subjective-to-objective sleep latency ratios from those four time points. The figure

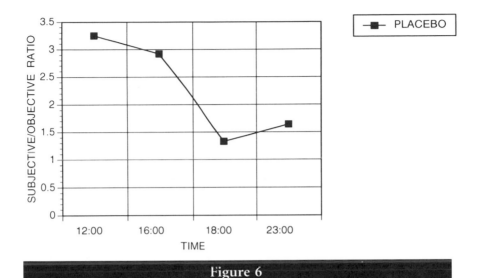

Figure 6

A comparison of subjective-to-objective sleep latency values for groups of young adults beginning sleep periods at four different circadian times.

generally supports the contention that there was a greater tendency to overestimate sleep onset in the afternoon compared with the evening and suggests a generally decreasing subjective-to-objective sleep latency ratio as arousal level declined toward the normal 2300-hr bedtime point.

As hypothesized, subjective-to-objective sleep latency ratios were greater after initial caffeine use compared with placebo and baseline and at the peak of the circadian rhythm compared with bedtime. Both types of evidence support the contention that going to sleep at a higher level of arousal will result in an increased estimate of sleep latency compared with EEG sleep latency.

CONTROLS

Do the data presented so far demonstrate the effect of varying levels of physiological arousal on the sleep-onset estimation, or can these data be explained as a mathematical artifact? It is clear in all of the examples that as the physiological level of arousal increases so do the EEG sleep latencies. Is there a means of determining whether longer periods of time (here time is defined as an unfilled interval) are more likely to be overestimated than are shorter periods of time? This issue was examined in a master's thesis (Moore, 1981) in which both insomniacs and NSs estimated various intervals at several times during the day. One set of intervals in each group was short ($M = 30$ s). In each group, there was also one 19-min interval (long). All the intervals were similar to sleep-onset periods in that they were unfilled, i.e., the subject was given a marker at the beginning and at the end, but no sound or task occurred between the markers. At the end of each interval, subjects simply estimated how long it had been since the initial stimulus had been given. The most consistent finding in the study was that both normal subjects and insomniacs overestimated the long intervals compared with the short intervals. Overall, the insomniacs' subjective-to-objective ratios for the unfilled short and long intervals were 1.18 and 1.59, respectively ($t = 6.82$, $p = .002$). Subjective-to-objective ratios in NSs for the unfilled short and long intervals were 1.02 and 1.38, respectively ($t = 2.72$, $p = .05$). It should be noted also that insomniacs overestimated both short and long intervals compared with the NSs. This difference, 1.18 versus 1.02 for short intervals and 1.59 versus 1.38 for long intervals, was small, but it was in the direction predicted by an increased level of arousal and was corrected for length of interval.

To what extent does the tendency to estimate long unfilled intervals disproportionately longer than short unfilled intervals account for the data that have already been presented? The availability of estimated data for short and long intervals made it possible to derive a specific equation to predict the degree of overestimation that should occur at various intervals of time. This equation was used to modify the estimated data presented earlier from the caffeine study in an attempt to estimate what proportion of the increase in the ratio could be attributed simply to estimating larger latency numbers. The caffeine data were chosen specifically because the sleep latencies were longer and thus more likely to be influenced by such scaling factors. Figure 7 presents the subjective-

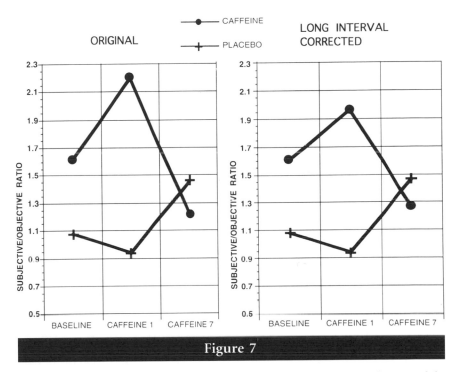

Figure 7

A comparison of subjective-to-objective sleep latency values for groups of young adults given placebo or caffeine (400 mg t.i.d.) for one week (left panel) and the same data controlled for the effect of estimating longer latencies on the caffeine nights (right panel).

to-objective ratios for the caffeine study as originally presented (on the left panel) and as modified by the equation (on the right panel). It can be seen that the long-interval effect indeed does reduce the amount of apparent overestimation at initial caffeine administration. However, even with this correction, an effect for degree of physiological arousal remains.

IMPLICATIONS

The data presented here support the contention that the perception of falling asleep is dependent on how long it takes to fall asleep and on the level of physiological arousal at sleep onset. Some of the findings presented were not directly testable by statistical methods or did not represent statistically significant differences, but the consistency of the findings over six independent studies with several designs presents a persuasive argument that estimates of sleep latency are dependent upon level of physiological arousal. Of 17 specific directional predictions that could be made in the six studies based on the physiological arousal hypothesis, 15 were in the predicted direction (binomial probability = .0011). However, it is also clear that the degree of overestimation of sleep latency depends additionally, to some extent, on the actual EEG latency.

These data support the idea that poor sleep or insomnia is a physiological phenomenon that can be controlled by varying the level of arousal. The data support the idea that decreasing the level of arousal by sleep deprivation or sedatives will decrease both sleep latency and overestimation of sleep latency. Similarly, increasing the level of arousal will increase both sleep latency and overestimation of sleep latency. The central idea is that poor sleep, whether it be acute or chronic, is a physiological (as opposed to a psychological) event that is amenable to physiological exploration and modification.

REFERENCES

Bonnet, M. H. (1991). The effect of varying prophylactic naps on performance, alertness and mood throughout a 52-hour continuous operation. *Sleep, 14,* 307–315.

Bonnet, M. H., & Arand, D. L. (1992). Caffeine use as a model of acute and chronic insomnia. *Sleep, 15,* 526–536.

Bonnet, M. H., Kramer, M., & Roth, T. (1981). A dose response study of the hypnotic effectiveness of alprazolam and diazepam in normal subjects. *Psychopharmacology, 75,* 258–261.

Bonnet, M. H., McNulty, T. B., & Arand, D. A. (1993). 24-hour metabolic rate in matched normals and insomniacs. *Sleep Research, 22,* 175.

Downey, R. D., & Bonnet, M. H. (1992). Sleep–wake discrimination in subjective insomnia improves as a function of sleep onset feedback. *Sleep, 15,* 58–63.

Frankel, B., Buchbinder, R., Coursey, R., & Snyder, F. (1973). Sleep patterns and psychological test characteristics of chronic primary insomniacs. *Sleep Research, 2,* 149.

Monroe, L. J. (1967). Psychological and physiological differences between good and poor sleepers. *Journal of Abnormal Psychology, 72,* 255–264.

Moore, S. E. (1981). *Estimates of sleep latency and of other temporal intervals in insomniac and normal sleepers.* Unpublished master's thesis, University of Cincinnati.

9

Home Monitoring of Sleep Onset and Sleep-Onset Mentation Using the Nightcap®

Robert Stickgold and J. Allan Hobson

INTRODUCTION

The question of how the brain controls mental activity remains an elusive one, despite the vast amount of research that has gone into the subject. Numerous approaches have been used to gain valuable insights into this issue. One of these approaches is the study of brain states. If altered brain states can produce altered mentation, and if we can understand the neurophysiological underpinnings of the changes in brain state, we can attempt to map these changes onto the parallel changes in mentation. The more obvious examples of parallel shifts in brain states and mental states include those resulting from the use of psychoactive drugs or from mental illness. But the most common, indeed ubiquitous, example is that of sleep.

For about 2 hr each night, during REM sleep, the brain enters a state in which the mind becomes formally psychotic. Wild and bizarre delusions are fed by visual and auditory hallucinations that can include other sensory modalities as well. The mind becomes hyperemotional, alternately terrified and ecstatic. Profound anxiety alternates with a sense of omnipotent grandiosity. Clearly, these profound shifts in mental state must result from the normal physiological changes that underlie REM sleep.

Since 1960, significant progress has been made in understanding the physiology of being awake, and of REM and non-REM (NREM) sleep. Anatomical, physiological, and biochemical systems within the brain stem all interact in a carefully orchestrated and well-documented sequence of changes as the body shifts from waking to NREM sleep and, then, to REM sleep. With specific reference to the neurophysiology of sleep onset, the reticular deactivation process that was first postulated by Moruzzi and Mogoun (1949) has now been further specified as involving most subsets of reticular neurons, including, significantly, the widely projective and ramifying cells of the noradrenergic locus coeruleus and of the serotonergic dorsal raphe nucleus, as well as more locally projecting elements, including the cholinergic subgroups that innervate the thalamus (Hobson & Steriade, 1986; Steriade & McCarley, 1990). Thus, sleep onset is associated with a massive and radical electrochemical deafferentation of the thalamocortical neurons that are believed to be the critical elements in the origins of consciousness.

Over the past decade, and more intensely in the past few years, we have been attempting to analyze reports of sleep mentation with an eye toward developing a bidirectional mapping between brain and mind.

In addition to sampling within well-established states, it is of interest to investigate the transitions between them. For example, it would be of interest to watch the changes in mentation and physiology that occur as a subject moves from NREM to REM sleep. In other words, how do dreams begin? We have been struck by the fact that in hundreds of reports of spontaneously recalled dreams, subjects never describe what they consider to be the *beginning* of a dream. The narrative is always picked up somehow along the way as if the dream were already in progress. Does this mean that subjects simply cannot remember dream onset, or does it mean that REM-sleep dreaming evolves seamlessly out of NREM sleep mentation?

This phenomenon might be studied more easily by examining the transition from wakefulness to sleep that occurs at sleep onset. Sleep-onset mentation bears important formal similarities to emergent REM-sleep mentation. At sleep onset, one can see the beginning of hypnagogic dreams and observe the transformation of presleep thoughts into the content of hypnagogic dreams. The study of sleep-onset mentation began in earnest with the French psychologists, Maury (1861) and d'Hervey de Saint-Denis (1867), who used self-observation to identify the basic characteristics of hypnagogic dreaming.

As a starting point, this study looks at the temporal development of such formal dream properties as bizarreness, hallucination, and hyperemotionality in hypnagogic dream reports, and examines whether dream features appear all at once or whether they develop in some orderly progression, by following the pioneering sleep laboratory work of Foulkes and Vogel (1965) and Vogel (1991). Preliminary pilot data illustrate the use of an inexpensive, home-based monitoring system, the Nightcap®, to obtain repeated measures from individual subjects. We emphasize that this is a demonstration project, not a completed, systematic study.

METHODOLOGICAL CONSTRAINTS

Methodologically, we set four requirements for this study. First, we wanted to conduct the study in a home environment because it is more natural and more cost effective than in a laboratory.

Second, we wanted to monitor the subject's sleep state during the period of dream collection. Although not requiring a full polysomnographic (PSG) recording, we needed a reliable indication of how far along in the sleep-onset process the subject was when a report was given.

Third, we wanted this monitoring to be totally passive, requiring no behavioral responses from the subject. We imposed this constraint because of the known sensitivity of the sleep-onset process to arousal, to thoughts, and even to the knowledge that dream reports were going to be collected. Thus, we wanted to avoid any unnecessary intrusions that might bias what the subjects were doing and thinking about as they fell asleep.

Fourth, we wanted the monitoring system itself to rouse the subjects for each report. Again, this was to relieve subjects from the necessity of constantly monitoring their thoughts in an attempt to identify sleep onset and awaken themselves.

All of these requirements were met by using our portable sleep-monitoring system known as the Nightcap (Mamelak & Hobson, 1989).

THE NIGHTCAP

The design of the Nightcap is based on several studies that indicate that body movement can be used to distinguish between wakefulness and sleep and that REM and NREM sleep can be distinguished by the presence or absence of rapid eye movements (Aaronson, Rashed, Biber, & Hobson, 1982; Helfand, Lavie, & Hobson, 1986; Webster, Kripke, Messin, Mullaney, & Wyborney, 1982). These characteristics are summarized in Table 1.

The Nightcap is a two-channel recording device that distinguishes wakefulness, REM sleep, and NREM sleep. One channel monitors eye

Table 1		
Basic State-Determining Algorithm		
State	Eye movements	Body movements
Wake	++	+
REM	+	−
NREM	−	−

NOTE: Wake is defined by very high numbers of eye movements and body movements. REM is defined by high numbers of eye movements with few or no body movements. NREM is defined by few or no eye movements or body movements.

movement, and the other monitors body movements. Eye movements are measured by an adhesive-backed, 25 mm × 7 mm piezoelectric film attached to the upper eyelid, which detects the passive deformation of the eyelid by movement of the eye. Body movements are measured by a cylindrical, multipolar mercury switch attached to the forehead, which produces a signal in response to a head rotation of 30°. These sensors are connected by 1-m cables to the main Nightcap unit, a 12 cm × 7 cm × 2.5 cm box containing signal detectors, A/D converters, a clock, an RS-232 serial port (for downloading data), and a microprocessor with 32 KB of RAM (Figure 1).

The Nightcap scores 250-ms epochs for eyelid and body movements and stores the number of epochs in each minute that have eyelid and body movements.

The data are then transferred to a computer and analyzed by a program called the NC Analyzer, which generates and graphically displays a hypnogram of sleep stages (Figure 2). The example shown in Figure 2 is from a subject who spent a night in the sleep laboratory wearing both the Nightcap and the standard array of electrodes for PSG. The hand scoring of the polygraph record is displayed along with the Nightcap data. Two features should be pointed out. First, the NC Analyzer identified all REM and NREM periods, as well as two nocturnal awakenings, scored from polygraph recordings. Only the precise timing of state transitions showed any discrepancies between the two scoring methods. Second, the time of sleep onset, as determined by the polygraph and the Nightcap, were within one min of each other. For this example (Figure 2), sleep onset was heralded by one minute with 130 eyelid movements and 38 head movements, a transitional minute with 15 eyelid movements and no body movements, and finally one minute with just 3 eyelid movements.

Several studies have validated the reliability and efficacy of the Nightcap. Mamelak and Hobson (1989) showed that a prototype of the Nightcap could successfully distinguish the wake, REM, and NREM states with an overall Nightcap–PSG agreement rate of 86%. Ajilore,

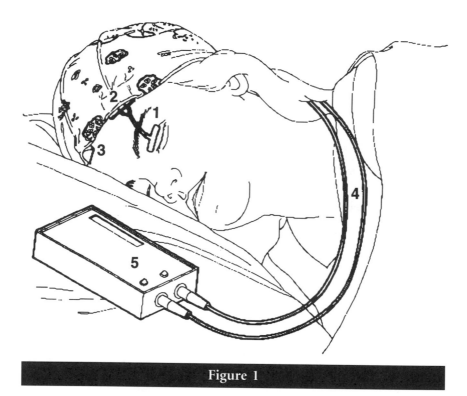

Figure 1

The Nightcap®. Line drawing made from a photograph of a subject sleeping with the Nightcap. The eye movement sensor (1) is applied to the left eyelid and attached to a mount (2) located under the bandanna. The head movement sensor (3) is on the right side of the forehead, under the bandanna. Leads from the two sensors (4) travel around the back of the subject's head to the battery-operated recording unit (5) lying on the bed covers next to the subject.

Stickgold, Rittenhouse, & Hobson (in press), using a portable version of the Nightcap, obtained 87% agreement between the two techniques based on 1-min epochs. They also demonstrated its efficacy and ease of use in the home. Pace-Schott, Kaji, Stickgold, & Hobson (in press) studied 21 good and poor sleepers in their home and showed that the Nightcap could distinguish between the two groups based on sleep latency and sleep efficiency. Both studies showed values for percentage of REM and NREM sleep in the home similar to those obtained in the

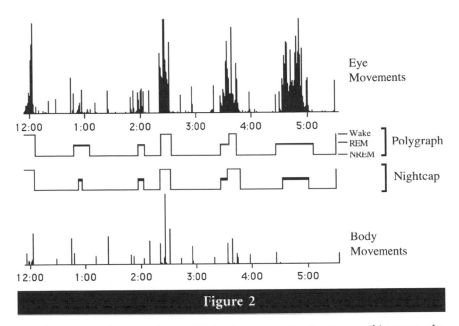

Figure 2

Sample output and analysis by the NC Analyzer program. Top trace = histogram plot of Nightcap-detected eyelid movements; second trace = hypnogram representing the manually scored PSG record; third trace = hypnogram of computer-scored Nightcap data; fourth trace = histogram plotting Nightcap-detected body movements. On all hypnograms, the top level represents wakefulness; the second, REM; and the third, NREM. Movement time is not shown. The lower axis indicates the time of night. Details of the scoring algorithm are given in Pace-Schott et al. (in press).

laboratory with PSG. Stickgold, Pace-Schott, & Hobson (1994) looked at spontaneous dream reports obtained after spontaneous REM and NREM awakenings in the home using the Nightcap and confirmed the correlation of REM awakenings with higher report frequencies and longer reports. All these studies confirm the ability of the Nightcap to identify polysomnographically scored periods of wakefulness and of REM and NREM sleep.

THE NIGHTCAP AT SLEEP ONSET

Although analyses such as that shown in Figure 2 are more than adequate for analyzing the overall sleep architecture of a night, they lack sufficient temporal resolution to look at the process of sleep onset. Greater resolution can be obtained by connecting the Nightcap to a computer during the night. In this case, the Nightcap sends out information after each 250-ms epoch, indicating whether an eyelid or body movement occurred during that epoch. The remainder of this chapter describes the preliminary results obtained through a self-study by one of the authors (Stickgold). The intent here is to demonstrate the feasibility of such an analysis for a group of subjects currently being studied.

FALLING ASLEEP IS A GRADUAL, INTERMITTENT PROCESS

Figure 3 shows the first 12.8 min of a night during which the subject attempted to rouse himself and give reports of sleep-onset mentation. Each pair of lines displays the eyelid and body movements detected in a 2-min period. Eyelid movments are shown on the upper line and body movements on the lower. During this study, the Nightcap was attached to a Macintosh computer, and the subject recorded the time of each report by pressing a key on the keyboard. The graph begins at the time at which the Nightcap was turned on. The arrow labeled 1, near the start of the record and drawn by the computer, indicates the time of a key press made immediately before the subject gave a verbal report of his name, the date, and the time. The arrow labeled 2, at the end of the display and also drawn by the computer, indicates the time of a key press immediately preceding the first mentation report. A transcript of the report is given below the graph. The time at the start of the transcript was obtained from a time stamp automatically multiplexed onto the audiotape at the time of the recording.

During the period shown in Figure 3, eyelid movements continued at a high rate, and there was no evidence of any change in eyelid movement frequency right up to the time of the report. By contrast, body movements were frequent during the first 10 min of the recording, but ceased approximately 3 min before the report (arrow 2 in the figure).

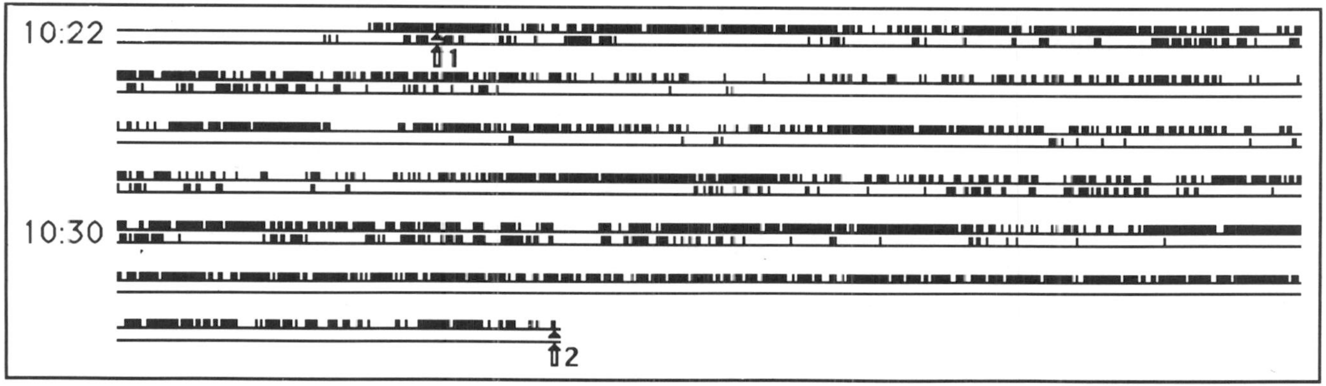

Report No. 2 (22:35). For the last minute or so, I've been slipping into sorta vivid prehallucinations, not true hallucinations. Ah. . .I wouldn't call them hypnagogic dreams, but ¨ think they're more intense than what I would normally experience when awake. Ah. . . One had to do with playing golf when I was a child in our backyard, and the other had something to do with thinking about the whole issue of . . . ah . . . whether it was hypnagogic or not. In retrospect, probably they were hypnagogic.

Figure 3

High-resolution display of Nightcap data and report. Top: Each pair of lines displays data for a 2-min interval, with eyelid movements marked on the upper line and body movements on the lower. Times of reports (registered by the subject's pressing the space bar on the keyboard) are marked below the lines with arrows and numbers. Bottom: Transcription of report dictated at the 2 mark. Time on transcript is read from dictaphone tape. Times on Nightcap data display taken from Nightcap.

The report explicitly stated that the subject considered the report to be a hypnagogic dream.

EYELID QUIESCENCE HERALDS THE HYPNAGOGIC EXPERIENCE

In the minutes following the report shown in Figure 3, the Nightcap output changed dramatically, as seen in Figures 4A and 4B. These two graphs and reports follow directly the period depicted in Figure 3. After each key press, eyelid movements returned as the subject dictated his report, but then disappeared abruptly within a minute of the initial key press. Interestingly, each cessation of eyelid movements was accompanied by 2 to 4 body movements, possibly reflecting the rolling of the head to the side as muscle tone was lost. The two reports were given following 2 to 4 min with almost no eyelid movements and clearly involved hypnagogic thoughts and imagery.

Figure 5 shows the correlation between the cessation of eyelid movements and the times of hypnagogic reports for each of 14 spontaneous arousals during a second night.

Each spontaneous arousal was preceded by at least 10 s of quiescence, and half the awakenings were preceded by less than 30 s of quiescence. In addition to these 14 arousals, each of 5 hypnagogic reports obtained during the night depicted in Figures 3 and 4 were preceded by at least 10 s of eye sensor quiescence. Eyelid movements normally recommenced about 5 s before the actual key press (Figure 5), presumably reflecting the arousal process itself. Thus, it appears that the initiation of eyelid movement quiescence detected by the Nightcap is tightly coupled with a shift of mental activity into the hypnagogic mode.

FORMAL FEATURES OF HYPNAGOGIC MENTATION

Hypnagogic reports can share many of the features of REM dreams listed in Table 2, including visual, auditory, and motor hallucinations,

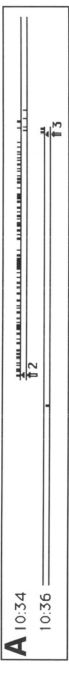

Report No. 3 (22:38). About 5 or 10 seconds ago, I was thinking about how the feature that I experienced in the last report was that I start to get some sort of floating sensation, and I was thinking about that and ... ah ... realized I was slightly hypnagogic when the phrase "prefrontal lobotomy" came into my train of thought. No idea why or what it was connected with.

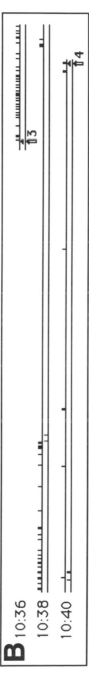

Report No. 4 (22:42). I don't remember what the story line was, but I did see hallucinations of some ... some men, I guess ... in uniforms ... similar to the ones worn by the royal guard at ... oh ... some palace we toured in London ... just with the fancy dress uniforms that they have ... and they were saying something, or I was thinking something, I am not sure which.

Figure 4

High-resolution analysis of sleep onset period. A: The period immediately following the time of report 2 (Figure 3). Report given at time of the arrow labeled "3" in the Nightcap display. B: The period immediately following the time of report 3 (Figure 4a). Report given at time of the arrow labeled "4" in the Nightcap display.

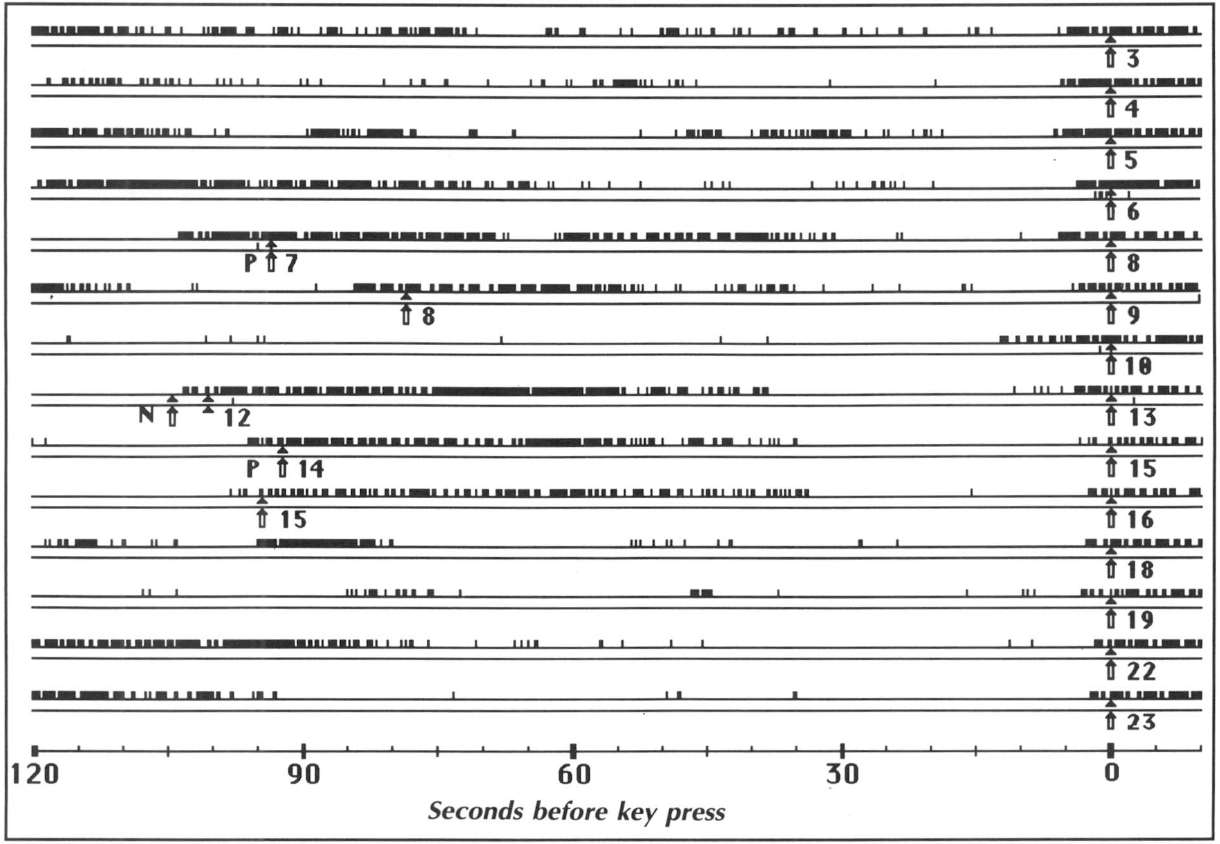

Figure 5

Nightcap output with aligned spontaneous arousals. Records from 14 spontaneous arousals during a single evening are aligned at the time of arousal, as indicated by a key press. Each behavioral response (key press) is preceded by 3 to 13 s of physiological arousal

Table 2

Formal Dream Properties

- Hallucination
- Visual imagery
- Auditory imagery
- Fictive motor activity
- Narrative plot
- Emotionality
- Bizarreness
- Self-representation

NOTE: See Hobson (1988) for discussion of formal dream features.

and hyperemotionality, bizarreness, and narrative structure. But these reports can also be surprisingly devoid of such features. Thus, some might be identified only by the presence of an inexplicably bizarre thought. One possible explanation for this variability is that these features become more prominent as the transition from waking to sleep proceeds.

In the pilot night shown in Figure 5 and described earlier, the subject roused himself 14 times in a 2-hr period to report hypnagogic thoughts or images. Each report was transcribed from an audio recording and subsequently scored for the presence or absence of the features listed in Table 2. Motor activity and narrative plot structure were scored whether they were hallucinated or merely reported as thoughts, whereas imagery and self-representation were scored only for hallucinations.

A significant positive correlation was found between the number of formal dream features present in a report and the length of the preceding period of eye sensor quiescence ($r = 0.58$, $df = 12$, $p < 0.02$; single-tailed Pearson's correlation test), with the average number of dreamlike features more than doubling as the period of quiescence increased from 10 s to 90 s. Thus, it would appear that these features do not appear all at once but, rather, develop over time, with the mentation taking on more and more features of REM sleep dreams as the period of eyelid movement quiescence lengthens. The number of features was also correlated with the time of night, but did not reach statistical significance. These results are in agreement with those reported by Foulkes and Vogel (1965), who reported an increase in the hallucinatory properties of reports as subjects' EEG patterns shifted from an alpha EEG to a spindling EEG.

This preliminary observation leads to the paradoxical hypothesis that eyelid movement is negatively correlated with dreamlike mentation at sleep onset but positively correlated with dreaming during emergent Stage 1 REM. To account for this paradox, we will need recourse to a model which acknowledges the rate of change of functions (such as eyelid movements, cortical activation, or input source), as well as their absolute levels and signs (Hobson, 1992).

COMPUTERIZED AWAKENINGS AT SLEEP ONSET

When the Nightcap is connected to a computer, the computer can analyze the data on line, identify sleep stages, and perform awakenings according to a specified protocol. For this study, a protocol was developed wherein awakenings were performed after varying intervals of eye sensor quiescence. When the waking criteria were met, a voice prompt was played and repeated every 5 s until the subject awoke and responded by pressing a key on the keyboard. The subject recorded on a dictaphone whether he thought he was awake or asleep and reported any thoughts, images, dreams, and so on that he could recall. While the subject recorded his reports on a dictaphone, the computer recorded all Nightcap data, the time that each waking prompt was begun, and the time at which the subject responded to each prompt. In a sample of six such awakenings, physiological responses (eyelid movements) occurred within 1 s to 2 s of the start of the voice prompt, and behavioral responses (key presses) were made within 3 s to 4 s.

PSG CORRELATES

What does the cessation of eyelid movements at sleep onset actually indicate about the underlying physiology of sleep onset? The Nightcap eye sensor is sensitive to all eyelid deformations, whether caused by movement of the eye beneath the lid or by blinks or eyelid twitches. It is clear from combined PSG–Nightcap studies such as those shown in Figure 2 that the Nightcap can detect eye movements as expected during wake and REM sleep, and does not detect them when not expected during NREM sleep. More detailed studies show the extent of this correlation.

The right panel of Figure 6 shows a PSG record from a subject wearing the Nightcap. The EOG-defined eye movements seen in channels 2 and 3 correlate well with the output of the Nightcap eyelid sensor shown in the bottom channel. For comparison, the left panel shows a

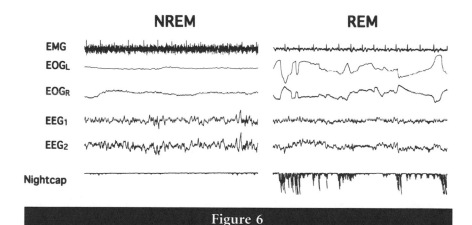

Figure 6

Nightcap eyelid sensor output and EOG in REM and NREM sleep. PSG recordings from a single night of simultaneous PSG and Nightcap recording. For each panel, top trace = submental EMG; traces 2 and 3 = left and right EOG recordings; traces 4 and 5 = EEG recordings; trace 6 = Nightcap eye sensor voltage. The left panel is taken from a period of NREM sleep, and the right panel from REM sleep. Each panel shows a 9-s recording period.

period of NREM sleep, with no eye movements obvious in either the EOG or Nightcap channels.

Although the EOG and the Nightcap show excellent agreement during REM and NREM sleep, the correlation is not nearly so obvious at sleep onset. Figure 7 shows a sample from one night of recording sleep-onset data with both PSG and the Nightcap. The panels in the figure show the combined PSG–Nightcap recording for the interval between reports 8 and 9 in Figure 5.

Although there is good correlation between EOG eye movements and Nightcap eyelid movements in the first panel, the second panel shows numerous Nightcap events with no obvious EOG correlates, as well as a slow eye movement detected by the EOG but not by the Nightcap. In the third panel, numerous slow eye movements go undetected by the Nightcap, whereas Nightcap events are marked at other times. This suggests that it is active twitching of the eyelid that is being detected at these times. Such an interpretation is supported by work suggesting that a decrease in eye blink rate may be an indicator of sleep onset (Allen & Krausman, 1993; Santamaria & Chiappa, 1987). Interestingly, the best correlation in the last two panels seems to be between Nightcap events and the alpha rhythm of the EEG. This appeared to be true throughout the 2-hr recording period; periods of alpha quiescence also appear to be periods with few or no Nightcap eye counts. This agrees with reports showing that hypnagogic mentation is often preceded by periods of depressed alpha waves (Davis, Davis, Loomis, Harvey, & Hobart, 1937; Liberson & Liberson, 1965). Again, we have only a general sense of this correlation, and systematic, quantitative studies will be necessary to determine the accuracy of this preliminary conclusion. The actual correlation between Nightcap eye sensor output and the various processes occurring at the time of sleep onset remains to be determined.

CONCLUSION

The studies reported here demonstrate that the Nightcap can passively detect a clear physiological boundary between periods of intense eyelid

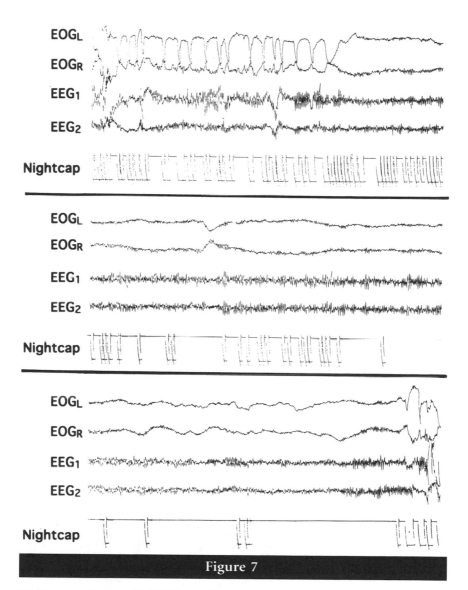

Figure 7

Nightcap correlation with EOG-detected eye movements at sleep onset. PSG recording for time interval between reports 8 and 9 in Figure 5. For each panel, top two traces = left and right EOG recordings; middle two traces = EEG recordings; bottom trace = Nightcap eyelid-movement events. Panels show consecutive 25-s intervals.

movement and periods of eyelid quiescence, and that this boundary occurs close to the time sleep-onset hypnagogic mentation begins. When the Nightcap is connected to a Macintosh computer, these transitions it identifies can be used to trigger the awakening of subjects for the collection of mentation reports.

Several preliminary results regarding sleep-onset mentation have been obtained. We feel that three in particular merit further attention.

First, we need to confirm the relationship between the cessation of eyelid movements as determined by the Nightcap and as determined by standard PSG measures. To what extent do Nightcap eyelid movement signals reflect movements of the eye? Do signals not correlated with obvious EOG peaks reflect lid twitches, or are they perhaps being triggered by micro-saccades? How do these signals correlate with the occurrence of alpha waves and spindles as seen in the EEG record? Can the apparent correlation with alpha waves be confirmed, and, if so, how strong is the correlation?

Second, we want to extend the collection of sleep-onset mentation reports at various time intervals after the cessation of eyelid movements, and the correlation of formal features of mentation reports with the duration of this time interval. Hopefully, this will lead to an extension of the early work of Foulkes and Vogel (1965) and provide a better understanding of the temporal development of the hypnagogic dream and clues as to how cognitive functions shift during the transition from wakefulness to sleep. In conjunction with these studies, it would be valuable to correlate the cessation of eyelid movements with the subjects' perceived state of wakefulness.

Third, we want to look carefully at the time of REM onset, again asking how sleep mentation develops. Whether this can be done with the Nightcap alone or whether it will require PSG monitoring remains to be determined. In either case, the results will allow a comparison of the brief hypnagogic dreams at sleep onset with the beginnings of REM dreams. Because these transitions are coming from opposite directions—down from wakefulness or up from deeper sleep—the similarities and differences might be both provocative and illuminating.

REFERENCES

Aaronson, S. T., Rashed, S., Biber, M. P., & Hobson, J. A. (1982). Brain state and body position: A time-lapse video study of sleep. *Archives of General Psychiatry, 39*, 330–335.

Ajilore, O., Stickgold, R., Rittenhouse, C., & Hobson, J. A. (in press). Nightcap: Laboratory and home-based evaluation of a portable sleep monitor. *Psychophysiology, 32.*

Allen, R. P., & Krausman, D. T. (1993). Spontaneous eye blink rate provides a leading indicator for the onset of sleepiness. *Sleep Research, 22*, 75.

Davis, H., Davis, P. A., Loomis, A. L., Harvey, E. N., & Hobart, G. (1937). Human brain potentials at the onset of sleep. *Journal of Neurophysiology, 1*, 24–37.

d'Hervey de Saint-Denis, J. M. L. (1867). *Les rêves et les moyens de les diriger* [Dreams and means of controlling them]. Paris: Amyot.

Foulkes, D., & Vogel, G. (1965). Mental activity at sleep onset. *Journal of Abnormal Psychology, 70*, 231–243.

Helfand R., Lavie, P., & Hobson, J. A. (1986). REM/NREM discrimination via ocular and limb movement monitoring: Correlation with polygraphic data and development of a REM state algorithm. *Psychophysiology, 23*, 334–339.

Hobson, J. A. (1988). *The dreaming brain.* New York: Basic Books.

Hobson, J. A. (1992). A new model of the brain–mind state: Activation level, input source, and mode of processing (AIM). In J. A. Antrobus & M. Bertini (Eds.), *Neuropsychology of sleep and dreaming* (pp. 227–245). Hillsdale, NJ: Erlbaum.

Hobson, J. A., & Steriade, M. (1986). Neuronal basis of behavioral control. In V. Mountcastle, F. E. Bloom, & S. R. Geiger (Eds.), *Handbook of physiology— The nervous system IV* (pp. 701–823) Bethesda, MD: American Physiological Society.

Liberson, W. T., & Liberson, C. W. (1965). EEG records, reaction times, eye movements, respiration, and mental content during drowsiness. *Recent Advances in Biological Psychiatry, 8*, 295–302.

Mamelak, A., & Hobson, J. A. (1989). Nightcap: A home-based sleep monitoring system. *Sleep, 12*, 157–166.

Maury, A. (1861). *Le sommeil et les rêves* [Sleep and dreams]. Paris: Amyot.

Moruzzi, G., & Mogoun, H. W. (1949). Brain-stem reticular formation and activation of the EEG. *Electroencephalography and Clinical Neurophysiology, 1*, 455–473.

Pace-Schott, E., Kaji, J., Stickgold, R., & Hobson, J. A. (in press). Nightcap measurement of sleep quality in self-described good and poor sleepers. *Sleep, 17.*

Santamaria, J., & Chiappa, K. H. (1987). The EEG of drowsiness in normal adults. *Journal of Clinical Neurophysiology, 4,* 327–382.

Steriade, M., & McCarley, R. (1990). *Brainstem control of wakefulness and sleep.* New York: Plenum Press.

Stickgold, R., Pace-Schott, E., & Hobson, J. A. (1994). A new paradigm for dream research: Mentation reports following spontaneous arousals from REM and NREM sleep recorded in a home setting. *Consciousness and Cognition, 3,* 16–29.

Vogel, G. (1991). Sleep-onset mentation. In S. J. Ellman & J. S. Antrobus (Eds.), *The mind in sleep: Psychology and psychophysiology* (2nd ed.). New York: Wiley.

Webster, J. B., Kripke, D. F., Messin, S., Mullaney, D. J., & Wyborney, G. (1982). An activity-based sleep monitor system for ambulatory use. *Sleep, 5,* 389–399.

10

Sleep Paralysis and Sleep-Onset REM Period in Normal Individuals

Kazuhiko Fukuda

SLEEP PARALYSIS

History of Sleep Paralysis as a Subject of Medicine

In 1880, Gelineau devised the term *narcolepsy* to describe patients who were suffering from long-lasting irresistible daytime sleepiness. Then, Wilson (1928) reported sleep paralysis in his narcoleptic patients, and L'hermitte and Tournay (1927) discovered the link between hypnagogic hallucinations and narcolepsy. Yoss and Daly (1957) considered that four symptoms, that is, sleep attacks, cataplexy, hypnagogic hallucinations, and sleep paralysis, formed a *narcoleptic tetrad*.

However, it had been known even much earlier that sleep paralysis and hypnagogic hallucinations could occur in normal individuals. (Sleep paralysis was described by Mitchell [1876], and hypnagogic hallucinations were identified by Maury [1848] in normal individuals.)

The major portion of this article is based on work done by the author in collaboration with Dr. Akio Miyasita, Dr. Kaneyoshi Ishihara, Mr. Maki Inugami, Ms. Yuka Sasaki, and Ms. Tomoka Takeuchi.

Incidence of Sleep Paralysis

Despite early references to sleep paralysis in normal individuals, it has been known mostly as a symptom of narcolepsy. Although many papers have reported occurrences in normal individuals, most were reports of a few cases of the phenomenon. However, a few works have surveyed its incidence in normal samples.

Goode (1962) has been most frequently cited for a survey of sleep paralysis in normal subjects. Indeed, leading classification manuals of sleep disorders (Association of Sleep Disorders Centers [ASDC], 1979; American Sleep Disorders Association [ASDA], 1990) have cited his work as describing the occurrence of sleep paralysis among normal individuals. Goode suggested that 4.7% of normal respondents had experienced this phenomenon at least once.

However, there are interesting discrepancies among the reported incidences of the phenomenon. Everett (1963) reported that 15.4% of 52 respondents had experienced sleep paralysis. Penn, Kripke, and Scharff (1981) found it in 16.3% of 80 college students. Moreover, there are other studies reporting even higher incidences. Bell et al. (1984) noted that sleep paralysis occurred in 40.7% of Black subjects. Ness (1978) surveyed the "old hag" phenomenon, which is symptomatically identical to sleep paralysis, and found a very high (62.3%) prevalence of it in a village in Newfoundland. Fukuda, Miyasita, Inugami, and Ishihara (1987) found that 39.8% of 635 university students in Japan had experienced the *kanashibari* phenomenon at least once. From descriptions provided, the terms *sleep paralysis, old hag,* and *kanashibari* refer to the same phenomenon. A number of hypotheses have been offered to explain the different incidences reported.

Factors Affecting Incidence of Sleep Paralysis

Factors that are considered to affect the incidence of sleep paralysis could be classified into two categories. Factors in the first category directly affect the incidence of the phenomenon itself, whereas those in the second influence the respondents' decision to report the experience or the memory of the experience.

Racial Factor

One of the possible factors affecting the occurrence of sleep paralysis is a racial factor. Bell et al. (1984) suggested that the high incidence found among blacks may be attributed to a racial factor because Goode (1962) had reported earlier a much lower incidence in a sample of whites. Moreover, he suggested that this racial factor could be interpreted as assumed hyperactivity in *locus coeruleus* in black subjects. However, as mentioned above, Ness (1978) reported a very high prevalence in a sample of Whites in Newfoundland, and Ohaeri, Odejide, Ikuesan, and Adeyemi (1989) found a lower incidence in Nigerian Black subjects than Bell et al. (1984) encountered. Therefore, it seems doubtful that the hypothesis of a biologically based racial factor can explain completely the discrepancy in prevalence in these reports.

Psychological or Psychoanalytic Interpretation

Several papers have suggested that psychological factors affect the occurrence of sleep paralysis. These reports are often based on the theory of psychoanalysis. Van der Heide and Weinberg (1945) presented two cases of combat fatigue in which the patients claimed frequent sleep paralysis experiences. The authors suggested that the sleep paralysis was related to a state of confusion as to emotion and intention, with resulting indecisiveness. Schonberger (1946) hypothesized that the episodes, which involved motor paralysis and intense anxiety, represented a punishment for and defense against his patient's sexual and aggressive fantasies of incestuous wishes. Schneck (1969b) reported four cases of isolated sleep paralysis and stressed the possibility that the paralysis was an expression of conflicts between passive and aggressive personality trends.

Although these reports are important for suggesting a possible relationship between the phenomenon and some personality factor, they are only anecdotal case reports. Hence, one cannot determine to what extent those characteristics could be generalized.

Bell, Dixie-Bell, and Thompson (1986) mailed out flyers containing a description of sleep paralysis and asked recipients to participate in a short phone interview about the phenomenon. They also used newspaper ads to recruit subjects who had experienced sleep paralysis. They reported that frequent episodes were associated with stress and that subjects with isolated sleep paralysis had an unusually high prevalence of panic disorder. They suggested that anxiety and stress play an important role in the occurrence of sleep paralysis. Furthermore, they speculated that sleep paralysis and panic disorder may be different clinical manifestations of the same disorder. Fukuda, Miyasita, Inugami, & Ishihara (1987) asked respondents with sleep paralysis about their physical and psychological conditions immediately before these experiences. Many of the subjects reported that they had experienced psychological or physical stress or an irregular sleep–wake pattern. Fukuda and Hozumi (1989) reported a minor, not statistically significant, positive correlation between the frequency of the attacks and the neuroticism score on the Maudsley Personality Inventory among psychiatric outpatients. Fukuda, Inamatsu, Kuroiwa, and Miyasita (1991) reported a small but statistically significant difference in the Minnesota Multiphasic Personality Inventory paranoia scores between university students experiencing sleep paralysis and those who were not. These facts suggest that some psychological factors are related with this symptom; however, these factors seem to be too weak to explain the mechanism of this phenomenon fully. At any rate, a construct like personality might not be so important for interpreting the mechanisms of the phenomenon in physiological terms, unless the physiological background of personality is understood. Moreover, one cannot assume that some studies were based on psychologically deviated "normal" subjects compared with other research and also assume that this could explain the discrepancy in the incidence.

Factors Affecting Apparent Incidence

Sleep paralysis has been well known in folklore: *kanashibari* in Japan (Fukuda, Miyasita, Inugami, & Ishihara, 1987), old hag in Newfoundland (Hufford, 1982; Ness, 1978), *kokma* in the West Indies (Ness, 1978), and *Hexendrücken* in some parts of Germany (Firestone, 1985). Liddon (1967) insists that sleep paralysis and hypnagogic hallucinations were treated as a part of nightmares in the last century throughout the Western world. Schneck (1969a) suggested that the painting *The Nightmare* (Figure 1) by Henry Fuseli (1741–1825) represents the phenomenon presently known as sleep paralysis. This picture shows several characteristics of the phenomenon.

Thus, cultural background might play a role in the reported incidence. In fact, it seems that surveys conducted in cultures where people know the phenomenon well as a nondisease, like old hag (Ness, 1978) or *kanashibari* (Fukuda, Miyasita, Inugami, & Ishihara, 1987), reported

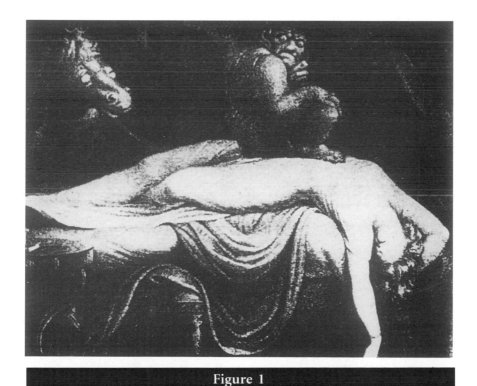

Figure 1

The Nightmare, painting by Johann Heinrich Füssli (Henry Fuseli), 1781.

higher incidences than other studies. Although Bell et al. (1984) reported a higher incidence using the medical term *sleep paralysis*, the fact that they interviewed all the subjects individually may have contributed to the higher incidence. In other studies, subjects were given only a medical description of the phenomenon and were administered a questionnaire. For these reasons, subjects could answer the question in the affirmative more easily in the former surveys than in the latter ones. Indeed, one of Everett's (1963) subjects at first contemplated answering "no" for fear that a "yes" answer might convey undesirable psychiatric implications.

Folklore names like *kanashibari* or old hag, even if they are precisely and adequately defined as sleep paralysis in the questionnaire, would likely facilitate some false positive answers from respondents with a knowledge of the name of the phenomenon. Fukuda (1993) surveyed the potential effect of the terminology for the phenomenon on the reported incidence of sleep paralysis. The study revealed that questionnaires differing in only one word (the name of the phenomenon) resulted in differences in the reported incidence too great to ignore. Use of the term *kanashibari* resulted in a higher rate of positive answers (39.3%), especially among female respondents, whereas use of the term *transient paralysis* resulted in a lower rate of positive answers (26.4%), also especially among the female respondents. The author suggested that a positive response rate of about 30% would be most probable because that figure was obtained when using the most neutral terminology, that is, when the term *condition* was used for the phenomenon.

Some Comments on the Incidence of Sleep Paralysis

Although there is still much to be done before one can state something conclusive on the matter, it is likely that the discrepancy is more apparent than real because the reported incidence of occurrence seems to be sensitive to both the expression used for the phenomenon and the procedures used for the survey. It may be recommended that the same procedure and terminology, preferably a neutral expression, be used to survey different racial or cultural environments to clarify these problems.

The ASDA has published the *International Classification of Sleep Disorders: Diagnostic and Coding Manual* [ICSD] (1990) in which sleep paralysis is treated as an independent clinical entity, rather than as just one of the symptoms of narcolepsy, by eliminating adjectives like "familial" or "isolated" that had been used in the previous edition of the manual (ASDC, 1979). Surprisingly, concerning the incidence of the phenomenon, the manual states that "isolated sleep paralysis occurs at least once in a lifetime in 40–50% of normal subjects." However, it simultaneously cites Goode's work (1962), which suggests only a 4.7% incidence in the normal population, making no comment on the wide discrepancy between these two statements.

A discrepancy in the reported incidence of sleep paralysis exists not only among the normal population but also among narcoleptic patients. Goode (1962) reported that only 17% of 146 narcoleptic patients had symptoms of sleep paralysis, whereas Hishikawa (1976) found it in 57% of 102 narcoleptics. Hishikawa assumed that this discrepancy could be attributed to the difference in the methods used for the surveys. He insisted that he found a rather high incidence because the patients were carefully questioned about the symptoms. He also suggested that his patients found the symptoms less troublesome compared with other major narcoleptic symptoms, such as sleep attacks and cataplexy, so they failed to report it when they were not carefully examined. Incidentally, the ICSD states that the incidence of sleep paralysis in narcoleptics is 17% to 40% (ASDA, 1990). These figures are hardly definitive and quite close to the reported incidence among normal subjects.

SLEEP-ONSET REM PERIOD (SOREMP)

SOREMP and Sleep Paralysis

It is well known that REM sleep occurs cyclically with a periodicity of about 90 min. The first REM sleep occurs about 60–100 min after sleep onset. However, under certain conditions or in some patients, REM sleep occurs at sleep onset. This unusual occurrence of REM sleep is called a *sleep-onset REM period* (SOREMP). SOREMPs are known to occur frequently in narcoleptic patients (Takahashi & Jimbo, 1963). In fact, SOREMPs were taken as sufficient criteria for diagnosing narcolepsy in earlier definitions in the classification manual edited by ASDC (1979). However, SOREMPs by themselves have been reassessed as an insufficient, but still important, criterion for narcolepsy in the more recent version of the diagnostic manual (ICSD) by the ASDA (1990). Many studies on narcolepsy have suggested that sleep paralysis occurs during SOREMP (Hishikawa & Kaneko, 1965; Hishikawa et al., 1978; Koida, Nan'no, & Hishikawa, 1971; Suzuki, 1966). Recently, Takeuchi, Miyasita, Sasaki, Inugami, and Fukuda (1992) succeeded in eliciting sleep paralysis in normal subjects by interrupting their sleep. They obtained electrophysiological data during these periods. The data suggest that most episodes of sleep paralysis occurred during SOREMP. One subject did not exhibit rapid eye movements, which is necessary for REM sleep by definition, during one of his two episodes of sleep paralysis, but other parameters (i.e., EEG and electromyogram [EMG]) showed the features of REM sleep. The subject also got out of the sleep paralysis by moving his body forcefully so that the episode could be regarded as an "unaccomplished REM period." Thus, it is reasonable to think that sleep paralysis occurs exclusively during SOREMPs.

SOREMP and Depression

SOREMPs are also considered to be a "biological marker" of certain forms of depression. Kupfer and Foster (1972) reported shortened mean REM sleep latency observed in the sleep of depressed patients. Schulz, Lund, Cording, & Dirlich (1979) found that this shortened REM sleep latency resulted from a bimodal distribution of REM sleep latencies with peaks at sleep onset and about 60 min later and also found that a peak with shorter latency (i.e., SOREMPs) disappeared after remission in their "endogenous" depressive patients (Figure 2).

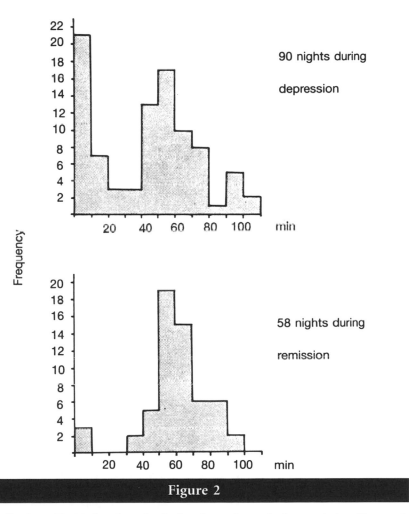

Figure 2

Distribution of REM sleep latencies during depression and after remission. The *x*-axis gives the latency, in minutes; the *y*-axis, the absolute frequency. Upper diagram: REM latency in 90 polysomnograms of six endogenous depressive patients. Lower diagram: REM sleep latency in 58 polysomnograms of four of these patients after remission. From Schulz et al. (1979). Reprinted with permission.

SOREMP in Altered Sleep Schedule

SOREMPs appear in connection with certain disorders and also with certain altered sleep schedules in normal individuals. Some studies report the occurrence of SOREMPs under conditions of acute reversal of the sleep and wakefulness cycle (Weitzman, Kripke, Goldmacher, McGregor, & Nogeire, 1970), ultradian sleep and wakefulness schedule (Carskadon & Dement, 1975; Weitzman et al., 1974), naps (Marron, Rechtschaffen, & Wolpert, 1964), and interruption of nocturnal sleep in normal individuals (Fukuda, Miyasita, & Inugami, 1987; Miyasita, Fukuda, & Inugami, 1989; Sasaki et al., 1993). Figure 3 indicates the distribution of stage REM latencies after a deliberate interruption of nocturnal sleep (Miyasita et al., 1989). This distribution is quite similar to that in depressive patients (Figure 2).

SOREMP in Early Infantile Period

In a very early period of life, human infants show very short REM sleep latencies (Schulz, Salzarulo, Fagioli, & Massetani, 1983). Schulz et al. found that although younger infants (less than 3 months old) manifested predominantly shorter REM latencies, older infants (4–13 months old) produced a bimodal distribution of short and long REM latencies. They also found that REM sleep with shorter latency occurred predominantly after shorter episodes of prior wakefulness. Ellingson and Peters (1980) found that active sleep onset, which could be considered to be the equivalent of SOREMP at that period of age, disappeared around the sixth to the eighth week after birth.

DISCUSSION

Conditions Conducive to SOREMP

As already mentioned, SOREMPs occur in many situations, such as in depressive states, altered sleep schedules, and the early infantile period. These situations might be summarized as sleep disruption or weakened amplitude of the circadian rhythm. Interruption of sleep (Fukuda, Mi-

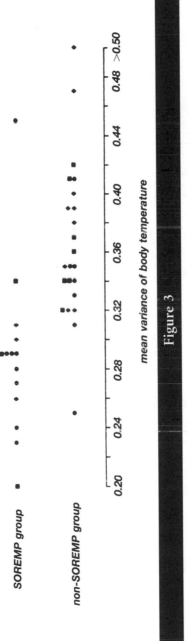

Figure 3

Distribution of the mean variance of body core temperature around the 24-hr mean value. Dots represent depressed patients ($n = 15$), rhombs represent patients in remission ($n = 12$), and rectangles represent control subjects ($n = 10$). From Schulz and Lund (1983). Reprinted with permission.

yasita, & Inugami, 1987; Miyasita et al., 1989; Sasaki et al., 1993) and a polyphasic sleep–wakefulness schedule (Carskadon & Dement, 1975; Weitzman et al., 1974) seem to be sufficient to produce a sleep disruption.

Although it was difficult to test the hypothesis in depressive patients, Schulz and Lund (1983) found smaller variations of body core temperature in depressive patients who presented SOREMPs (Figure 4). It is also difficult to investigate this hypothesis in infants. Schulz et al. (1983) found a difference in the distribution of REM sleep latencies between infants under and those over 3 months of age. Ellingson and Peters (1980) found a decrease in the rate of active sleep (REM sleep) onset from 6 to 8 weeks after birth. During the first few weeks of life, human infants showed scattered episodes of sleep over the 24 hr of the day. Eventually, the sleep episodes began to be consolidated during nighttime. Recently, Fukuda (1992) and Fukuda and Ishihara (1993) found a discontinuous change in infants' circadian rhythm of sleep and wakefulness around the seventh week after birth. This coincidence in these timings seems to suggest that the amplitude of the circadian rhythm or consolidation of sleep might be related to the distribution of stage REM latencies (i.e., with or without SOREMP).

Conditions Conducive to Sleep Paralysis

Some investigations have found evidence that sleep paralysis is likely to appear in disruptive sleep schedules. Ness (1978) stated that his subjects with sleep paralysis experienced it very frequently during lumber camp work, which requires exhausting labor and sleep loss. Snyder (1983) reported two normal individuals who experienced sleep paralysis during "jet-lag" syndrome. Folkard, Condon, and Herbert (1984) clearly showed that a considerable number of nurses experience sleep paralysis during their night shifts and that the incidence increases over consecutive night shifts. Fukuda, Miyasita, Inugami, & Ishihara (1987) revealed that a large number of the students with sleep paralysis reported physical or psychological stress or disturbed sleep and wakefulness cycles immediately before their attacks (Figure 5). Thus, some

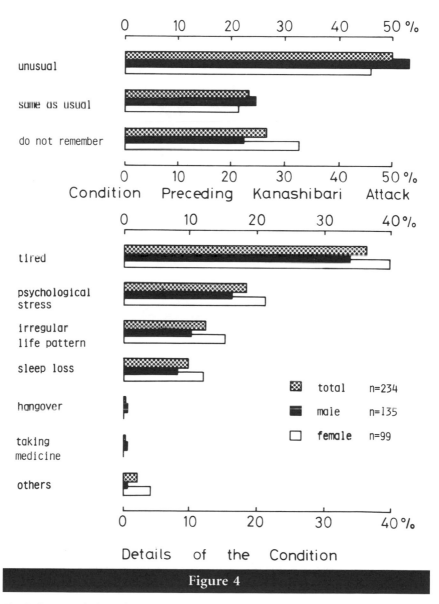

Figure 4

Physical or psychological condition preceding *kanashibari* attack. From Fukuda, Miyasita, Inugami, & Ishihara (1987). Reprinted with permission.

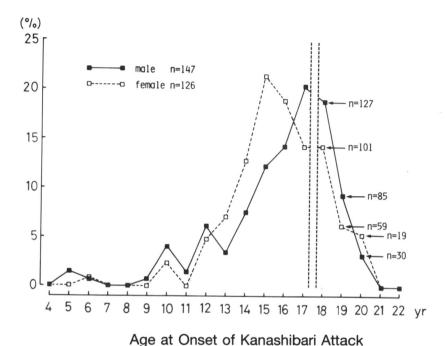

Age at Onset of Kanashibari Attack

Figure 5

Distribution of age at onset of *kanashibari* attack. Over 18 years, subjects younger than or equal to each age were eliminated. Number of subjects at each age is shown. From Fukuda, Miyasita, Inugami, & Ishihara (1987). Reprinted with permission.

physiological process concerned with stress, tiredness, and sleep disruption, which might weaken the circadian rhythm of sleep and wakefulness, probably plays a role in causing sleep paralysis.

Folkard et al. (1984) found clear age-related changes in the experience of sleep paralysis. The symptom is most likely to occur at ages 30 years and under. Fukuda, Miyasita, Inugami, & Ishihara (1987) reported the distribution of victims' ages at the time of the first episode, which showed that the distribution for men peaked in late adolescence, whereas that for women peaked a little earlier (Figure 6).

Although it is unclear why the phenomenon tends to occur more at this stage of life, it might be related to increased sleepiness at this

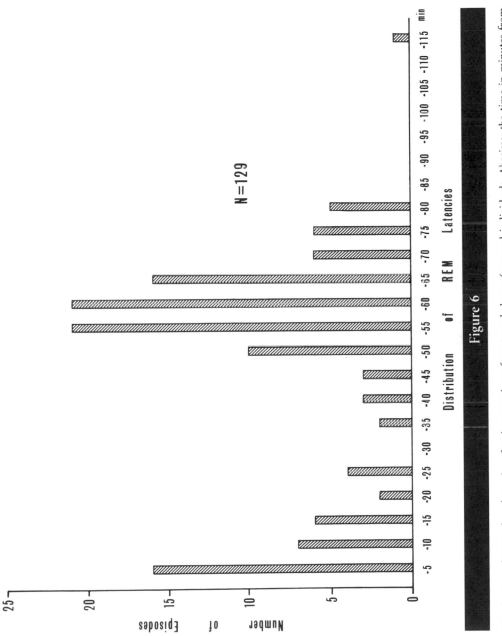

Figure 6

Distribution of REM sleep latencies after interruption of nocturnal sleep of normal individuals. Abscissa: the time in minutes from sleep onset to REM onset after returning to sleep. From Miyasita et al. (1989). Reprinted with permission.

later period of adolescence. Carskadon and Dement (1987) conducted a longitudinal study of sleepiness over the course of seven years during the students' adolescence and suggested that the need for sleep increased with age during the adolescent period.

CONCLUSION

Sleep-onset REM periods occur in many situations that have in common either some sleep disruption or weakened amplitude of circadian rhythm. Similarly, sleep paralysis tends to occur during situations concerned with the disruption of sleep. It is not known how these conditions affect the occurrence of this phenomenon. Slow wave sleep (SWS) is known to be correlated with the amount of preceding wakefulness (Endo et al., 1981). Reduced SWS pressure, which should have been caused by disruption of sleep, might be important for the occurrence. Schulz et al. (1983) found that, in infants, REM sleep with shorter latency occurred predominantly after shorter episodes of prior wakefulness.

Reduced sleep latency or some kind of sleepiness might also be important. Fukuda, Miyasita, & Inugami (1987) showed that SOREMPs were found only after sleep interruption in short sleepers, whose sleep latencies were shorter than those of long sleepers, who presented no SOREMPs. It is well known that narcoleptics show short sleep latencies (Montplaisir, 1976). Carskadon and Dement (1987) found that sleepiness correlated positively with the amount of stage REM during the subsequent sleep period in the 90-min schedule of the sleep–wakefulness cycle. Broughton and Aguirre (1987) found greater sleepiness immediately before SOREMP compared with usual non-REM (NREM) onset of sleep. As for the mechanisms for these phenomena, more investigations and arguments are needed before firm conclusions can be drawn, but it seems that sleep paralysis and SOREMPs are likely to occur in many kinds of situations related to sleep disruption, including narcolepsy.

Further Comments on Sleep Onset

Although this is still a controversial and speculative issue, the author suggests that the SOREMP is a frequently encountered sleep pattern when circadian rhythmicity is somewhat weakened. This can be seen first as the rhythm develops in early childhood. The REM–NREM cycle order is the original cycle order that is destroyed by the later intrusion of SWS into sleep onset. During maturation, NREM onset of sleep would be a by-product of the establishment of adult circadian rhythm; it squeezes SWS into the sleep-onset period in place of the ontogenetically earlier REM sleep (SOREMP). So, some residue of this first REM sleep (SOREMP) may be found in ordinary NREM onset of sleep, and this may help to explain why various subjective experiences were reported exclusively during this hypnagogic NREM period.

REFERENCES

American Sleep Disorders Association. (1990). *ICSD–International classification of sleep disorders: Diagnostic and coding manual.* Rochester, MN: Author.

Association of Sleep Disorders Centers. (1979). *Diagnostic classification of sleep and arousal disorders* (1st ed.). *Sleep, 2,* 1–137.

Bell, C. C., Dixie-Bell, D. D., & Thompson, B. (1986). Further studies on the prevalence of isolated sleep paralysis in Black subjects. *Journal of the National Medical Association, 78,* 649–659.

Bell, C. C., Shakoor, B., Thompson, B., Dew, D., Hughley, E., Mays, R., & Shorter-Gooden, K. (1984). Prevalence of isolated sleep paralysis in Black subjects. *Journal of the National Medical Association, 76,* 501–508.

Broughton, R., & Aguirre, M. (1987). Differences between REM and NREM sleepiness measured by event-related potentials (P300, CNV), MSLT, and subjective estimate in narcolepsy–cataplexy. *Electroencephalography and Clinical Neurophysiology, 67,* 317–326.

Carskadon, M. A., & Dement, W. C. (1975). Sleep studies on a 90-minute day. *Electroencephalography and Clinical Neurophysiology, 39,* 145–155.

Carskadon, M. A., & Dement, W. C. (1987). Sleepiness in the normal adolescent. In C. Guilleminault (Ed.), *Sleep and its disorders in children* (pp. 53–66). New York: Raven Press.

Ellingson, R. J., & Peters, J. F. (1980). Development of EEG and daytime sleep patterns in normal full-term infants during the first 3 months of life: Longitudinal observations. *Electroencephalography and Clinical Neurophysiology, 49*, 112–124.

Endo, S., Kobayashi, T., Yamamoto, T., Fukuda, H., Sasaki, M., & Ohta, T. (1981). Persistence of the circadian rhythm of REM sleep: A variety of experimental manipulations of the sleep cycle. *Sleep, 4*, 319–328.

Everett, H. C. (1963). Sleep paralysis in medical students. *Journal of Nervous and Mental Disease, 3*, 283–287.

Firestone, M. (1985). The "old hag": sleep paralysis in Newfoundland. *Journal of Psychoanalytic Anthropology, 8*, 47–66.

Folkard, S., Condon, R., & Herbert, M. (1984). Night shift paralysis. *Experientia, 40*, 510–512.

Fukuda, K. (1992). Nyujiki ni okeru suimin-kakusei rhythm no hattatsu: Tokuni seigo 2 kagetsu chu ni mitomerareru hirenzokuteki henka ni tsuite [Development of sleep–wake rhythm during early infancy: Discontinuous change in the second month of life]. *Japanese Journal of Medical and Psychological Study of Infants, 1*, 29–37. (in Japanese with English abstract)

Fukuda, K. (1993). One explanatory basis for the discrepancy of the reported prevalences of sleep paralysis among healthy respondents. *Peceptual and Motor Skills, 77*, 803–807.

Fukuda, K., & Hozumi, N. (1989). Some aspects of *kanashibari* phenomenon (sleep paralysis) may have minor association with some variables concerning anxiety within a sample of psychiatric outpatients. *Bulletin of Faculty of Education, Fukushima University, 47*, 45–53.

Fukuda, K., Inamatsu, N., Kuroiwa, M., & Miyasita, A. (1991). Personality of healthy young adults with sleep paralysis. *Perceptual and Motor Skills, 73*, 955–962.

Fukuda, K., & Ishihara, K. (1993). Developmental change of human sleep and wakefulness rhythm during the first six months of life: Discontinuous changes at the 7th and 12th week after birth. *Sleep Research, 22*, 405.

Fukuda, K., Miyasita, A., & Inugami, M. (1987). Sleep onset REM period observed after sleep interruption in normal short and normal long sleeping subjects. *Electroencephalography and Clinical Neurophysiology, 67*, 508–513.

Fukuda, K., Miyasita, A., Inugami, M., & Ishihara, K. (1987). High prevalence of isolated sleep paralysis: *kanashibari* phenomenon in Japan. *Sleep, 10*, 279–286.

Goode, G. B. (1962). Sleep paralysis. *Archives of Neurology*, 6, 228–234.

Hishikawa, Y. (1976). Sleep paralysis. In C. Guilleminault, P. Passouant, & W. C. Dement (Eds.), *Advances in sleep research: Vol. 3. Narcolepsy* (pp. 97–124). New York: Spectrum.

Hishikawa, Y., & Kaneko, Z. (1965). Electroencephalographic study on narcolepsy. *Electroencephalography and Clinical Neurophysiology*, 18, 249–259.

Hishikawa, Y., Koida, H., Yoshino, K., Wakamatsu, H., Sugita, Y., Iijima, S., & Nan'no, H. (1978). Characteristics of REM sleep accompanied by sleep paralysis and hypnagogic hallucinations in narcoleptic patients. *Waking and Sleeping*, 2, 113–123.

Hufford, D. (1982). *The Terror That Comes in the Night*. Philadelphia: University of Pennsylvania Press.

Koida, H., Nan'no, H., & Hishikawa, Y. (1971). Some characteristics of the paradoxical phase of sleep in narcoleptic patients. *Electroencephalography and Clinical Neurophysiology*, 31, 187.

Kupfer, D. J., & Foster, F. G. (1972). Interval between onset of sleep and rapid eye-movement sleep as an indicator of depression. *Lancet*, 2, 684–686.

L'hermitte, J., & Tournay, A. (1927). Rapport sur le sommeil normal et pathologique [Report on normal and pathological sleep]. *Revue Neurologique*, 1, 751–822; 885–887.

Liddon, S. C. (1967). Sleep paralysis and hypnagogic hallucinations. *Archives of General Psychiatry*, 17, 88–96.

Marron, L., Rechtschaffen, A., & Wolpert, E. A. (1964). Sleep cycle during napping. *Archives of General Psychiatry*, 11, 503–508.

Maury, A. (1848). Les hallucinations hypnagogiques (ou les erreurs des sens dans l'état intermédiaire entre la veille et le sommeil) [Hypnagogic hallucinations (or sensory errors in the intermediary state between waking and sleeping)]. *Annales MédicoPsychologiques*, 11, 26–40.

Mitchell, S. (1876). On some of the disorders of sleep. *Virginia Medical Monthly*, 2, 769–781.

Miyasita, A., Fukuda, K., & Inugami, M. (1989). Effects of sleep interruption on REM–NREM cycle in nocturnal human sleep. *Electroencephalography and Clinical Neurophysiology*, 73, 107–116.

Montplaisir, J. (1976). Disturbed nocturnal sleep. In C. Guilleminault, W. C. Dement, & P. Passouant (Eds.), *Advances in Sleep Research: Vol. 3. Narcolepsy* (pp. 43–56). New York: Spectrum.

Ness, R. C. (1978). The old hag phenomenon as sleep paralysis: A biocultural interpretation. *Culture, Medicine and Psychiatry, 2,* 15–39.

Ohaeri, J. U., Odejide, A. O., Ikuesan, B. A., & Adeyemi, J. D. (1989). The pattern of isolated sleep paralysis among Nigerian medical students. *Journal of National Medical Association, 81,* 805–808.

Penn, N. E., Kripke, D. F., & Scharff, J. (1981). Sleep paralysis among medical students. *Journal of Psychology, 107,* 247–252.

Sasaki, Y., Miyasita, A., Takeuchi, T., Inugami, M., Fukuda, K., & Ishihara, K. (1993). Effects of sleep interruption on body temperature in human subjects. *Sleep, 16,* 478–483.

Schneck, J. M. (1969a). Henry Fuseli, nightmare, and sleep paralysis. *Journal of American Medical Association, 207,* 725–726.

Schneck, J. M. (1969b). Personality components in patients with sleep paralysis. *Psychiatric Quarterly, 43,* 343–348.

Schonberger, S. (1946). A clinical contribution to the analysis of the nightmare-syndrome. *Psychoanalytic Review, 33,* 44–70.

Schulz, H., & Lund, R. (1983). Sleep onset REM episodes are associated with circadian parameters of body temperature: A study in depressed patients and normal controls. *Biological Psychiatry, 18,* 1411–1426.

Schulz, H., Lund, R., Cording, C., & Dirlich, G. (1979). Bimodal distribution of REM latencies in depression. *Biological Psychiatry, 14,* 595–600.

Schulz, H., Salzarulo, P., Fagioli, I., & Massetani, R. (1983). REM latency: Development in the first year of life. *Electroencephalography and Clinical Neurophysiology, 56,* 316–322.

Snyder, S. (1983). Isolated sleep paralysis after rapid time zone change (jet lag) syndrome. *Chronobiologia, 10,* 377–379.

Suzuki, J. (1966). Narcoleptic syndrome and paradoxical sleep. *Folia Psychiatrica et Neurologica Japonica, 20,* 123–149.

Takahashi, Y., & Jimbo, M. (1963). Polygraphic study of narcoleptic syndrome, with special reference to hypnagogic hallucinations and cataplexy. *Folia Psychiatrica et Neurologica Japonica, 7* (Suppl.), 343.

Takeuchi, T., Miyasita, A., Sasaki, Y., Inugami, M., & Fukuda, K. (1992). Isolated sleep paralysis elicited by sleep interruption. *Sleep, 15,* 217–225.

Van der Heide, C., & Weinberg, J. (1945). Sleep paralysis and combat fatigue. *Psychosomatic Medicine, 7,* 330–334.

Weitzman, E. D., Kripke, D. F., Goldmacher, D., McGregor, P., & Nogeire, C. (1970). Acute reversal of the sleep–waking cycle in man. *Archives of Neurology*, 22, 483–489.

Weitzman, E. D., Nogeire, C., Perlow, M., Fukushima, D., Sassin, J., McGregor, P., Gallagher, T., & Hellman, L. (1974). Effects of a prolonged 3-hour sleep–wakefulness cycle on sleep stages, plasma cortisol, growth hormone and body temperature in man. *Journal of Clinical Endocrinology and Metabolism*, 38, 1018–1030.

Wilson, S. (1928). The narcolepsies. *Brain*, 51, 63–77.

Yoss, R. E., & Daly, D. D. (1957). Criteria for the diagnosis of the narcoleptic syndrome. *Proceedings of the Staff Meetings of the Mayo Clinic*, 32, 320–328.

PART FOUR

EEG Changes

11

Period Analysis of Sleep Onset in Depressed Outpatients and Normal Control Subjects

Roseanne Armitage, Angela Hudson, Thomas Fitch, and Paula Pechacek

Despite the interest in determining the precise instant of sleep on-set, few studies have attempted to delineate characteristic changes in central nervous system functions that accompany the transition from wakefulness to sleep. The difficulty may be due, in part, to the current theoretical position that sleep physiology can be organized into discrete stages, a carry-over from attempts to standardize visual sleep-stage scoring in the late 1960s.

Visual sleep-stage scoring techniques identify the global organization of sleep, but are too imprecise and use too wide a sampling window (30 s) to characterize the transition from wakefulness to sleep or from one sleep stage to another. In addition, visual scoring prohibits the identification of events that are shorter than 15 s, the rule

This research was supported by NIMH-RO1-46886 and NIMH-P50-MH-4115.

We thank Kenneth Z. Altshuler, MD, chair, Department of Psychiatry (University of Texas) for administrative support of this work. We also gratefully acknowledge the technical support team of the Sleep Study Unit, under the supervision of Darwynn D. Cole, and thank Doris Burton for secretarial support. We are indebted to the Mental Health Clinical Research Center under the direction of A. John Rush, MD, for expert recruitment, diagnosis, and follow-up of clinical patients.

for assigning a stage score to a 30-s epoch (Rechtschaffen & Kales, 1968).

QUANTITATIVE SLEEP EEG ANALYSIS

An alternative strategy is to evaluate the electroencephalogram (EEG) frequency characteristics that underlie sleep onset and transitions between sleep events. The two most popular EEG frequency analyses are fast Fourier transforms (FFTs), also called power spectral analysis, and period analysis (PA; Hoffmann, Moffitt, Shearer, Sussman, & Wells, 1979; Pigeau, Hoffmann, & Moffitt, 1981). FFT power values reflect both the incidence and amplitude of a given frequency. A decrease in power may reflect either a decrease in the number of waves of any one frequency, a decrease in the amplitude of the waves, or both. It is this issue that has given rise to controversy over the use of FFTs in quantifying EEG (Feinberg, 1989). In clinical populations such as the depressed, for whom decreased delta activity has been reported (Kupfer, 1989; Kupfer, Grochocinski, & McEachran, 1986; Kupfer, Reynolds, & Ehlers, 1989), it is important to know whether what has occurred is a reduction in the amount of delta activity or simply a reduction in the amplitude. Similarly, one of the reported effects of aging on sleep is a reduction in delta activity, although it is unclear whether decreased amplitude or incidence or both result. Some studies suggest that only the amplitude is reduced in the elderly (Feinberg, 1989). These events are likely to result from different neurophysiological or neuropsychological substrates, caused by a failure to recruit neurons to fire in synchrony or from a reduction in the strength of firing rates, or both (Armitage, Roffwarg, et al., 1992). These issues can be addressed with period-analytic measurement of sleep EEG, but not FFTs (Armitage, Calhoun, Rush, & Roffwarg, 1992; Armitage, Hoffmann, Loewy, & Moffitt, 1989; Armitage, Roffwarg, et al., 1992; Feinberg, 1989; Hoffmann et al., 1979; Ktonas, 1987).

There is considerable controversy over the choice of FFTs or PA to quantify the sleep EEG (see Armitage, Roffwarg, et al., 1992; Geering,

Achermann, Eggimann, & Borbély, 1993), although controversy may be stronger than empirical investigation can support. Nevertheless, computer-analytic strategies have become more popular in clinical research.

QUANTITATIVE ANALYSIS IN DEPRESSION

Sleep studies with depressed patients and more than 90% of the current work in this area rely on visual stage-scoring of polygraphic records. A number of macroarchitectural abnormalities have been reported in these patients (Reynolds & Kupfer, 1987). Prolonged sleep onset, increased Stage 1 sleep, short REM latency, decreased slow wave sleep (SWS), and intermittent wakefulness have all been linked to depression. Although few studies report the percentage of patients with these characteristics, data from the University of Texas Southwestern Sleep Study Unit suggest that about 60% of unipolar depression patients show these abnormalities. The macroarchitectural differences between depressed subjects and normal controls are less consistent than computer-quantified differences.

Increased fast-frequency activity, particularly in the right hemisphere, appears to differentiate reliably the depressed from control subjects (Armitage, Roffwarg, et al., 1992; Armitage, Roffwarg, & Rush, 1993). Furthermore, reduced interhemispheric EEG coherence is present in depression. Both of these abnormalities seem to persist in the state of remission, suggesting that there may be traitlike electrophysiological features of depression. Decreased delta activity has also been reported in several studies from Kupfer and colleagues (see Armitage, in press, for a review). None of these studies, however, has focused on the interval around sleep onset, and all have been conducted on half- or one-minute epochs. Two epochs can receive the same stage score, yet there may be considerable variability within each epoch. Stage-scoring procedures may, in fact, obscure sleep EEG differences in depressed and normal subjects and perhaps in other clinical groups as well (Armitage, Roffwarg, et al., 1992).

The purpose of this study was to compare period-analyzed EEG frequency distributions around the interval of sleep onset in a group of symptomatic depression outpatients and of normal control subjects.

METHODS

Subjects

Eight healthy, normal volunteers (22–33 years of age) participated in the study. Individuals with personal and family histories of psychopathy among first-degree relatives were excluded from the study. The depressed subjects consisted of 28 unipolar outpatients (22–35 years of age) who met *DSM-III-R* (American Psychiatric Association, 1987) criteria for major depression, diagnosed by using structured clinical interviews (Spitzer, Williams, & Gibbons, 1986). A minimum score of 17 on the 17-item Hamilton Rating Scale (Hamilton, 1960) was required for entry. All subjects were medication-free for a minimum of two weeks at the time of the study and completed a five-day home diary to verify regularity of bed- and rise times. Caffeine and alcohol intake was restricted for 5 days prior to the study.

PROCEDURE

Each subject spent two consecutive nights in the University of Texas Southwestern Sleep Study Unit. All subjects were screened for independent sleep disorders, such as narcolepsy, sleep apnea, and myoclonus, using a full electrode montage (nasal–oral thermistors, leg leads, chest and abdomen respiration bands) on the first night of study.

EEG activity was recorded from C3 and C4 placements referenced to linked-ear lobes. Electrooculograms (EOGs) were recorded from the left and right outer ridges of the eye. Electromyograms (EMGs) were recorded from a chin–cheek bipolar montage. Impedances were maintained below 2 Kohms. All electrophysiological signals were amplified on Grass P511 A/C amplifiers. EEG sensitivity was set at 5 Hz, with half-amp, low-frequency filters set at 0.1 Hz and high filters at 30 Hz.

Polygraphic data were digitized at 250 Hz on a 486 50-MHz micro-computer using a 16-bit Microstar A/D board. Data were stored on optical disk for off-line visual stage-scoring and PA.

Period Analysis Algorithm

The PA algorithm was based on the early work of Hoffmann and colleagues (Hoffmann et al., 1979; Moffitt et al., 1982; Sussman, Moffitt, Hoffmann, Wells, & Shearer, 1979). Details of the period analysis algorithm are presented elsewhere (Armitage, Roffwarg, et al., 1992; Hoffmann et al., 1979). Briefly, PA is a time-domain EEG-quantification technique that includes measurement of half- and full-wave zero-cross, first derivative and amplitude in 5 EEG frequency bands: beta, 16–32 Hz;[1] sigma, 12 to < 16 Hz; alpha, 8 to < 12 Hz; theta, 4 to < 8 Hz; and delta, 0.5 to < 4 Hz, usually in 30-s epochs. A zero-cross event is a polarity change from positive to negative or vice versa. Full-wave analyses detect only negative changes in polarity. Zero-cross analyses are preferentially sensitive to slower frequencies. Full-wave, first-derivative analysis is preferentially sensitive to fast-frequency EEG activity, detecting small negative inflections in the signal that do not necessarily cross zero volts. The amplitude, or power estimate, reflects the squared area under the half-wave zero-crosses in each frequency band and is equivalent to μV^2. The algorithm detects the length of time between successive events, thereby determining the EEG frequency. A time-in-frequency category is accumulated, and, at the end of each 30-s epoch, the percentage of total zero-cross time in each frequency is computed. Similarly, a time-in-frequency category accumulator is incremented for the first-derivative analyses, and at the end of each epoch, the percentage of first-derivative time in each frequency is computed. Each of the half-wave zero-cross, full-wave zero-cross, and first-derivative measures sums to 100, independently, across frequency bands. Power is de-

---

[1]Frequencies as high as 70 Hz will be detectable, using a sensitivity of 5, because of amplifier–filter roll-off.

rived from the cumulative voltage of zero-crosses in each frequency category. For the purposes of this study, all period analyses were conducted on 2-s epochs. The sleep records were also scored visually, according to standard Rechtschaffen and Kales (1968) criteria, by personnel trained at greater than 90% interrater agreement.

Averaging across half a minute around sleep onset does not provide information about the EEG frequency distributions associated with the instant of sleep onset. Between-group differences that may emerge at the moment of sleep onset are lost in this type of analysis. To compensate for this problem, between-group differences were assessed at each 2-s epoch within the half-minute interval of sleep onset. The 2-s epoch in which delta half-wave zero-cross and power showed a sharp, sustained 30% or greater increase over baseline was arbitrarily deemed to be the instant of sleep onset. As the change in delta was used strictly as a cut-point, without regard for the degree of increase, delta measures were also included in subsequent statistical evaluations. The procedure permitted a comparison of between-group differences in the degree of delta change and interhemispheric differences because the delta change at sleep onset was identified from C3 alone and only from the half-wave delta measure.

The data were then coded for group (depressed or control), and a mixed-model multivariate analysis of variance (MANOVA) was computed. EEG frequency band (five levels), hemisphere (two levels), and night (two levels) were treated as repeated measures. Group was used as a two-level between factor. Half-wave zero-cross, full-wave zero-cross, first derivative, and power were treated as four separate dependent variables. As this was a preliminary analysis without specific hypotheses, Bonferroni correction factors for probability levels were not used. However, univariate analyses were performed only if a significant overall MANOVA was obtained and a significant repeated-measures analysis of variance (ANOVA) of each PA measure was revealed. A significant Group × Hemisphere × Frequency Band × Measure interaction was obtained using a MANOVA, $F(4,31) = 38.9$, $p < .001$.

RESULTS

Half-Wave Zero-Cross

The data from two representative subjects are presented in Figure 1 (normal at top, depressed at bottom). Note that delta half-wave zero-cross was higher in the normal control subjects than in the depressed patients, particularly in the right hemisphere. The instance of sleep onset was more clearly defined in the normal control subjects and was

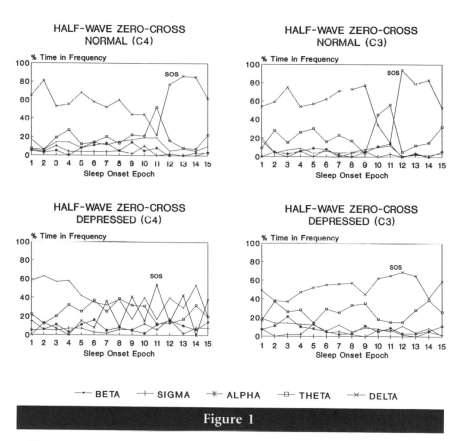

Figure 1

Half-wave zero-cross data in the 2-s × 2-s analysis of sleep onset in a representative normal control subject (top) and a depressed patient (bottom).

191

preceded by a phasic increase in theta activity. The depressed subjects showed striking hemispheric asymmetries, without a sharp transition to sleep onset in the right hemisphere. Beta activity was also elevated in the depressed subjects, primarily in the right hemisphere. Furthermore, there was no sustained increase in delta in the right hemisphere of the depressed patients.

An ANOVA revealed significant Group × Frequency Band and Hemisphere × Frequency Band interactions, F (4,136) = 22.0, $p < .001$; F (4,136) = 13.2, $p < .001$, respectively, along with several main effects. Significant between-group differences were obtained in all five frequency bands from univariate comparisons. The most dramatic group differences were evident in beta and sigma zero-cross, as seen in Figure 2. Beta activity was higher in the depressed group throughout the sleep-onset epoch. Sigma activity was generally higher in the depressed group, particularly in the left hemisphere. Alpha activity was also higher overall in the depressed group, especially in the left hemisphere. Theta in the right hemisphere was higher in the normal control subjects at sleep onset, whereas delta was lower in the depressed patients in both hemispheres.

First Derivative

A significant Group × Hemisphere × Frequency Band interaction was found, F (4,136) = 12.51, $p < .00$, along with several main effects. Beta in the right hemisphere and sigma and alpha in the left hemisphere showed significant group differences. Beta in the right was generally higher in the depressed patients, echoing the finding in half-wave zero-cross measures. Sigma and alpha in the left hemisphere were higher in the normal control subjects at some, but not all, 2-s epochs. Sigma and alpha first derivatives in the right hemisphere did not differentiate the two groups, accounting for hemisphere interaction.

Full-Wave Zero-Cross

A marginally significant group effect, F (1,34) = 3.9, $p < .06$, and a Hemisphere × Frequency Band interaction, F (4,136) = 6.5, $p < .001$,

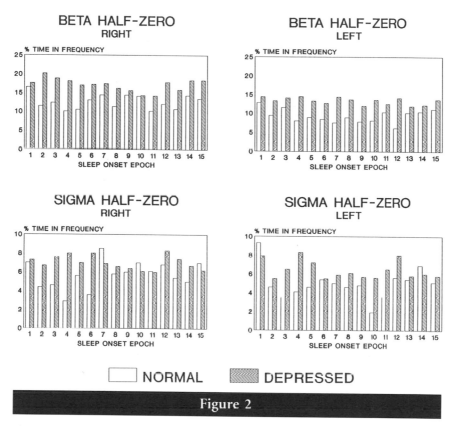

Figure 2

Significant group differences in the 2-s × 2-s analysis of sleep onset, beta half-wave zero-cross (top) and sigma half-wave zero-cross (bottom).

were obtained for full-zero data. However, only beta full-zero showed a significant group difference from univariate analyses. The depressed patients showed large asymmetries in this measure, with twice as much beta in the right than in the left hemisphere during some 2-s epochs. The normal controls showed small interhemispheric differences on the order of 3%. They also showed larger asymmetries prior to sleep onset, whereas the depressed patients showed larger asymmetries after sleep onset.

Power

A Group $\times$ Frequency Band interaction, F (4,136) = 4.7, p < .001, and a Hemisphere $\times$ Frequency Band interaction, F (4,136) = 15.0, p < .001, were found for power measures. These effects are illustrated in the group means presented in Figure 3. The normal subjects had higher delta power overall than did the depressed subjects. Both groups had higher delta in the right than in the left hemisphere. Theta power was higher in the control subjects in both hemispheres at the instant of and following sleep onset than was evident in the depressed subjects.

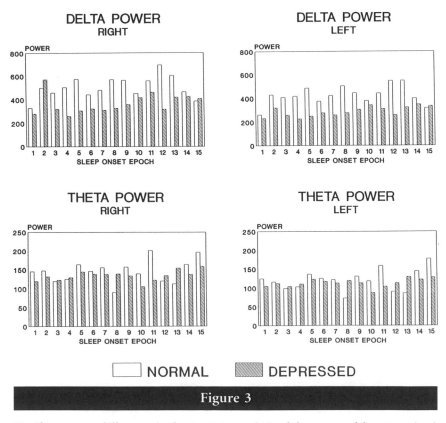

Significant group differences in the 2-s $\times$ 2-s analysis of sleep onset, delta power (top) and theta power (bottom).

DISCUSSION

Analysis of the sleep-onset period in 2-s intervals revealed striking group differences, evident in both incidence and amplitude measures. Again, fast-frequency activity was elevated in the group with depression, particularly in the right hemisphere, with the exception of beta full-wave zero-cross. Slower frequencies were elevated in the normal group, particularly among amplitude measures. The pattern of hemispheric asymmetries was, however, strikingly different for the two groups. It should be noted that not all PA group differences persisted throughout the sleep onset epoch, further enhancing the notion that sleep onset is part of a continuous process rather than a discretely bounded event. This point may be particularly relevant in groups of depressed patients, and perhaps in other clinical populations among whom the transition to sleep may be a more gradual and more highly variable process.

Depression has long been associated with functional abnormalities in the right hemisphere (Ross, 1981), based primarily on the assumption that emotions, in general, and response to emotional stimuli, are mediated by the right hemisphere. This popular view has been supported by recent electrophysiological data that indicate elevated fast-frequency activity in the right hemisphere of depressed patients in wakefulness (Pollock & Schneider, 1989) and during sleep (Armitage, in press; Armitage et al., 1993). Furthermore, elevated right-hemisphere beta is maximal in REM sleep and may be related to abnormal REM macroarchitecture in depression, although increased right-hemisphere activity persists throughout NREM stages (Armitage et al., 1993).

More recently, affective disorders have been linked to hypothalamic–pituitary–adrenal (HPA) abnormalities (Ehlers & Kupfer, 1987; Holsboer, 1989). Corticotropin-releasing factor (CRF) has been implicated in the production and regulation of acetylcholine and in a variety of neuroendocrine functions. Although highly speculative, it is not unreasonable to suggest that modulation of CRF may affect the regulation of cortical EEG activity. The definitive proof rests in the discovery of a preferential pathway between the HPA axis and the right hemisphere. Serotonergic asymmetries have recently been described, and more imipramine binding sites have been documented in the right than in the left hemisphere (Arato, Frecska, Tekes, & MacCrimmon, 1991). Serotonergic abnormalities have also been described in depression (Rush et al., 1991), and the hypothalamus has been implicated in the control of serotonin during sleep (Jones, 1989), further enhancing the notion of a preferential link to the right hemisphere in depression.

The data reported here suggest that elevated fast-frequency activity characterizes the interval around sleep onset. It is compelling that some measures of right-hemisphere beta are maximally different from controls, at the instant of sleep onset. One might be tempted to interpret these data as simple hyperarousal in depression. However, slower frequencies are also elevated in the right hemisphere in depression, although significantly lower than those found in control subjects. This finding suggests that *both* increased fast- and slow-EEG activity are present in the right hemisphere of depressed patients. These data do not fit a simple hyperarousal explanation but may be indicative of more general interhemispheric dysregulation, as suggested previously (Armitage, Roffwarg, et al., 1992; Armitage et al., 1993).

Our data also suggest that the initiation and maintenance of sleep onset are different in depressed subjects. In all the control subjects in this study, sleep onset, as characterized by a sharp, sustained increase in delta activity, was preceded directly by an increase in theta activity. This EEG change was evident in only two of the depressed subjects. If replicated, this periodic increase in theta may be necessary for sustained initiation of sleep. It is interesting that a sharp increase in theta activity is usually observed in REM sleep, in both depressed and normal control subjects (Armitage, Roffwarg, et al., 1992). In fact, changes in theta activity in REM sleep may be greatest in the depressed patients. Increased phasic EEG activity, including theta bursts, are prevalent in depressed subjects in REM sleep. At sleep initiation, however, increased theta activity is not observed in this group.

Depression has also been linked to a supersensitive cholinergic system with increased REM "pressure" during the night. If dysregulation of this particular neurotransmitter is the driving force behind depression, one might expect *increased*, not decreased, theta activity at sleep onset relative to that in the control group. It is, however, possible that increased cholinergic activity in depression occurs only after sleep initiation. Perhaps more important, the depressed patients showed only about 10% less delta incidence than the control group, although the amplitude of delta activity was lower in the depressed group. We also computed delta power relative to total power (because power measures are arbitrary units) and found significantly lower amplitude in the depressed group. Thus, the depressed subjects failed to "generate" delta waves of the same magnitude as the normal subjects, even though the incidence of delta was only slightly lower than that of normal subjects. The link to specific neurotransmitter systems is, however, speculative. The mechanisms that underlie sleep EEG abnormalities in depression remain unknown.

Subjective complaints of difficulty in falling sleep are common in depression. The results from this study suggest that some EEG characteristics, normally associated with sleep onset, are absent in depressed outpatients. Perhaps future research may identify unique EEG abnormalities in those depressed patients who specifically report sleep-onset insomnia complaints.

REFERENCES

American Psychiatric Association (1987). *DSM-III-R: Diagnostic and statistical manual of mental disorders* (3rd ed., rev.). Washington, DC: Author.

Arato, M., Frecska, E., Tekes, K., & MacCrimmon, D. J. (1991). Serotonergic interhemispheric asymmetry: Gender differences in the orbital cortex. *Acta Psychiatrica Scandinavica, 84,* 110–111.

Armitage, R. (in press). Microarchitectural findings in sleep EEG in depression: Diagnostic implications. *Biological Psychiatry, 36.*

Armitage, R., Calhoun, J. S., Rush, A. J., & Roffwarg, H. P. (1992). Comparison of the delta EEG in the first and second non-REM periods in depressed adults and normal controls. *Psychiatry Research, 41,* 65–72.

Armitage, R., Hoffmann, R., Loewy, D., & Moffitt, A. (1989). Variations in period-analysed EEG asymmetry in REM and NREM sleep. *Psychophysiology, 26,* 329–336.

Armitage, R., Roffwarg, H., & Rush, A. J. (1993). Digital period analysis of EEG in depression: Periodicity, coherence, and interhemispheric relationships during sleep. *Progress in Neuro-Psychopharmacology and Biological Psychiatry, 17,* 363–372.

Armitage, R., Roffwarg, H., Rush, A. J., Calhoun, J. S., Purdy, D., & Giles, D. (1992). Digital period analysis of sleep EEG in depression. *Biological Psychiatry, 31,* 52–68.

Ehlers, C. L., & Kupfer, D. J. (1987). Hypothalamic peptide modulation of EEG sleep in depression: A further application of the S-process hypothesis. *Biological Psychiatry, 22,* 513–517.

Feinberg, I. (1989). Effects of maturation and aging on slow-wave sleep in man. In A. Wauquier, C. Dugovic, & A. Radulovacki (Eds.), *Slow-wave sleep: Physiological, pathophysiological, and functional aspects* (pp. 31–48). New York: Raven Press.

Geering, B., Achermann, P., Eggimann, F., & Borbély, A. (1993). Period–amplitude analysis and power spectral analysis: A comparison based on all-night sleep EEG recordings. *Journal of Sleep Research, 2,* 121–129.

Hamilton, M. (1960). A rating scale for depression. *Journal of Neurological and Neurosurgical Psychiatry, 23,* 56–62.

Hoffmann, R. F., Moffitt, A. R., Shearer, J. C., Sussman, P. S., & Wells, R. B. (1979). Conceptual and methodological considerations towards the development of computer-controlled research on the electrophysiology of sleep. *Waking and Sleeping, 3,* 1–16.

Holsboer, F. (1989). Psychiatric implications of altered limbic–hypothalamic–pituitary–adrenocortical activity. *European Archives of Psychiatry and Neurological Science, 238,* 302–322.

Jones, B. (1989). Basic mechanisms of sleep–wake states. In M. Kryger, T. Roth, & W. C. Dement (Eds.), *Principles and practice of sleep medicine* (pp. 121–138). Philadelphia: Saunders.

Ktonas, P. (1987). Period–amplitude EEG analysis [Editorial comment]. *Sleep, 10,* 505–507.

Kupfer, D. J. (1989). Neurophysiological factors in depression: New perspectives. *European Archives of Psychiatry and Neurological Science, 238*, 251–258.

Kupfer, D. J., Grochocinski, V. J., & McEachran, A. B. (1986). Relationship of awakening and delta sleep in depression. *Psychiatry Research, 19*, 297–304.

Kupfer, D. J., Reynolds, C. F., III, & Ehlers, C. L. (1989). Comparison of EEG sleep measures among depressive subtypes and controls in older individuals. *Psychiatry Research, 27*, 13–21.

Moffitt, A., Hoffmann, R., Wells, R., Armitage, R., Pigeau, R., & Shearer, J. (1982). Individual differences among pre- and post-awakening EEG correlates of dream reports following arousals from different stages of sleep. *Psychiatric Journal of the University of Ottawa, 7*, 111–125.

Pigeau, R., Hoffmann, R., & Moffitt, A. (1981). A multivariate comparison of two EEG analysis techniques: Period analysis and fast Fourier transforms. *Electroencephalography and Clinical Neurophysiology, 52*, 656–658.

Pollock, V. E., & Schneider, L. S. (1989). Quantitative, waking EEG research on depression. *Biological Psychiatry, 27*, 757–780.

Rechtschaffen, A., & Kales, A. (1968). *A manual of standardized terminology, techniques and scoring system for sleep-stages of human subjects.* Washington, DC: U.S. Government Printing Office.

Reynolds, C. F., & Kupfer, D. J. (1987). Sleep research in affective illness: State-of-the-art circa 1987. *Sleep, 10*, 199–215.

Ross, E. (1981). The aprosodias: Functional–anatomical organization of the affective components of language in the right hemisphere. *Archives of Neurology, 20*, 561–580.

Rush, A. J., Cain, J. W., Reese, J., Stewart, R. S., Waller, D. A., & Debus, J. D. (1991). Neurological bases for psychiatric disorders. In R. N. Rosenberg (Ed.), *Comprehensive Neurology* (pp. 555–603). New York: Raven Press.

Spitzer, R. L., Williams, J. B. S., & Gibbons, M. (1986). *The structured clinical interview for DSM-III-R (SCID).* New York: State Psychiatric Research Institute.

Sussman, P. S., Moffitt, A. R., Hoffmann, R. F., Wells, R. B., & Shearer, J. (1979). The description of structural and temporal characteristics of tonic electrophysiological activity during sleep. *Waking and Sleeping, 3*, 279–290.

12

Fluctuations in Single-Hertz EEG Activity During the Transition to Sleep

Pietro Badia, Kenneth P. Wright, Jr., and
Albert Wauquier

M ost polygraphic sleep studies focus on electroencephalogram (EEG) characteristics and the various EEG changes that occur across the night. Fewer studies have focused on EEG changes occurring specifically during the relatively short transition period between wakefulness and sleep. This study does the latter and documents the various EEG changes that occur during the transition period. Although these EEG changes are of interest in themselves, they may also be related to parallel changes in other measures that have been reported during sleep, such as (a) general reduction in sensory awareness and responsiveness (e.g., Ogilvie, Wilkinson, & Allison, 1989), (b) loss of memory (amnesia) for new events (e.g., Badia, 1990), (c) absence of elicited skin conductance responses (e.g., Johnson, 1970), (d) drop in body temperature and change in temperature set point (e.g., Barrett, Lack, & Morris, 1993; Wehr, 1990), and (e) respiratory changes (e.g., Colrain, Trinder, Fraser, & Wilson, 1987; Naifeh & Kamiya, 1981).

For addressing most questions concerning sleep, standard sleep-scoring criteria using broadband EEG activity (alpha, beta, theta) and long, 30-s epochs are acceptable. However, for studying short time periods, such as the transition from wakefulness to sleep, standard sleep-scoring procedures have limitations. The main one is epoch size. An analysis using 30-s epochs is insensitive to fluctuations that occur over shorter time periods and, thus, is too crude and imprecise for tracking EEG changes during the relatively brief transition period. Therefore, to detect possible short-term fluctuations in EEG activity during the transition period, the current study placed emphasis on 5-s epochs.

In addition to the problem posed by epoch duration, the analysis of broadband EEG changes can also present certain problems in regard to assessing the transition period. The standard sleep-scoring procedure generally focuses on broadband EEG activity. Focusing on the activity of the alpha (8–12 Hz), beta (14–30 Hz), and theta (4–7 Hz) bands rather than on single-hertz activity assumes that the frequencies within each EEG band respond (change) in a similar way during the transition. A broadband analysis does not permit identifying possible differential effects for each EEG frequency. This problem can be addressed easily by means of fast Fourier transform (FFT) and power spectral analysis to decompose the EEG signal and to assess changes in single-hertz activity during the transition period.

In this study, we focused on EEG changes that occur during the transition to sleep. To this end, we used short, 5-s epochs and a single-Hertz EEG analysis (3–25 Hz), along with traditional measures, to document EEG changes at three recording sites (F3, C3, and O1).

METHOD

Subjects

Undergraduate students ($N = 14$) enrolled at Bowling Green State University served as subjects (9 women and 5 men, of age 18 to 21 years; $M = 19.1$ years). They were selected from a larger group of 68 subjects, who had been instructed simply to fall asleep (see *Procedure* section). The 14 subjects selected from this group were those showing a smooth transition from wakefulness to sleep (i.e., awake followed by three continuous, 30-s epochs of sleep without a wake–sleep fluctuation).

Apparatus

We used Grass 7P511L AC amplifiers (Model 7F polygraph) to record EEG, electrooculogram (EOG), and electromyogram (EMG) signals. Sleep was recorded by means of the standard electrode montage. We used Compaq 386 computers for spectral analysis of EEG data recorded from J6 of the Grass amplifiers. The EEG data were sampled and stored at a rate of 128 samples per second per channel with a 12-bit DTACQ A/D board (Model DT-2821). Beckman biopotential electrodes were used for the EEG (16 mm in diameter), EOG, and EMG (each 11 mm in diameter) recordings.

Procedure

Subjects arrived at the Sleep and Psychophysiology Laboratory at either 1000 or 1300 hr, at which time they received a description of the procedure and gave informed consent. Electrodes were secured for recording EOG (outer canthi, above and below the midline), EMG (supra- and submental), and EEG (F3, C3, O1, left and right mastoids). Subjects were then escorted to the bedroom and were asked simply to fall asleep. Sleep onset was defined as three consecutive 30-s epochs of any stage of sleep. If the subject did not fall asleep within a 20-min period, the session was terminated. Subjects slept in an electrically shielded, sound-attenuated bedroom. White noise (65-dB sound pressure level) was generated by a Grason Stadler 455 G noise generator during the entire nap period.

Sleep Scoring

Changes in broadband and single-Hertz EEG power for each site were examined for 3 min of continuous EEG activity during the transition from wakefulness to sleep (i.e., the last three 30-s epochs of wakefulness [W1, W2, and W3], followed by the first three 30-s epochs of stage 1 sleep [S1, S2, and S3]). Sleep and wakefulness activity for the 30-s analysis was scored according to the guidelines of Rechtschaffen and Kales (1968). In addition to a 30-s epoch analysis, changes in EEG activity across the 3-min period were also examined in 5-s epochs. The 5-s epochs were scored for wake–sleep activity by means of the following criteria. The number of EEG peaks for each 1-s period was tabulated, and 1-s epochs with 7 or fewer peaks (7 Hz or less) were scored as sleep, whereas 1-s epochs with 8 or more peaks (8 Hz or more) were scored as wakefulness. If the majority of 1-s epochs (3 or more of the 5) were scored as sleep, then the entire 5-s epoch was scored as sleep; otherwise it was scored as wakefulness. The reliability of the sleep scoring exceeded .90 among scorers.

Spectral Analysis

We assessed EEG data for changes in amplitude by submitting the acquired data to an FFT analysis over a frequency range of 3–25 Hz. The analysis of EEG data included both relative and absolute power for the broadbands (3–7 Hz, 8–12 Hz, 13–25 Hz) and for the single-Hertz values from 3 to 25 Hz. Delta activity below 3 Hz was not examined, because artifacts from slow eye movement during the transition to sleep may be indistinguishable from low-frequency EEG activity (Coburn & Moreno, 1988).

RESULTS

Our first analysis deals with both broadband EEG activity and single-Hertz EEG activity across traditional 30-s epochs. This is then followed by an analysis of single-hertz activity across 5-s epochs. Preliminary analysis suggested few differences in EEG patterning between relative and absolute power analyses. Therefore, only the relative power analyses are presented.

Thirty-Second Epochs

Figure 1 displays the data across the three 30-s epochs of wake and the three 30-s epochs of sleep for the 3–7-Hz, 8–12-Hz and 13–25-Hz ranges at each cortical site. As shown in the figure, EEG changes at each brain site begin to occur before sleep onset (S1) and are charac-

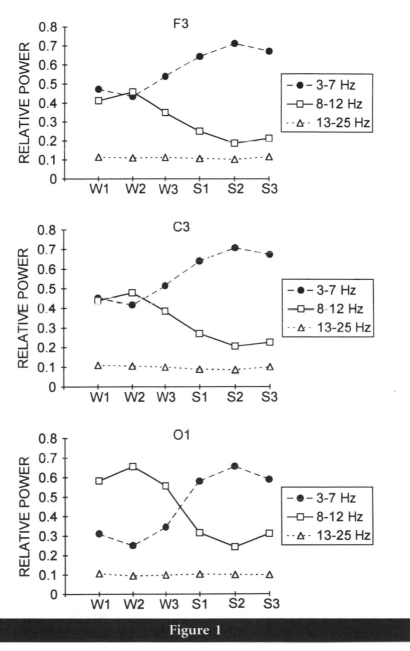

Figure 1

Broadband changes in EEG power across the last three 30-s epochs of wakefulness (W1, W2, and W3) and the first three 30-s epochs of sleep (S1, S2, and S3); $n = 14$.

terized by increases in 3–7-Hz activity and decreases in 8–12-Hz activity. Overall, the figure shows that decreases in 8–12-Hz activity and increases in 3–7-Hz activity occur before visually scored sleep onset (from W2 to W3). In general, 8–12-Hz activity is relatively high during wakefulness, and 3–7-Hz activity is relatively high during sleep. There was little change in activity within the 13–25-Hz range. Figure 1 also reveals that the EEG activity at F3 and that at C3 tend to be more similar to each other than to activity at O1. Statistical analyses of some of these relationships are as follows.

The 3–7-Hz range

One-way analyses of variance (ANOVAs) for each brain site revealed a significant main effect for all sites across time. Planned comparisons for each brain site were then computed across time periods to determine which comparisons were significant. Significant increases in spectral power for 3–7 Hz from W2 to W3 were observed 30 s before visually scored sleep onset at all brain sites: For F3, $F(1, 13) = 8.45$, $p < .01$; for C3, $F(1, 13) = 6.57$, $p < .02$; for O1, $F(1, 13) = 11.30$, $p < .005$. Significant increases in 3–7-Hz activity were also observed at the point of visually scored sleep onset from W3 to S1 at all brain sites: For F3, $F(1, 13) = 10.87$, $p < .006$; for C3, $F(1, 13) = 14.99$, $p < .002$; for O1, $F(1, 13) = 94.44$, $p < .0001$.

The 8–12-Hz range

One-way ANOVAs for each brain site revealed that significant main effects occurred for time at each site. Planned comparisons were then computed, and they revealed that significant decreases in spectral power for the 8–12-Hz range occurred from W2 to W3 at each site before visually scored sleep onset: For F3, $F(1, 13) = 8.52$, $p < .01$; for C3, $F(1, 13) = 5.95$, $p < .03$; for O1, $F(1, 13) = 9.16$, $p <. 01$. In addition, significant decreases in spectral power were seen at the point of visually scored sleep onset from W3 to S1: For F3, $F(1, 13) = 7.81$, $p < .015$; for C3, $F(1, 13) = 10.57$, $p < .006$; for O1, $F(1, 13) = 62.7$, $p < .0001$.

The 13–25-Hz range

One-way ANOVAs across individual brain sites revealed no significant differences in 13–25-Hz activity during the transition from wakefulness to sleep.

Single-Hertz Activity

Figures 2 and 3 display the data for single-Hertz activity (3–12 Hz) across 30-s epochs for each brain site.

Changes in single-Hertz activity within the 3–7-Hz range during the transition to sleep varied considerably. The observed transition changes were due mostly to the large increases in power observed at 3 and 4 Hz. Systematically smaller increases in power were observed at 5, 6, and 7 Hz (see Figure 2). In fact, with the exception of Site O1, there was little change in EEG activity from wakefulness to sleep at 7 Hz. This pattern was generally consistent at each of the brain sites.

As shown in Figure 3, changes in single-Hertz activity within the 8–12-Hz range during the transition revealed that the single-Hertz differences between wakefulness and sleep were greatest at 10 Hz. The next greatest decrease occurred at 9 and 11 Hz. Very little change in EEG activity occurred at either 8 Hz or 12 Hz during the transition to sleep.

Similarly to the broadband analysis, none of the single-Hertz values within the 13–25-Hz range showed a significant change during the transition.

Five-Second Epochs

Table 1 contains the sleep-scoring data of the 5-s epochs for 6 of the 14 subjects. These subjects are representative of the entire group. Wake (0) and sleep (1) scoring for each of the thirty-six 5-s epochs (i.e., a 3-min wake–sleep period) at each brain site is shown. These data reveal that the transition to sleep is not the smooth shift suggested by the 30-s epoch analysis. A 5-s epoch analysis reveals many fluctuations be-

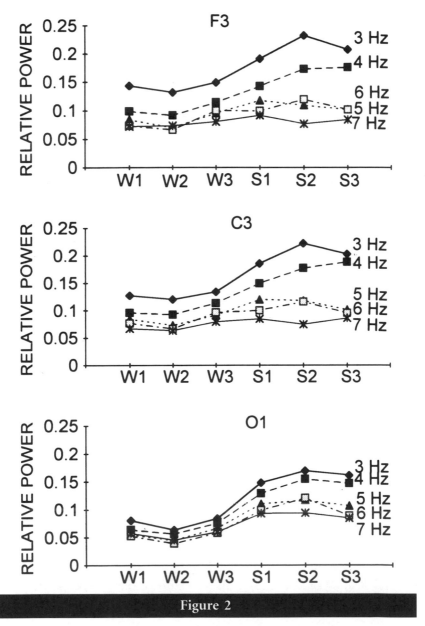

Figure 2

Single-Hertz changes in relative EEG power from 3–7 Hz across the last three 30-s epochs of wakefulness (W1, W2, and W3) and the first three 30-s epochs of sleep (S1, S2, and S3); $n = 14$.

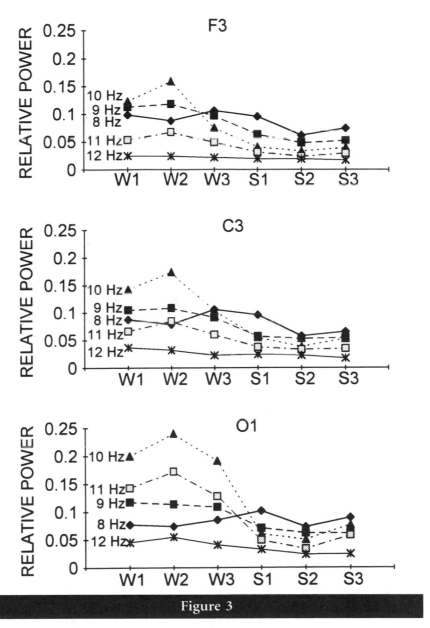

Figure 3

Single-Hertz changes in relative EEG power from 8–12 Hz across the last three 30-s epochs of wakefulness (W1, W2, and W3) and the first three 30-s epochs of sleep (S1, S2, and S3); $n = 14$.

Table 1

Data Showing Whether Individual Subjects Were Awake (0) or Asleep (1) Across Each of the Thirty-Six 5-s Epochs for Each Brain Site

Brain Site	1	2	3	4	5	6	7	8	9	10	11	12	13	14	15	16	17	18	19	20	21	22	23	24	25	26	27	28	29	30	31	32	33	34	35	36
Subject 307																																				
F3	0	0	0	1	0	0	0	1	0	0	0	0	0	0	0	0	0	0	0	0	1	1	1	0	0	0	1	0	1	0	1	1	1	1	0	0
C3	0	1	0	1	0	1	1	0	0	0	0	0	0	0	0	0	0	0	0	0	1	1	0	0	0	1	0	1	0	0	1	1	0	0	0	0
O1	0	0	0	1	0	1	1	0	0	0	0	0	0	0	0	0	0	0	0	0	1	1	1	1	0	0	1	1	1	1	1	1	0	0	0	0
Subject 310																																				
F3	0	0	0	0	0	0	0	0	0	0	0	0	0	0	0	0	0	1	1	0	0	1	1	1	1	1	1	1	1	1	1	1	0	1	1	1
C3	0	0	0	0	0	0	0	0	0	0	0	0	0	0	0	0	0	1	0	1	0	1	1	1	1	0	1	0	1	1	1	0	0	0	1	1
O1	0	0	0	0	0	0	0	0	0	0	0	0	0	0	0	0	0	1	1	0	0	1	1	1	1	1	1	0	1	1	1	0	0	0	1	1
Subject 327																																				
F3	0	1	1	1	1	0	1	1	0	1	1	1	1	1	0	1	1	1	1	0	1	1	1	1	1	0	1	1	1	1	0	1	0	1	1	1
C3	0	0	0	0	0	0	0	0	0	0	0	0	0	0	0	0	0	0	0	0	1	1	1	1	0	0	1	1	1	1	0	0	0	0	0	1
O1	0	0	1	0	1	0	0	1	1	0	1	1	1	0	0	0	0	1	0	0	1	0	0	1	0	0	0	0	1	1	1	0	0	0	1	1
Subject 337																																				
F3	0	0	1	1	0	1	0	0	0	0	0	0	0	0	0	0	0	0	0	0	0	1	0	1	0	1	0	1	0	0	1	1	1	1	1	1
C3	0	1	1	1	1	0	1	0	0	0	0	0	0	0	0	0	0	1	1	1	1	1	1	1	1	0	1	1	1	1	1	1	1	1	1	1
O1	0	0	0	1	0	1	1	1	0	0	0	0	0	0	0	0	0	1	1	1	1	1	1	1	1	0	0	1	0	1	0	1	1	1	1	1
Subject 338																																				
F3	0	0	0	0	0	0	1	1	0	0	0	0	1	1	1	0	1	0	0	0	0	0	1	0	1	1	1	1	1	1	1	0	1	0	1	1
C3	0	0	0	0	0	1	1	1	0	0	0	0	1	1	1	1	0	0	1	0	0	0	0	0	1	1	1	1	1	1	1	1	1	1	0	0
O1	0	0	0	0	0	0	0	0	0	0	0	0	0	0	1	0	1	0	0	0	0	0	0	0	0	1	1	1	1	1	1	1	0	0	0	1
Subject 402																																				
F3	1	1	0	0	0	0	1	1	1	1	0	0	0	0	0	0	0	1	1	1	1	1	1	1	1	1	1	1	1	1	1	1	1	1	1	1
C3	1	1	0	0	0	0	1	0	1	0	0	0	0	0	0	0	0	1	1	1	1	1	1	1	1	0	1	1	0	1	1	1	0	1	1	1
O1	1	1	0	0	0	0	1	0	1	1	0	0	0	0	1	0	1	1	1	1	1	1	1	1	1	1	0	0	0	1	1	0	0	0	0	0

NOTE: For brain site, F = frontal, C = central, O = occipital.

tween wakefulness and sleep during the transition period and suggests that the shift from wakefulness to sleep is more abrupt than gradual. These data also show brain-site differences during the transition to sleep. As Table 1 shows, it is not uncommon for one brain site to exhibit wake activity while another exhibits sleep activity. In this regard, EEG activity at brain sites F3 and C3 were more similar to each other than they were to O1.

The 3–7-Hz range

Figure 4 provides an example of changes in EEG activity in Subject 307 during the transition to sleep as seen with a 5-s epoch analysis. Activity at 3 Hz tends to track fluctuations both to sleep and back to wakefulness during the transition period. This frequency was selected to depict the transition to sleep because it showed the largest positive point-biserial correlation between EEG power and sleep. In general, the majority of subjects showed low EEG power at 3 or 4 Hz, or both, during wakefulness and high power at these frequencies during sleep (see Table 2).

Figure 5a displays the degree of increase in relative power between wakefulness and sleep for the 3–7-Hz range (averaged EEG power during sleep minus averaged EEG power during wakefulness). Increases at 3 and 4 Hz are predominant during the transition to sleep, with smaller increases at 5 and 6 Hz and very little change at 7 Hz. This pattern was consistent across all brain sites except for the O1 site, which did show a small but significant increase at 7 Hz.

The top half of Table 2 contains the number of subjects and the specific EEG frequency showing the largest increase in relative power when going from wakefulness to sleep for each brain site. Some individual differences are apparent, but the table shows that the majority of subjects exhibited the largest increases in EEG power at 3 and 4 Hz during the transition from wakefulness to sleep. Brain-site differences are also apparent, in that some subjects exhibited the largest increases in EEG power at 5 and 6 Hz at brain site O1 (see chapters 13 and 14, this volume).

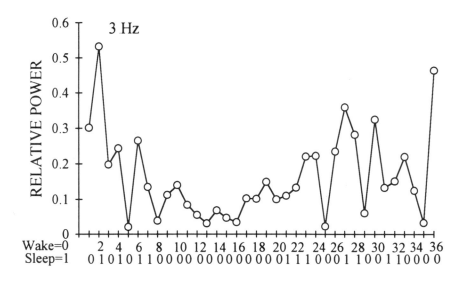

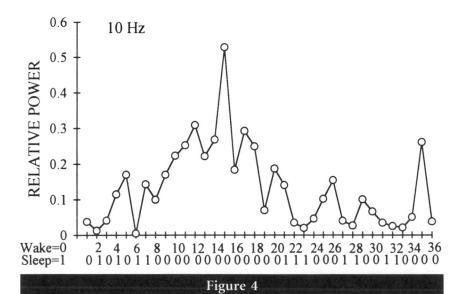

Figure 4

Data for Subject 307 at C3, during the last 90 s of wakefulness and the first 90 s of sleep, across thirty-six 5-s epochs, showing that activity at 3 Hz tended to track the relatively rapid fluctuations to both wakefulness and sleep during the transition, whereas activity at 10 Hz tracked primarily the transition to sleep.

Table 2

EEG Frequencies and Number of Subjects Showing the Largest Change at Those Frequencies During the Transition to Sleep for Each Brain Site

Freq. in Hz	F3	C3	O1
		Largest relative power increase	
3	8	8	3
4	5	5	6
5	0	0	3
6	1	1	2
7	0	0	0
		Largest relative power decrease	
8	2	2	1
9	6	2	3
10	5	7	7
11	0	3	3
12	1	0	0

NOTE: EEG = electroencephalogram, F = frontal, C = central, O = occipital.

The 8–12-Hz range

Figure 4 also shows that activity at 10 Hz tracks the transition to sleep, but unlike what happens at 3 or 4 Hz, very little change occurs at 10 Hz in response to brief awakenings once sleep has begun; increases in activity are usually seen instead at 8 or 9 Hz. In general, the majority of subjects show high EEG power at 10 Hz during wakefulness and low power during sleep. Figure 5b displays the degree of decrease in relative power (averaged power during wakefulness minus averaged power during sleep) between wakefulness and sleep for the 8–12-Hz range. These data show that decreases at 10 Hz are predominant during the transition to sleep, with smaller decreases at 9 and 11 Hz, and even smaller decreases at 8 and 12 Hz. This pattern was consistent across all brain

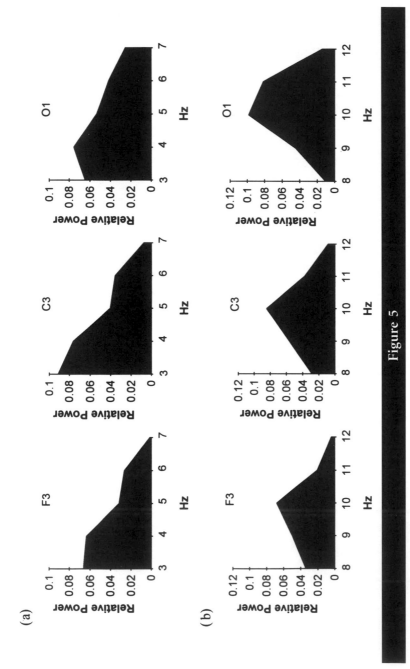

Figure 5

Single-Hertz relative EEG power differences between wakefulness and sleep for (a) 3–7 Hz, and (b) 8–12 Hz at each recorded brain site across 5-s epochs; *n* = 14.

sites. Activity at brain sites F3 and activity at brain site C3 appear to be more similar to each other than to activity at O1.

The bottom half of Table 2 contains the number of subjects and the specific EEG frequency showing the largest decrease in relative power, for each brain site, when going from wakefulness to sleep. The data show that the majority of subjects exhibited the largest decreases in EEG power at 10 Hz and then at 9 and 11 Hz during the transition from wakefulness to sleep. Brain-site differences are also apparent. Brain site F3 appears to have more subjects showing the largest decreases in the slower frequencies compared with brain sites C3 and O1.

CONCLUSION

These results demonstrate that a single-Hertz analysis of the EEG across 5 s epochs provides additional information concerning changes in brain activity during the transition from wakefulness to sleep. During the transition, the majority of subjects showed the largest increases in brain activity at 3 or 4 Hz and the largest decreases in brain activity at 10 Hz. Furthermore, the 5-s analysis revealed that the transition to sleep is not smooth. In fact, frequent fluctuations between wakefulness and sleep EEG activity were observed for all subjects during the transition. These fluctuations from wakefulness to sleep and from sleep to wakefulness tended to be tracked best by changes observed at 3 or 4 Hz. Changes in EEG activity at 10 Hz tracked the transition to sleep better than the transition to brief awakenings. In this regard, the data also show that EEG activity within the broadbands was differentially affected by the transition. Specifically, a nearly symmetrical, decremental gradient of EEG activity occurred on either side of 10 Hz.

These results are in agreement with the broadband changes reported in previous studies of the transition from wakefulness to sleep. Studies using visual scoring of the EEG report decreases in alpha activity with concomitant increases in theta activity as the transition from wakefulness to sleep is made (e.g., Davis, Davis, Loomis, Harvey, & Hobart,

1937, 1938; Dement & Kleitman, 1957; Rechtschaffen & Kales, 1968). Computer analyses of the EEG during the transition confirm increases in theta activity and decreases in alpha activity (Azekawa, Sei, & Morita, 1990; Hori, 1985; Hori, Hayashi, & Morikawa, 1990) during the transition. Increases in delta activity (Hori, 1985) and decreases in beta activity (Merica, Fortune, & Gaillard, 1991) have also been reported. Unfortunately, experiments using computer analysis techniques do not all agree on the precise moment of EEG change. Specifically, the aforementioned studies show EEG changes to occur before and after the onset of Stage 1 sleep. The present study also observed temporal EEG changes before sleep onset. The disparity among studies in pinpointing the moment of sleep onset may be due to methodological differences among the studies (e.g., epoch length, differences in the computer analysis performed, and brain site observed).

Brain-site differences during the transition from wakefulness to sleep were also observed in the present study. Sleep or wake activity did not always occur concurrently at the frontal, central, and occipital brain regions (see Table 1). In addition, individual differences were observed in that the specific EEG frequency showing the largest changes in power varied according to site and individual. Differences among brain sites make it particularly troublesome to define a precise moment of sleep onset. The difficulty in defining sleep onset is not a new phenomenon. In fact, Davis et al. (1938) stated the following:

> Only if we choose to define sleep in terms of response to a particular stimulus or a particular change in the potential record from a particular area of the cortex—only then can a moment of falling asleep be precisely defined. Otherwise the problem is just as vague and difficult as that of determining the exact moment of death. (p. 35)

The findings of the present study provide further support for their statement.

In closing, the use of a single-Hertz analysis across short-duration epochs provides further information about brain functioning during the transition from wakefulness to sleep. The single-hertz analysis revealed that the greatest changes in EEG power were observed at 3 or 4 Hz and also at 10 Hz. The use of short-duration epochs revealed that frequent fluctuation between wakefulness and sleep occurred during the transition, and whether one was judged asleep or awake often depended on the cortical site measured.

REFERENCES

Azekawa, T., Sei, H., & Morita, Y. (1990). Continuous alteration of EEG activity in human sleep onset. *Sleep Research, 19,* 7.

Badia, P. (1990). Memories in sleep: Old and new. In R. R. Bootzin, J. F. Kihlstrom, & D. L. Schacter (Eds.), *Sleep and cognition* (pp. 67–87). Washington, DC: American Psychological Association.

Barrett, J., Lack, L., & Morris, M. (1993). The sleep-evoked decrease of body temperature. *Sleep, 16,* 93–99.

Coburn, K. L., & Moreno, M. A. (1988). Facts and artifacts in brain electrical activity mapping. *Brain Topography, 1,* 37–45.

Colrain, I. M., Trinder, J., Fraser, G., & Wilson, G. V. (1987). Ventilation during sleep onset. *Journal of Applied Physiology, 63,* 2067–2074.

Davis, H., Davis, P. A., Loomis, A. L., Harvey, E. N., & Hobart, G. (1937). Changes in human brain potentials during the onset of sleep. *Science, 86,* 448–450.

Davis, H., Davis, P. A., Loomis, A. L., Harvey, E. N., & Hobart, G. (1938). Human brain potentials during the onset of sleep. *Journal of Neurophysiology, 1,* 24–38.

Dement, W., & Kleitman, N. (1957). Cyclic variations in EEG during sleep and their relation to eye movements, body motility, and dreaming. *Electroencephalography and Clinical Neurophysiology, 9,* 673–690.

Hori, T. (1985). Spatiotemporal changes of EEG activity during waking–sleeping transition period. *International Journal of Neuroscience, 27,* 101–114.

Hori, T., Hayashi, M., & Morikawa, T. (1990). Topography and coherence analysis of the hypnagogic EEG. In J. Horne (Ed.), *Sleep '90: Proceedings of the 10th European Congress on Sleep Research, Strausberg, May 1990* (pp. 10–12). Bochum, Federal Republic of Germany: Pontenagel Press.

Johnson, L. C. (1970). A psychophysiology for all states. *Psychophysiology, 6,* 501–516.

Merica, H., Fortune, R. D., & Gaillard, J. M. (1991). Hemispheric temporal organization during the onset of sleep in normal subjects. In M. G. Terzano, P. L. Halasz, & A. C. Declerck (Eds.), *Phasic events and dynamic organization of sleep* (pp. 73–83). New York: Raven Press.

Naifeh, K. H., & Kamiya, J. (1981). The nature of respiratory changes associated with sleep onset. *Sleep, 4,* 49–59.

Ogilvie, R. D., Wilkinson, R. T., & Allison, S. (1989). The detection of sleep onset: Behavioral, physiological, and subjective convergence. *Sleep, 12,* 458–474.

Rechtschaffen, A., & Kales, A. (1968). *A manual of standardized terminology, techniques and scoring system for sleep stages of human subjects* (NIH Publication No. 204). Los Angeles: University of California.

Wehr, T. A. (1990). Effects of wakefulness and sleep on depression and mania. In J. Montplaisir & R. Godbout (Eds.), *Sleep and biological rhythms: Basic mechanisms and applications to psychiatry* (pp. 42–86). Oxford, England: Oxford University Press.

13

Quantitative Topographic EEG Mapping During Drowsiness and Sleep Onset

Joel Hasan and Roger Broughton

Although the polysomnographic patterns of drowsiness and sleep onset are well documented, the electroencephalogram (EEG) component has generally been recorded by using a limited number of scalp electrodes. Consequently, even if the temporal EEG sequences are well known, their spatial (topographical) aspects are not. The standard scoring manual of Rechtschaffen and Kales (1968) recommends only a pair of referential central EEG leads, to which some authors have added a backup contralateral central or an occipital derivation (or both), the latter for better documentation of the alpha rhythm. Others have used a variety of monopolar and bipolar montages. Santamaria and Chiappa (1987) unquestionably provide the most detailed description available of the EEG events during sleep onset. Most quantitative EEG studies of drowsiness and sleep onset have similarly used a very restricted num-

J. Hasan was supported by funds from Tampere University Hospital, the Academy of Finland, and the Finnish Social and Medical Board. The study was supported by a grant from the Medical Research Council of Canada to R. Broughton. Amy Smith, Ray Wolfe, Kathy Lutley-Borland, Michel Castonguay, and Manon Lafrenière were involved in the recordings. Martin Rivers wrote the conversion program. The Bio-logic System Corporation kindly loaned the Brain Atlas program.

ber of electrode positions (e.g., Hasan, Hirvonen, Värri, Häkkinen, & Loula, 1993; Hori, 1985; Matousek & Petersen, 1983; Ogilvie & Simons, 1992).

We know of no published studies on drowsiness or sleep onset in which full EEG scalp coverage has been used even for purely nonquantified descriptive reasons. Nor are we aware of any comprehensive topographical analysis of these patterns using referential quantified data. Both approaches are necessary to obtain a fuller understanding of the physiology and phenomenology of drowsiness and sleep onset. Previous topographic EEG studies have, in general, used relatively long epochs for analysis, typically 30 s. Thus, the short-term fluctuations have also largely been missed. We report here preliminary findings using full-scalp computerized topographical EEG analysis (EEG mapping), both of the EEG transients and of quantified (spectral) EEG.

METHODS

Patients referred for routine diagnostic EEGs ($N = 10$) or Multiple Sleep Latency Tests (MSLTs; $N = 9$) to the Ottawa General Hospital, and who showed EEG signs of sleepiness or sleep, were assessed. Mean age was 38 years (range 17–77 years). Ten were women. Patients referred for an EEG underwent a 20- to 30-min recording, using routine hospital montages with hyperventilation and photic stimulation supplemented by a 10-min recording with the 19-channel montage (see later) required for brain mapping. Patients referred for MSLTs were recorded with the same montage throughout a 4- and 5-nap test period. In this group, one to three naps from each patient were selected for analysis. The criteria for epoch selection included absence of artifacts and the need to obtain as many different EEG vigilance stages as possible from each subject.

A 19-channel coronal referential EEG montage was recorded from all patients: Fp1, Fp2; F7, F3, Fz, F4, F8; T3, C3, Cz, C4, T4; T5, P3, Pz, P4, T6; and O1 and O2, each referred to a common link-ear reference with a 10-kOhm resistor between A1 and A2. All recordings were made digitally in a sound-attenuated, dimly lit room. In routine EEG recordings, a 22-channel Nihon Kohden electroencephalograph amplified the signals for a Bio-logic Ceegraph digital EEG system (Bio-logic System Corp., Muldenheim, IL). The sampling rate was 200 Hz. The sleep data were collected by a 21-channel Grass polygraph connected to a Bio-logic Sleepscan system at a sampling rate of 100 Hz. In both, the time constant (0.3) and filterings were set to ensure a flat frequency response between 0.5 and 25 Hz. A 50-μV square wave signal was used for calibration. The MSLT recordings were converted to a data format accepted by the brain mapping program using local software.

Data analysis used Bio-logic's Brain Atlas, version 2.35, brain-mapping program. Amplitude maps of peaks and troughs of transients were made for raw data screened in 7-s epochs. Spectral frequency maps were constructed using manually chosen 2-s epochs representative of different EEG events, stages, and waveforms. These short epochs were treated by fast Fourier transform (FFT) with the Hanning window enabled. The frequency range obtained was 0.5–31.5 Hz, with a resolution of 0.5 Hz.

Samples for spectral analysis were taken from segments of presleep wakefulness, Stage 1A (diffuse and slowed alpha), low- and medium-voltage Stage 1B (prespindle mixed-frequency activity), and Stage 2, using the criteria of Valley and Broughton (1983). Stages 1A and 1B correspond closely to the original stages A and B of Loomis, Harvey, and Hobart (1937).

RESULTS

The Alpha Rhythm

EEG rhythms must be distinguished from other EEG activities. To constitute an EEG rhythm—for instance, the alpha rhythm—an activity must exhibit three principal characteristics: a frequency range, location, and specific reactivity (International Federation of Societies for Electroencephalography and Clinical Neurophysiology, 1974). Other EEG patterns in the alpha range are grouped as alpha activities.

During drowsiness and sleep onset, changes occurred both in the alpha rhythm and in other alpha activities. A small portion of our subjects showed the frequently described slowing (by 0.5–1.5 Hz) and anterior diffusion of the alpha rhythm into the central, temporal, and even frontal areas that characterizes Stage A of Loomis et al. (1937) or Stage 1A (Valley & Broughton, 1983). A few subjects at this time showed a maximum amplitude in the centro-parietal areas. In others, simple progressive disappearance of the alpha rhythm occurred, occasionally after a brief period of enhanced amplitude during which it would remain posteriorly. On arousal from drowsiness (Stage 1B) or sleep (Stage 2), the alpha rhythm often reappeared with a more focal and, at times, very asymmetrical distribution.

Alpha Activities

In most subjects, the first EEG sign of drowsiness was the appearance of a more anterior alpha activity with a typical field maximum in the frontal and central areas, falling off in the parietal, temporal, and occipital regions (Figure 1). Its frequency was about 0.5–2.0 Hz slower than the posterior alpha rhythm and never was higher than that. This "anterior alpha of drowsiness" typically occurred independently of the alpha rhythm and indeed was associated, in most cases, with marked attenuation or disappearance of the latter. At other times, the slower, more anterior alpha activity and the alpha rhythm coexisted. Source dipole analysis (Scherg & Picton, 1991) of their fields at such times documented different equivalent-source dipole locations and orientations for the two types of alpha activities (Figure 2). The appearance and disappearance of the two alpha phenomena were often so rapid that alpha distribution varied from one moment to the next. These fluctuations in amplitude were often asynchronous, so that alpha activities appeared to be waxing and waning independently in various

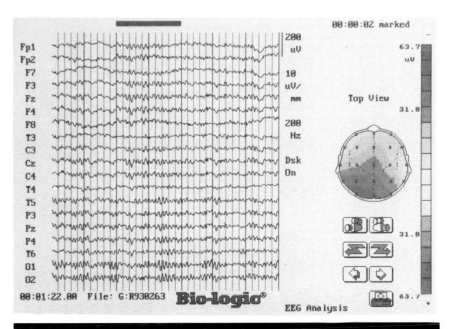

Figure 1a

Raw data (*1a*) and topographic colored spectral maps (*1b*) showing posterior alpha rhythm of mainly 9.5–10 Hz with alternating frontocentral alpha activity of 7–8 Hz typical of Stage 1A. Horizontal bar on top of *1a* indicates the 2-s segment analyzed. Although both types of alpha appear simultaneously on the maps, they are temporally independent, as shown by the raw data. The duration of the change in the EEG pattern is shorter than the shortest segment length available.

EEG channels, and showed moment-to-moment hemispheric asymmetries.

A different pattern of frontocentral maximum alpha activity was sometimes seen. This consisted of brief 1–2-s paroxysmal bursts of alpha that was 1–2 Hz slower than the alpha rhythm and occasionally became even slower to blend into the frontocentral theta bursts described below. Alpha activity could also be recorded in the temporal regions. Mostly, it appeared to represent temporal spread of the alpha

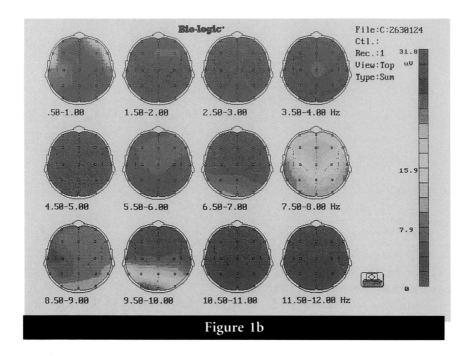

Figure 1b

rhythm or of the anterior slow alpha activity, rather than being a separate activity maximum in these areas.

Theta (3–7 Hz) Activities

Theta activities varied in frequency, amplitude, and rhythmicity throughout Stages 1B and 2. On spectral mapping, various patterns could be distinguished. Rhythmic 4–5-Hz theta activity was usually centrally distributed. On EEG mapping, such theta activity typically had a square "table distribution," being evenly present all over the scalp with the exception of the frontopolar, temporal, and often also the occipital areas (Figure 3). Bursts of theta activity in the 5–7-Hz range occurred, usually short lasting (1 s or less) and often with a frontal maximum distribution. At times, slower rhythmic 3-Hz activity could be observed, mainly in the central regions. These three patterns were consistent with

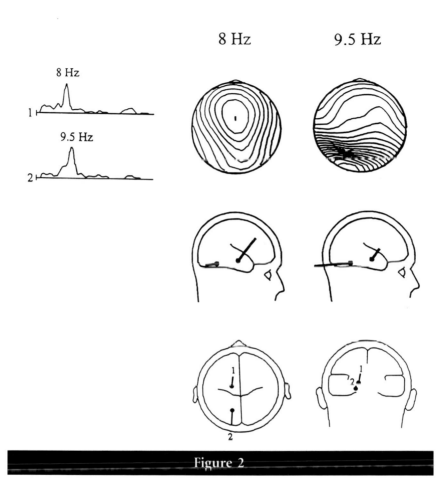

Figure 2

Equivalent source dipoles of the two alpha activities. The posterior alpha rhythm has an equivalent dipole deep in the occipital regions and horizontally oriented; that of the anterior slow alpha of drowsiness is more anterior, deep in the center of the brain, and oriented antero-superiorly. The lateralization somewhat to the left is an artifact from the use (unrecommended for this type of signal analysis) of the linked-ear reference.

the descriptions by Häkkinen (1972). Theta activities, like those in the alpha range, could simultaneously exhibit different frequencies in different locations. At times, theta was most prominent occipitally. At other moments, Stage 1B consisted of low-amplitude, mixed, slow frequencies without any rhythmic component.

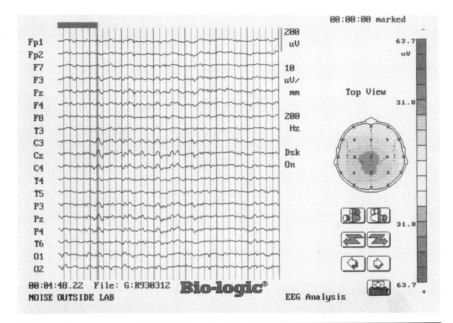

Figure 3

Voltage map showing a vertex sharp wave of Stage 1B with a field evenly distributed between Cz and Pz electrodes. Note the lower amplitude in the parasagittal areas compared to the midline.

Vertex Sharp Waves, Sawtooth Waves, and Isolated Anterior Delta Waves

Vertex sharp waves are nonspecific evoked potentials typically consisting of a smaller positive deflection followed by a larger negative wave, both having a steep field with very focal maximum at the midline central electrode, Cz. An occasional third, small, positive deflection also usually had this distribution. At times, the complex was more widespread and could become equipotential between electrodes C2 and Fz or electrodes Cz and Pz (Figure 4). In some subjects, repeated vertex sharp waves appeared, each with the same field. Two patients studied by MSLT showed REM sleep with typical sawtooth waves. Their maximum was at Cz or Cz–Pz, with both the waveform and field shape appearing

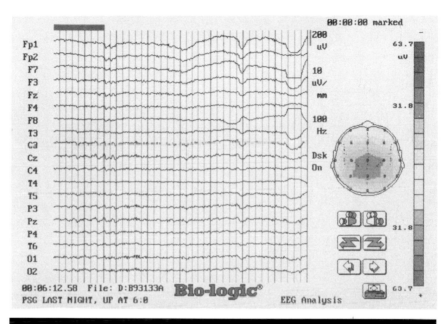

Figure 4

Voltage map of a sawtooth wave of Stage REM showing a field nearly identical to the vertex sharp wave shown in Figure 3.

identical to vertex sharp waves (Figure 5). Other transient waves in Stage 1B differed from the vertex sharp waves by being slower, having a more prominent positive component, being more parietally located, and being superimposed on slower background activity.

High-amplitude, mainly negative waves were often encountered in Stage 1B (and Stage 2) that had a frontopolar–frontal maximum at times with a steep field posteriorly (Figure 6). These were clearly distinguishable from both ocular artifacts and vertex sharp waves by their shape and topographic criteria. They nearly always occurred in isolation rather than as two or more in succession. Their presence was independent of vertex sharp waves, although, occasionally, they seemed to be loosely coupled to the latter or even to K-complexes.

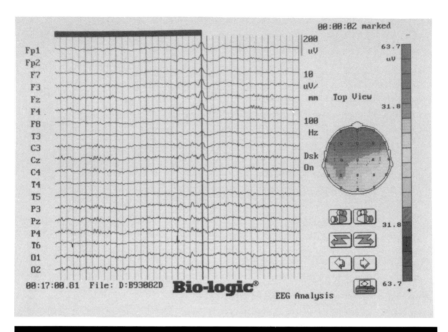

Figure 5

Voltage map showing an isolated frontal delta wave of Stage 1B. The amplitude of the waves in the central and parietal regions is notably lower. As with the vertex waves, the maximum is in the midline (also seen in the spectral color map in Figure 6). The duration of the frontal wave is much longer compared with that of the vertex wave of Figure 3.

Sleep Spindles and K-Complexes

Sigma spindles had a somewhat variable topographic distribution. The maximum amplitude was most often across the central regions, and for very low amplitude spindles (especially the first ones after sleep onset) the field could be restricted to Cz. However, at times, the maximum was parietal or equipotential between the parietal and central sites; on other occasions, the maximum was frontal. Some subjects showed independent spindle maximum in both the cental and parietal regions, usually with a somewhat more rapid frequency anteriorly. Asymmetries were occasionally encountered.

K-complexes most typically consist of the combination of a vertex

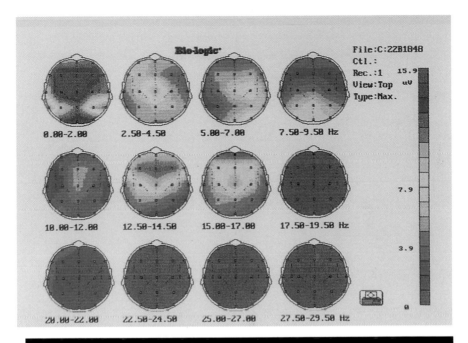

Figure 6

sharp wave, a slow wave lasting up to about 1 s, and a spindle (Roth, Shaw, & Green, 1956). At times, one of the three basic components was missing. In our voltage maps, the vertex sharp wave and spindle components had similar distributions, being maximum in the central regions. Most often, the slow wave was similarly distributed. At other times, however, it had the much more anterior distribution typical of isolated anterior delta waves and appeared to represent incorporation of the latter into the complex.

Limitations of a Single Central EEG Lead

It was instructive to reassess our results obtained with all 19 electrode sites to determine the information that would be lost if only the single central referential EEG lead recommended by the Rechtschaffen & Kales (1968) manual were used. It became obvious that the loss would be considerable. For example, the alpha rhythm was often localized to the occipital or parieto-occipital regions and absent centrally. In such instances, it would be undetected. Vertex sharp waves were frequently more or less exclusively present at midline central electrode Cz and not at parasagittal electrode C3 or C4. This was also sometimes true of sawtooth waves and even, at times, for low-amplitude spindles. Similarly, the anterior isolated negative delta waves could have such a steep field posteriorly that they were little, if at all, present in the central areas.

DISCUSSION

The most striking feature discovered was the high degree of complexity, diversity, and volatility of the EEG patterns from wakefulness through drowsiness to Stage 2 sleep. Alpha activities were particularly variable. It has been generally assumed that the widespread rhythmic activity in the alpha range during Stage 1A is due to anterior diffusion of the parieto-occipital alpha rhythm. Although this can occur, much more frequently the anterior alpha in drowsiness reflected the appearance of activity independent from the alpha rhythm. This conclusion is based on the distinguishing properties of the anterior alpha activities: frequency, topographic distribution, and temporal independence. The only previous distinction between these activities appears in a one-sentence description by Santamaria and Chiappa (1987). We could not confirm their finding of higher amplitude in the central than in the frontal areas.

The use of a single central referential lead makes that distinction impossible. Moreover, a single bipolar parieto-occipital lead (e.g., Hasan et al., 1993; Matousek & Petersen, 1983) can lead to false attribution of the anterior activity to the alpha rhythm, because, at times, it would record the higher amplitude parietal fringe of the anterior alpha activity against a low-amplitude nonalpha occipital EEG. In bipolar anterior–posterior chain derivations (e.g., Matousek & Peterson, 1983), the anterior alpha activities will tend to cancel from common mode, although incompletely because of the asynchronous waxing and waning of the activities.

Three different theta-burst patterns were isolated. The flat "table distribution" of 4–5-Hz activities appears previously undescribed, whereas the frontal maximum 5–7-Hz bursts further define the activity described as "episodic anterior drowsy theta in adults" by Janati, Kidawi, and Nowack (1986).

Quantitative mapping of vertex sharp waves confirmed their typical extremely steep field with a fine peak at Cz and a much lower amplitude or absence at neighboring electrodes, with occasionally more anterior or more posterior midline maxima, confirming Bancaud, Bloch, and Paillard (1953) and Gastaut (1953). Two ancillary findings were made: First, although the biparietal humps described by Gibbs and Gibbs (1950) using a montage lacking midline and central parasagittal electrodes undoubtedly often reflected pickup at their parietal electrodes of vertex sharp waves (Niedermeyer, 1987), we found that other parietal-maximum transients do exist. Their waveform and background activity are different from vertex sharp waves, and they appear more similar than do the vertex waves to the illustrations of Gibbs and Gibbs (1950). Second, the topography of vertex sharp waves was found to be very similar to that of the sawtooth waves of REM sleep (Jouvet, Michel, & Mounier, 1960; Schwartz, 1962).

The isolated anterior delta waves had a field distribution essentially identical to Brazier's (1949) description for some ongoing delta waves of sleep with a frontal maximum. Because of a different field, wave shape, and duration, they apparently represent a different phenomenon than the vertex waves. The findings that these isolated delta waves did not repeat in succession as do those of SWS, and that they sometimes appeared incorporated into K-complexes, may also reflect a different neurophysiological mechanism from the delta activity showing field similarities.

Our quantitative mapping of sleep spindles supports their description as reviewed by Jankel and Niedermeyer (1985). In particular, different frequencies and spatial distributions were documented. Further clarification was obtained concerning the K-complex. Some controversy concerns whether the three constituents (vertex sharp wave, slow wave, spindles) have different fields. We found that the slow wave could either show a central maximum like vertex sharp waves and spindles or be maximum much more anteriorly, the latter seemingly incorporating an isolated anterior delta wave into the complex.

Different fields of similar waveforms require the existence of different underlying neural generators. The anterior alpha activity of drowsiness and the alpha rhythm are fundamentally different and so must arise in different generators. This is supported by source dipole analysis. The anterior slow cycle of drowsiness may reflect anterior cortical–subcortical oscillations involving a deep thalamic center possibly in the area involved in human sleep initiation (Lugaresi et al., 1986).

Correspondingly, the similarity in the wave shapes and field distributions of the vertex sharp waves and the sawtooth waves of REM sleep suggests that they may represent the same phenomenon. Vertex sharp waves are a frequent association of startle responses in drowsiness. Correspondingly, the bursts of phasic activity in REM sleep could represent repetitive startle responses, the motor expression of which is blocked by the atonia of that state (Glenn, 1985).

Some restrictions and limitations exist for the techniques used. Voltage mapping is relatively straightforward, and if allowance is made for the DC offset in various channels from ocular and other causes, the findings can reasonably be taken at face value. On the other hand, FFT is arguably not the best method for quantifying short-lasting events. The approach is based on the assumption that the signals remain stationary. This prerequisite could not always be fulfilled, because the shortest epoch length available in the system of 2 s is longer than that of many events studied. On the other hand, the use of shorter epoch lengths would result in decreased resolution for the slower frequencies. One approach for overcoming the problem of nonstationarity would be to use adaptive segmentation (Bodenstein & Praetorius, 1977; Värri, Hirvonen, Hasan, Loula, & Häkkinen, 1992). For segments below 1 s in duration, approaches other than FFT (e.g., period–amplitude analysis) would appear preferable.

REFERENCES

Bancaud, J., Bloch, V., & Paillard, J. (1953). Contribution EEG à l'étude des potentiels évoqués chez l'homme au niveau du vertex [EEG contribution to the study of evoked potentials in man at the vertex level]. *Revue Neurologique, 89,* 399–418.

Bodenstein, G., & Praetorius, H. M. (1977). Feature extraction from the electroencephalogram by adaptive segmentation. *Proceedings IEEE, 65,* 642–652.

Brazier, M. A. B. (1949). The electrical fields at the surface of the head during sleep. *Electroencephalography and Clinical Neurophysiology, 1,* 195–204.

Gastaut, H. (1953). Les pointes négatives évoqueés sur le vertex: Leur signification psychophysiologiques et pathologique [Negative points evoked on the vertex: Their psychophysiological and pathological meaning]. *Revue Neurologique, 89,* 382–389.

Gibbs, F. A., & Gibbs, E. (1950). *Atlas of electroencephalography: Vol. 1. Methods and controls.* Reading, MA: Addison-Wesley.

Glenn, L. L. (1985). Brainstem and spinal control of lower limb motoneurons with special reference to phasic events and startle reflexes. In J. McGinty, R. Drucker-Colin, A. Morrison, & P. L. Parmeggiani (Eds.), *Basic mechanisms of sleep* (pp. 81–95).

Häkkinen, V. (1972). *EEG vigilance measurement and lucidness discrimination in humans during drowsy states.* Unpublished doctoral dissertation, Institute of Physiology, University of Helsinki, Finland.

Hasan, J., Hirvonen, K., Värri, A., Häkkinen, V., & Loula, P. (1993). Validation of computer analysed polygraphic patterns during drowsiness and sleep onset. *Encephalography and Clinical Neurophysiology, 87,* 117–127.

Hori, T. (1985). Spatiotemporal changes of EEG activity during waking–sleeping transition period. *International Journal of Neuroscience, 27,* 101–114.

International Federation of Societies for Electroencephalography and Clinical Neurophysiology. (1974). A glossary of terms commonly used by clinical electroencephalographers. *Electroencephalography and Clinical Neurophysiology, 376,* 538–548.

Janati, A., Kidawi, S., & Nowack, W. J. (1986). Episodic anterior drowsy theta in adults. *Clinical Electroencephalography, 17,* 135–138.

Jankel, W. R., & Niedermeyer, E. (1985). Sleep spindles. *Journal of Clinical Neurophysiology, 37,* 538–548.

Jouvet, M., Michel, F., & Mounier, D. (1960). Analyse électroencéphalographique comparée du sommeil physiologique chez le chat et chez l'homme [Comparative electroencephalographic analysis of physiological sleep in the cat and in man]. *Revue Neurologique, 103,* 189–204.

Loomis, A. L., Harvey, E. N., & Hobart, G. A. (1937). Cerebral states during sleep, as studied by human brain potentials. *Journal of Experimental Psychology, 21,* 127–144.

Lugaresi, E., Medori, R., Montagna, O., Baruzzi, A., Cortelli, P., Lugaresi, A., Tinuper, P., Zucconi, M., & Gambetti, P. (1986). Fatal familial insomnia. *New England Journal of Medicine, 315,* 997–1003.

Matousek, M., & Petersen, I. (1983). A method for assessing alertness fluctuations from the EEG spectra. *Electroencephalography and Clinical Neurophysiology, 55,* 108–113.

Niedermeyer, E. (1987). Sleep and EEG. In E. Niedermeyer & F. Lopes da Silva (Eds.), *Electroencephalography: Basic principles, clinical applications and related fields* (pp. 119–132). Baltimore and Munich: Urban & Schwarzenberg.

Ogilvie, R. D., & Simons, I. (1992). Falling asleep and waking up: A comparison of EEG spectra. In R. J. Broughton & R. D. Ogilvie (Eds.), *Sleep, arousal and performance* (pp. 73–87). Boston: Birkhauser.

Rechtschaffen, A., & Kales, A. (1968). *A manual of standardized terminology, technique and scoring for sleep stages of human subjects.* Los Angeles: Brain Information Service/Brain Research Institute.

Roth, M., Shaw, J., & Green, J. (1956). The form, voltage, distribution and physiological significance of the K complex. *Electroencephalography and Clinical Neurophysiology, 8,* 385–402.

Santamaria, J., & Chiappa, K. H. (1987). *The EEG of drowsiness.* New York: Demos Publications.

Scherg, M., & Picton, T. W. (1991). Separation and identification of event-related potential components by brain electric sources analysis. In C. M. H. Brunia, G. Mulder, & M. N. Verbaten (Eds.), *Event-related potentials of the brain* (pp. 24–37). Amsterdam: Elsevier.

Schwartz, B. (1962). EEG et mouvements oculaires dans le sommeil de nuit [EEG and eye movements in night sleep]. *Electroencephalography and Clinical Neurophysiology, 14*, 126–128.

Valley, V., & Broughton, R. (1983). The physiological (EEG) nature of drowsiness and its relation to performance deficits in narcoleptics. *Electroencephalography and Clinical Neurophysiology, 55*, 243–251.

Värri, A., Hirvonen, K., Hasan, J., Loula, P., & Häkkinen, V. (1992). A computerized analysis system for vigilance studies. *Computer Methods and Progress in Biomedicine, 39*, 113–124.

14

Topographical EEG Changes and the Hypnagogic Experience

Tadao Hori, Mitsuo Hayashi, and Toshio Morikawa

The hypnagogic period is one of the most interesting states for psychologists to study because of (a) the occurrence of dreamlike mentation, (b) the poor agreement between standard electroencephalogram (EEG) stages of sleep and the subjective experience of being asleep, and (c) the discrepancies between the EEG stages of sleep and behavioral responses.

Foulkes and Vogel (1965) observed that dreamlike reports occurred even during a presleep awake period with an EEG alpha rhythm. Their observations suggested that the onset of the hypnagogic period might precede Stage 1 onset (as identified by a modified version of the Dement–Kleitman [1957] criteria). Stage 2 sleep, scored by standard criteria (Rechtschaffen & Kales, 1968), is often used as the objective marker of "true" sleep. Yet, even in this stage, considerable discrepancies appear between subjective reports and polygraphic recordings (Foulkes & Vogel, 1965; Kamiya, 1961; Sewitch, 1984) and between the behavioral responses and the EEG stages of sleep (Ogilvie & Wilkinson, 1984, 1988). The former set of studies suggests that the hypnagogic effects on the subjective process probably continue after Stage 2 onset, so that subjective sleep onset may be delayed beyond Stage 2 onset. On the other hand, the latter set of studies suggests that the behavioral sleep process may start in the period of sleep Stage 1. These observations suggest that the hypnagogic state is a neurophysiologically and psychophysiologically complex and even paradoxical state, and that the standard sleep stage criteria, especially for Stage 1, are too vague to define when the convergence of behavioral, subjective, and polygraphical measures in the hypnagogic state is of interest.

We studied the topographic map of 12-channel EEGs during the wake–sleep transition period (Hori, Hayashi, & Morikawa, 1990). Seven characteristic patterns were distinguished in the topographies from the sampled period. These patterns were similar to those described by Shiotsuki, Ichino, and Shimizu (1954), which was a revision of the Gibbs and Gibbs atlas (1950). The Shiotsuki criteria were modified for short epoch scoring (5 s for point S/W [sleep–wake] stage judgments; Ogilvie, Wilkinson, & Allison, 1989). We then assessed the point of convergence between behavioral (reaction time [RT], Hori, Hayashi, & Kato, 1991) and subjective (hypnagogic imagery [HI], Hori, Hayashi, & Hibino, 1992) measures on the nine EEG stages of the hypnagogic period. It was found that the relationships between these measures and EEG stages were a linear function for the former (RT) and a nonlinear function for the latter (HI, Hori et al., 1991, 1992).

We also studied a laterality index (LI) and an anterior/posterior (A/P) ratio as topographical parameters of EEG measurement. Significant relationships were observed between the EEG topographical measures and the behavioral–subjective measures.

METHOD

Subjects

Fifty-seven right-handed, unpaid volunteer subjects (27 male, 30 female), about 21 to 26 years of age ($M = 22.5$, $SD = 1.24$), participated in the study. Seven were graduate students taking a course in human behavior at Hiroshima University (Japan). The subjects had previously been adapted to the recording chamber.

The subjects were screened at three phases of the experiment. At the first, 12 subjects were excluded from further analysis because of an insufficient number of total trials in one or more of the EEG stages (criterion: more than 10 trials for each EEG stage); at the second, 15 subjects were excluded because their recall rate of HI did not reach criterion (more than 20% in total trials); and at the third, 5 subjects were excluded because they did not reach criteria for artifact-free EEG data (more than 7 of 10 epochs per EEG stage). Thus, only the data of 26 subjects (14 male, 12 female), 21 to 24 years of age ($M = 22.2$, $SD = 0.86$), were used in further analysis.

Apparatus

An 18-channel NEC San-Ei Model lA97 electroencephalograph was used for the continuous polysomnograms. Surface electrodes were placed on 12 scalp areas (Fp$_1$, Fp$_2$, F$_7$, F$_8$, Fz, C$_3$, C$_4$, Pz, O$_1$, O$_2$, T$_5$, T$_6$), referenced to the ipsilateral earlobes (EEG), on the right and left outer canthi (electrooculogram [EOG]), each referenced to ipsilateral mastoids for slow eye movement ($\tau = 3.2$ s), on the chin (mentalis: electromyogram [EMG]), referenced to each other, and on the forehead for the body ground. In addition, respiration movements were monitored by two sets of pneumographs (carbon strain gage) for thoracic and abdominal movements. Stimulus onset and the subject's responses were also recorded. The electroencephalograph ran at a paper speed of 10 mm/s. The EEG data and stimulus-response marker were simultaneously recorded by FM tape recorder (TEAC, SR-50).

A NEC computer (PC-9801VX2) was programmed to generate and present 1000-Hz tones to the subject and to record and file the reaction times (RTs). Each tone (50 dB) was delivered through a speaker located 1.5 m above the subject's pillow for a maximum of 5 s. The off switch was relocated in a grip apparatus (14 mm × 72 mm) that the volunteer could hold comfortably in the dominant hand. A weight of 130 g was required to activate the switch. The intertone interval varied pseudo-randomly between 30 s and 2 min.

The sleeper's room was 3 m × 3 m (electrically shielded and sound attenuated). After the room light was off, the subject's behavior was monitored by an infrared TV system. The verbal responses by subjects were recorded on videotape as well as on audio cassette tape.

Procedure

Each subject was studied for two nonconsecutive nights. The interval between two experimental nights was one to two weeks. The sampling protocol for all subjects consisted of five trials on each of nine EEG stages for each experimental night. Thus, 90 samples in total were obtained for each subject. A trial was defined as a tone presentation in response to which the subjects had been instructed to press the microswitch and verbally identify their perceived behavioral state just before hearing the tone by stating whether they had been awake or asleep. When subjects failed to respond within 5 s, an experimenter awakened them by calling their name and requesting that they state their behavioral state just before the awakening. At each awakening, the subjects were also requested to state what was going through their mind just before the awakening.

The categories of hypnagogic experiences used to assess the hypnagogic mentation were those referred to by Foulkes and Vogel (1965): (a) usual thinking, (b) unusual thinking, (c) visual imagery, (d) auditory imagery, (e) bodily imagery, (f) olfactory imagery, (g) miscellaneous, (h) no experience, (i) very feeble or forgotten.

The nine EEG stages were defined as follows (see Figure 1):

Stage 1. Alpha wave train: Epoch composed of a train of alpha activity with a minimum amplitude of 20 μV.
Stage 2. Alpha wave intermittent (A): Epoch composed of a train of more than 50% of alpha activity with a minimum amplitude of 20 μV.
Stage 3. Alpha wave intermittent (B): Epoch contained less than 50% of alpha activity with an amplitude of 20 μV.
Stage 4. EEG flattening: Epoch composed of suppressed waves less than 20 μV.

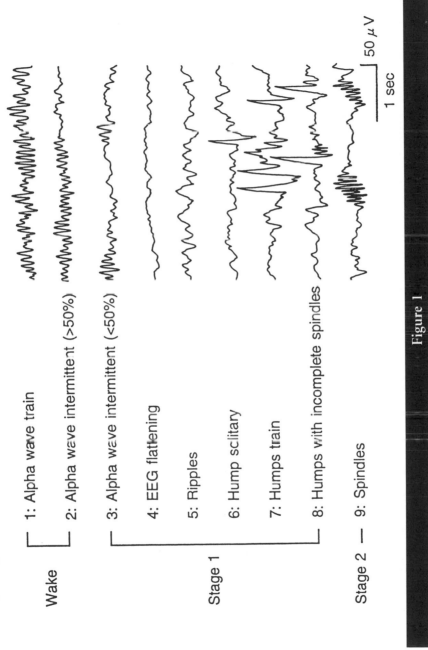

Sleep Stages   EEG Stages

Wake   1: Alpha wave train

2: Alpha wave intermittent (>50%)

3: Alpha wave intermittent (<50%)

4: EEG flattening

Stage 1   5: Ripples

6: Hump solitary

7: Humps train

8: Humps with incomplete spindles

Stage 2 — 9: Spindles

1 sec

50 μV

Figure 1

EEG recordings illustrating nine EEG stages and correspondence to standard sleep stages.

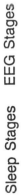

Stage 5. Ripples: Epoch composed of low-voltage theta wave (20 μV $< 0 < 50$ μV) burst suppression.

Stage 6. Vertex sharp wave solitary: Epoch contained one well-defined vertex sharp wave.

Stage 7. Vertex sharp wave train or bursts: Epoch contained at least two well-defined vertex sharp waves.

Stage 8. Vertex sharp wave and incomplete spindles: Epoch contained at least one well-defined vertex sharp wave and one incomplete spindle: duration < 0.5 s, amplitude < 20 μV, > 10 μV).

Stage 9. Spindles: Epoch contained at least one well-defined spindle at least 0.5 s in duration and 20 μV in amplitude.

Stages 1 and 2 correspond to Stage W in standard criteria (Rechtschaffen & Kales, 1968), Stages 3 to 8 correspond to standard Stage 1, and Stage 9 corresponds to standard Stage 2.

The scoring epoch was 5 s in duration. Each record (C_3 or C_4) was scored entirely by one scorer during the experiment. After the experiment, two scorers rescored the EEG records and corrected the initial judgments.

EEG Analysis

The tape-recorded EEG signals obtained for 5 s prior to the onset of each tone stimulus were played back into a NEC San-Ei, Model 7T18A signal processor, with a sampling rate of 200/s. For a 5-s epoch, artifact-free 2.5-s segments were submitted to a fast Fourier transform in conjunction with a Hanning window. Averaging over the two segments yielded a magnitude spectrum in microvolts from 1 to 20 Hz. Artifacts were screened by visual inspection, and rejection decisions were made blindly with regard to subject and EEG stage. Average magnitude in the alpha (7.6–13.2 Hz) band was computed for 12 EEG channels.

Next, the left hemispheric power (LHP $= Fp_1 + F_7 + C_3 + O_1 + T_5$) and the right hemispheric power (RHP $= Fp_2 + F_8 + C_4 + O_2 + T_6$) were computed. Then, the EEG laterality index (LI) was computed by using the formula $[(LHP - RHP)/(LHP + RHP)] \times 100$. For the anterior–posterior EEG ratio, the anterior power (AP: $Fp_1 + Fp_2 + Fz + F_7 + F_8$) and the posterior power (PP: $Pz + O_1 + O_2 + T_5 + T_6$) were computed, and an A/P ratio was obtained by using the formula AP/PP.

Statistical Analysis

For each analysis of variance (ANOVA), significance levels were determined following the conservative Greenhouse–Geisser approach for repeated observations (see Winer, Brown, & Michels, 1991). Only significant results are presented.

Because the incidence of HI was not enough to test the relationships between EEG samples with and without HI for the nine EEG stages, the data were pooled for adjoining stages. The pooled data sets were Stage I (alpha dominant: Stages 1 + 2), Stage II (alpha suppression: Stages 3 + 4), Stage III (ripples: Stage 5), Stage IV (vertex sharp wave: Stages 6 + 7 + 8), and stage V (spindles: Stage 9).

RESULTS

Gross Analysis of Data Set

A total of 1,996 artifact-free data sets (data collection rate: 85.3%) and 751 hallucinatory reports (HI recall rate: 37.6%) were obtained from 2,340 trials of 26 subjects.

Analysis of the Awake–Asleep Dimension

Reaction Time in the Nine EEG Stages

The left column of Table 1 shows the means of RT across 26 subjects as a function of EEG stage. The RT in Stage 9 is 2.7 times as long as the RT in Stage 1. A significant stage effect was obtained $F(1,25) = 11.59$, $p < .01$. Post hoc testing (Tukey-b test: Winer et al., 1991) further indicated that the RT of the nine EEG stages could be divided into four subgroups (i.e., [Stage 1, 2, 3, 4] < [Stage 5, 6, 7] < [Stage

Table 1

Means of Reaction Time (RT) to the Tone Stimulus and Anterior–Posterior EEG Ratio (A/P) in Alpha Band Across All Subjects ($N = 26$) for Nine EEG Stages

Stage	RT ± *SE*	A/P ± *SE*
1	711.1 ± 45.3	0.464 ± 0.044
2	842.9 ± 49.5	0.527 ± 0.045
3	960.7 ± 54.7	0.579 ± 0.046
4	996.0 ± 48.2	0.703 ± 0.052
5	1121.8 ± 56.9	0.714 ± 0.057
6	1237.8 ± 61.3	0.734 ± 0.055
7	1386.6 ± 91.0	0.757 ± 0.056
8	1579.8 ± 106.2	0.789 ± 0.060
9	1936.9 ± 135.3	0.839 ± 0.063

NOTE: *SE*: Standard error (SD/$\sqrt{N}$).

8] < [Stage 9]). These groups almost corresponded to (a) the disappearance of alpha activity, (b) the theta and vertex sharp wave mixture, and (c) the vertex sharp wave and incomplete spindles mixture and the appearance of well-defined sleep spindles.

Subjective Assessment of Behavioral State

Table 2 shows the mean percentages of three subjective assessments (SAs) (i.e., "awake," "asleep," and no response [including "forget" and "very feeble"]) for EEG stages. Because the distribution of those responses was skewed, the proportions (p) were transformed using the transformation $z = \arcsin \sqrt{p}$ (Winer et al., 1991), averaged across subjects and converted back to proportions. The proportion of "awake" responses decreased in association with the progress of EEG stages. The response rate was highest in Stage 1 and lowest in Stage 9. From Stage 6 (appearance of vertex sharp waves), the percentages of "awake" response decreased to less than 50%. Although the Stage 8 EEG included partial spindle components, the "awake" response in this stage was

Table 2

Mean Percentages of Three Subjective Assessments (SAs) for Nine EEG Stages

Stage	W%	S%	N%	Total
1	82.5	7.2	10.3	100.0
2	82.2	7.6	10.2	100.0
3	77.1	8.1	14.8	100.0
4	64.5	19.7	15.8	100.0
5	51.2	24.0	24.8	100.0
6	50.0	28.3	21.7	100.0
7	45.5	28.6	25.9	100.0
8	41.8	31.3	26.9	100.0
9	26.2	43.7	30.1	100.0

NOTE: W%: awake response %; S%: asleep response %; N%: no response %, including "forget" and "very feeble."

41.8%, which was almost twice as much as in Stage 9. Contrary to the "awake" judgments, "asleep" responses increased from Stage 1 to Stage 9. It should be noted that the "asleep" judgments did not exceed 50% in spite of the judgments being made within 5 s of the appearance of well-defined spindles. Similarly to the "asleep" response, the percentages of "no response" also increased from Stage 1 to Stage 9. The ANOVA (EEG stages × SA categories) yielded a main effect for EEG stages ($F[1, 25] = 5.21$, $p < .05$), for SA categories ($F[1, 25] = 4.83$, $p < .05$), and the interaction between EEG stages and SA categories ($F[1, 25] = 4.56$, $p < .05$). The results of post hoc testing revealed four subgroups among the nine EEG stages (i.e., [Stages 1, 2, 3], [Stage 4], [Stages 5, 6, 7, 8], [Stage 9]). These groups each corresponded to a characteristic EEG pattern, that is, (a) alpha waves, (b) EEG suppression, (c) theta wave and vertex sharp wave mixture, and (d) spindle bursts. These findings demonstrate that there is a clear relationship between S/W judgments and the nine sleep-onset EEG stages.

Anterior–posterior EEG Ratio

The right column of Table 1 shows the average A/P ratios in alpha band for the nine EEG stages. The A/P ratios increased from Stage 1 to Stage 9 as a function of EEG stage. The ratio in Stage 9 was twice the Stage 1 ratio. The ANOVA indicated a main effect for the EEG stages ($F[1, 25] = 9.95$, $p < .01$). Post hoc testing revealed two sub-groups of EEG stages (i.e., [Stages 1, 2, 3], [Stages 4, 5, 6, 7, 8, 9]). The main changes of the A/P ratio appeared between Stages 3 and 4. These results show that the A/P ratio is a simple way of detecting changes at early phases of the sleep-onset period.

Analysis of Hypnagogic Imagery (HI)

Recall Rate in the Nine EEG Stages

The average recall rates of HI for the nine EEG stages are shown in the second column of Table 3. The distribution of recall rate shows an inverted V shape with a peak at Stage 5. The ANOVA indicated a significant effect of the EEG stages ($F[1, 25] = 5.14$, $p < .05$). The results of post hoc testing revealed three subgroups (i.e., [Stages 1, 2] < [Stages 3, 4, 6, 7, 8, 9] < [Stage 5], whereas the difference between Stages 5 and 6 was not significant). The average distribution of HI for each sensory modality across EEG stages is shown in the right columns of Table 3. As Foulkes and Vogel (1965) showed in their early study, our present data also clearly reveal that HI are primarily visual in character. The visual imagery increased gradually from Stage 1 to Stage 6 and remained high in the other stages. Percentages of auditory and bodily imagery were less than 15% and showed a steady decline from Stage 1 to Stage 6. The ANOVA (EEG stages × imagery modalities) indicates a main effect for EEG stages ($F[1, 25] = 5.41$, $p < .05$) and for imagery modality ($F[1, 25] = 8.18$, $p < .01$), but not for an (EEG stages × imagery modality) interaction. Post hoc testing revealed the two sub-groups of the visual imagery ([Stages 1, 2, 3, 4] < [Stages 5, 6, 7, 8, 9]), but not for the other two modalities of imagery. Because the dis-

246

Table 3

Average Recall Rate of Hypnagogic Imagery (HI%) and Average Distribution of HI for Each Sensory Modality Across EEG Stages

EEG Stage	HI%	Sensory modalities of HI				Total
		VIS	AUD	BOD	MS	
1	23.3 (1.1)[a]	73.6	12.5	12.7	1.2	100.0
2	25.8 (1.3)	75.3	14.5	8.3	1.9	100.0
3	33.5 (1.4)	77.2	14.5	7.3	1.0	100.0
4	37.7 (1.5)	82.4	12.6	5.0	0.0	100.0
5	45.7 (2.3)	91.4	5.0	3.6	0.0	100.0
6	39.8 (1.9)	95.2	2.4	2.4	0.0	100.0
7	38.7 (1.8)	93.1	3.1	3.0	0.8	100.0
8	34.6 (1.7)	90.5	2.1	7.4	0.0	100.0
9	31.9 (1.5)	91.0	1.4	7.6	0.0	100.0
Mean	34.6	85.5	7.6	6.4	0.5	100.0
SE	2.2	2.6	1.8	1.0	0.2	

NOTE: VIS: visual imagery; AUD: auditory imagery; BOD: bodily imagery; MS: miscellaneous.
[a]Figures in parentheses are standard errors (SEs).

tributions of both auditory and bodily imageries were skewed, a nonparametric ANOVA was conducted for these two data sets separately. The Friedman statistic (FS) was significant for auditory imagery (FS = 21.23, $df = 8$, $p < .01$), but not for bodily imagery.

Relationship Between EEG Laterality and HI Recall Rate

To compare EEG laterality indexes (LIs) with and without recall of HI, EEG samples were pooled for five EEG stages (see "Method" section). Table 4 shows the comparisons of the LIs between the EEG samples with and without recall of HI for the five EEG stages.

The ANOVA (EEG stages × LIs) indicated a significant difference between LIs with and without HI ($F[1, 25] = 11.56$, $p < .01$). Post

Table 4

Comparisons of Average Rate of Hypnagogic Imagery (HI%) and EEG Laterality Indexes With (LI–H) and Without (LI–N) Recall of HI for Five EEG Stages

Stage	HI%	LI–H	LI–N	H versus N
I	24.6 (1.3)[a]	−0.45 (1.01)	0.60 (1.00)	ns
II	35.6 (1.0)	−0.63 (1.18)	−0.39 (1.06)	ns
III	45.7 (1.0)	−3.19 (1.27)	−0.32 (0.77)	$p < .10$
IV	37.7 (0.9)	−2.85 (1.11)	1.11 (1.03)	$p < .05$
V	31.9 (0.8)	−1.64 (1.39)	3.54 (1.23)	$p < .05$

NOTE: H versus N: t-tests between LI–H and LI–N conditions.
[a]Figures in parentheses are standard errors (SEs).

hoc testing revealed that the LIs with HI recall (LI–H) were lower than those without HI recall (LI–N, see Table 4). A significant effect for EEG stage was also observed ($F[1, 25] = 6.24$, $p < .05$). The post hoc testing revealed that the LI–Hs in Stages III, IV, and V (in 5 EEG stages) were significantly lower than those in Stages I and II, whereas the LI–Ns were higher than those in other stages. The means of HI recall rate are shown in the second column of Table 4 for comparison of LIs among the five EEG stages. A significant relationship between HI rates and LIs was observed only in the condition with HI recall ($r = -0.816$, $p < .05$), whereas the condition without HI recall was not significant ($r = -0.370$, NS).

DISCUSSION AND CONCLUSION

Awake–Asleep Dimension and Sleep-Onset Period

This study demonstrated that parameters related to the awake–asleep dimension (RT, SA, and A/P ratio) changed as a function of the nine EEG stages. Discriminated subgroups of EEG stages for each parameter were not exactly coincident with each other. The statistically unstable stages were Stage 4 (EEG flattening) and Stage 8 (vertex sharp waves and incomplete spindles mixture). These two stages were equivalent to the early and the late portions of standard sleep Stage 1 (Rechtschaffen & Kales, 1968). Ogilvie and Wilkinson (1984) introduced the concept of a sleep-onset period (SOP), defined as the transition between relaxed, drowsy wakefulness and unresponsive sleep. So although the SOP may have standard Stage 1 at its center, it clearly overlaps into Stage W and Stage 2, scored by standard criteria (Ogilvie & Wilkinson, 1988). Our present data agree with their concept of a SOP. Behavioral and neurophysiological arousal was lower in the early portion of standard Stage 1 than in wakefulness and was significantly lower again in standard Stage 2 than when measured during late Stage 1.

The A/P ratio in this study clearly changed between Stage 3 (alpha intermittent, <50%) and Stage 4 (EEG flattening). These results suggest that the ratio is sensitive enough to detect the start of a SOP, and that it could be used as an objective indicator to gage the approach of "true" sleep onset without interrupting the natural hypnagogic process.

Sleep spindles or standard Stage 2 (our Stage 9) have long been used as the objective marker of true sleep. Webb (1980) reported that the proportion of "asleep" responses in Stage 2 was 66.7% on the first night and 85.0% on the second night. On the other hand, Kamiya (1961) obtained only 25.5% of "asleep" judgments out of early Stage 2 (first sleep spindle). Although Foulkes and Vogel (1965) did not report exact percentages of "asleep" responses, all of their subjects ranked themselves as having been awake even in Stage 2. Clearly, there are considerable discrepancies among reports of the proportion of "asleep" responses in Stage 2.

In this study, the proportion of "asleep" responses was 43.7% in standard Stage 2. The present results are very similar to the findings of Sewitch (1984), who obtained 45% "asleep" responses in standard Stage 2. The "awake" response rates were, however, dissimilar: 55% in the Sewitch study and 26.2% in our study. Although methodological differences must be considered, the appearance of sleep spindles probably neither so sharply enhances the "asleep" response nor leads to an extreme underestimation of SA, as reported in early studies. The present data demonstrate a gradual increase in no-responses, to 30.1 % in Stage 9 (standard Stage 2). When no-responses could be regarded as "not awake" responses and were included in the "asleep" category, the total "asleep" index became 73.8%. This percentage is similar to the findings of Webb (1980). It may be, however, that "no responses" and lengthened RT are a reflection of a subject's conflict or opposition in the organization of SA. Beginning in Stage 6 (vertex sharp waves), the "awake" percentages dropped below 50%. The hypnagogic inhibitory effect exerted on cognitive function and judgments after Stage 6 would produce vagueness. In this context, the appearance of the well-defined spindles might be necessary for a remarkable diminution of the "awake" response. In any case, one could expect increased perception of having slept in Stage 2 in normal young adults.

Hypnagogic Imagery (HI) and EEG Laterality

Foulkes and Vogel (1965) reported that the incidence of dramatic hallucinatory episodes occurred most frequently during Stages 1 and 2; alpha REM: 31%; alpha SEM: 43%; Stage 1: 76%; and Stage 2: 71%. Although the recall rates in their study were higher than in the present study, the results of our study fundamentally confirmed these tendencies. Furthermore, the present study demonstrates that the distribution of HI percentages shows an inverted V shape with a peak at Stage 5 (theta-wave burst suppression). From Stages 3 to 9 (standard Stages 1 and 2), HI recall rate is significantly higher than from Stages 1 and 2 (standard Stage W). These findings are quite important. They clearly demonstrate that the SOP overlaps with standard Stage 1 and is centered at Stage 5. It might be thought that the intrusions of daydreams (Kripke & Sonnenschein, 1978) into standard Stage W (our Stages 1 and 2), and of NREM dreams (Foulkes & Schmidt, 1983) into standard Stage 2 (our Stage 9), occur on both the ends of standard Stage 1. The fantastic production during Stage 1, however, could be considered as the characteristic HI.

In this study, the alpha band LI, which derived from the EEG samples without HI, increased positively (left hemisphere dominance) with the progression of EEG stages (Table 4). However, the LIs derived from EEG samples with HI did not show a positive shift; rather, they shifted toward negative after Stage III (theta-wave burst suppression) up to spindle stage (Stage V). As a result, the discrepancy of LIs between with and without HI conditions grew larger after Stage III.

Alpha band activity rapidly decreases just before the onset of standard Stage 1 and, then, subsequently increases in spite of the fact that apparent alpha waves disappear completely (Hori, 1985). The negativity of the LI means that the alpha band power of the right hemisphere was larger than that of the left hemisphere. It is well known that the alpha band activity has dual meanings. When the alpha band power increases during the low arousal state, the increase means neurophysiological arousal. On the contrary, when the alpha band power increases during the higher arousal state, the increase signals dearousal. Therefore, the increase in alpha band activity during the theta-wave burst-suppression state (Stage 5, or III) or vertex sharp wave state (Stages 6 to 8, or IV) could be interpreted as neurophysiological arousal. The negative shift of LI during SOP reflects the arousal of right hemisphere function. In this context, HI would be produced in those states in which the right hemisphere function is relatively aroused.

In conclusion, evidence has been presented that supports the contention that the SOP is a unique period that cannot be accurately categorized as either wake or sleep. Moreover, the SOP has unique behavioral, electrophysiological, and subjective characteristics. Further topographical analysis of the EEG might supply useful information to distinguish the SOP from both wake and sleep and to understand the psychophysiological structure of the SOP and its function.

REFERENCES

Dement, W. C., & Kleitman, N. (1957). Cyclic variations in EEG during sleep and their relation to eye movements. *Electroencephalography & Clinical Neurophysiology, 9,* 673–690.

Foulkes, D., & Schmidt, M. (1983). Temporal sequence and unit composition in dream reports from different stages of sleep. *Sleep, 6,* 265–280.

Foulkes, D., & Vogel, G. (1965). Mental activity at sleep onset. *Journal of Abnormal Psychology, 70,* 231–243.

Gibbs, F. A., & Gibbs, E. L. (1950). *Atlas of electroencephalography* (Vol. 1). Reading, MA: Addison-Wesley.

Hori, T. (1985). Spatiotemporal changes of EEG activity during waking–sleeping transition period. *International Journal of Neuroscience, 27,* 101–114.

Hori, T., Hayashi, M., & Hibino, K. (1992). An EEG study of the hypnagogic hallucinatory experience. *International Journal of Psychology, 27,* 420.

Hori, T., Hayashi, M., & Kato, K. (1991). Changes of EEG patterns and reaction time during hypnagogic state. *Sleep Research, 20,* 20.

Hori, T., Hayashi, M., & Morikawa, T. (1990). Topography and coherence analysis of hypnagogic EEG. In J. Horne (Ed.), *Sleep '90* (pp. 10–12). Bochum, Germany: Pontenagel Press.

Kamiya, J. (1961). Behavioral, subjective and physiological aspects of drowsiness and sleep. In D. W. Fiske & S. R. Maddi (Eds.), *Functions of varied experience* (pp. 145–175). Homewood, IL: Dorsey Press.

Kripke, D. F., & Sonnenschein, D. (1978). A biological rhythm in waking fantasy. In S. P. Kenneth & L. S. Jerome (Eds.), *The stream of consciousness* (pp. 321–332). New York: Plenum.

Ogilvie, R. D., & Wilkinson, R. T. (1984). The detection of sleep onset: Behavioral and physiological convergence. *Psychophysiology, 21,* 510–520.

Ogilvie, R. D., & Wilkinson, R. T. (1988). Behavioral versus EEG-based monitoring of all-night sleep/wake patterns. *Sleep, 11,* 139–155.

Ogilvie, R. D., Wilkinson, R. T., & Allison, S. (1989). The detection of sleep onset: Behavioral, physiological, and subjective convergence. *Sleep, 12,* 458–474.

Rechtschaffen, A., & Kales, A. (Eds.), (1968). *A manual of standard terminology, techniques and scoring system for sleep stages of human subjects.* Los Angeles: UCLA Brain Research Institute.

Sewitch, D. E. (1984). The perceptual uncertainty of having slept: The inability to discriminate electroencephalographic sleep from wakefulness. *Psychophysiology, 21,* 243–259.

Shiotsuki, M., Ichino, Y., & Shimizu, K. (1954). Changes in the electroencephalogram during whole night natural sleep. *Journal of the Surgical Society of Japan, 55,* 322–331.

Webb, W. B. (1980). The natural onset of sleep. In L. Popoviciu, B. Aşgian, & G. Badia (Eds.), *Sleep 1978. Fourth European Congress on Sleep Research* (pp. 19–23). Tîrgu-Mureş, Rumania, & Basel, Switzerland: S. Kager.

Winer, B. J., Brown, D. R., & Michels, K. M. (1991). *Statistical principles in experimental design* (3rd ed.). New York: McGraw-Hill.

15

Sleep EEG Characteristics After a Spontaneous Awakening

Teresa Paiva and Agostinho Rosa

The definition of sleep onset is a complex issue. It has been difficult to determine the variables involved in the sleep-onset process, to access validly the behaviors heralding the transitions from awake to asleep, and to evaluate the exact borders between awake and asleep. The electroencephalogram (EEG), the electromyogram (EMG), and the electrooculogram (EOG) present typical changes; however, they are not always coincident in time and exhibit different relations with the subjective evaluation of falling asleep (Carskadon & Dement, 1989). The sleep latency of the major sleep episode (i.e., the time of sleep onset) is a landmark of normal and pathological sleep: It may be increased, as happens in insomnia; it may be abnormally reduced, as occurs in sleep apnea; or it may occur in an abnormal fashion, as is the case in narcolepsy. There are, however, other transitions from awake to asleep

This project was supported in part by the Junta Nacional de Investigação Científica—JNICT Projects No. 87423/MIC and PMCT/C/SAU/764/90.

We thank Prof. Filipe Arriaga for selecting the patients, Eng. Rogério Largo for his help in transition analysis, and Prof. Nunes Leitão for his comments and criticisms. Mrs. Antonia Seixas typed the manuscript.

because sleep is usually reestablished after spontaneous awakenings that supervene during the major sleep episode.

The interrelations between awake and other sleep stages have been studied in normal subjects, especially in Stage 4 non-REM (NREM; Merica, Blois, & Gaillard, 1990) sleep. These authors showed that cycles interrupted by excessive amounts of wakefulness have a reduction of slow wave sleep (SWS). The characteristics of the transitions, including awake in normal subjects, have also been studied, both by means of transition probabilities (Merica & Gaillard, 1985) and by the use of transition rates (Kemp, 1987; Kemp & Kamphuisen, 1986). The relation of awake to other sleep stages, when described in terms of stage transitions especially with regard to evolution across the sleep night, must be significantly changed in patients complaining of insomnia. It is well recognized that pathological sleep often includes excessive amounts of awake, which strongly affect subjective sleep evaluation. Such features are particularly relevant in psychiatric patients with insomnia.

Sleep disruption may also be related to transient events such as microarousals. *Microarousals* are defined as short-lasting events (no longer than 3 s) occurring in stable sleep; however, their exact meaning has not been fully clarified (American Sleep Disorders Association, 1992). Some authors hold that normal sleepers have recurrent periods of spontaneous arousals, *phases d'activation transitoire* (Muzet, Schieberg, Ehrhart, & Lienhard, 1973); others have suggested that microarousals constitute a landmark of normal sleep, because they are reduced in pathological cases (Paiva, Arriaga, Rosa, & Leitão, 1993); and some others describe paroxysmal arousals with periodic occurrence (Montagna, Sforza, Tinuper, Cirignotta, & Lugaresi, 1990). Such transient arousals of short duration must be distinguished from awakenings of longer duration; indeed, nocturnal awakenings have different behavioral consequences because they are more easily remembered and have stronger consequences for subjective sleep quality (Beersma, van den Hoofdakker, & Dijk, 1987).

The rules of sleep reinitiation deserve particular attention because it is important to know whether there is an organized fashion of re-falling asleep. Knowledge about the phenomena preceding an awakening might conceal information about its characteristics and disclose possible forerunners. Furthermore, the sleep difficulties of some pathological entities, namely of those presenting a sleep maintenance insomnia, might be explained in terms of abnormalities of the awakening-related events. Given this, we decided to investigate spontaneous awakenings in normal subjects and in dysthymic patients. Dysthymic patients were chosen because their sleep disturbance is characterized by an increased percentage of wakefulness and a reduction of slow-wave sleep (SWS), together with subjective complaints of poor sleep quality (Arriaga, Rosado, & Paiva, 1990; Paiva et al., 1988).

To evaluate the features associated with the awake stage in both groups, we investigated the mechanisms of transition from awake to other stages and from other stages to awake. In addition to the EEG, changes occurring before and after an awakening were studied and analyzed.

METHODS

Two population groups, normal (Nor) and dysthymic subjects (Dyst), were investigated, each including 23 Caucasian individuals. The normal subjects selected had no complaints about sleep, no past history of neurological or psychiatric disorder, no chronic medical disturbance, no family history of psychiatric disorder, no history of drug or medication consumption (except for oral contraceptives), and no irregular sleep habits. The patients selected met the *DSM-III-R* (1987) criteria for dysthymia. During the period of study, medications were not allowed (except for oral contraceptives). The sleep of the patients was recorded after a two-week placebo treatment to allow washout from previous medication. The normal subjects included 6 men and 17 women with a mean age of 34.1 years ($SD = 8.9$); the patients were all female with a mean age of 38.3 ($SD = 7.2$).

The sleep-recording procedure included three consecutive nights in the sleep laboratory; the last two were used for analysis. Recordings took place in a sound-attenuated room with temperature control. Video monitoring of the subjects with an infrared camera was routine.

Polysomnography included nine EEG channels (F_4, F_z, F_3, C_4, C_z, C_3, O_2, O_z, O_1) using, as reference, the linked ears, EOG at the outer canthus of both eyes, submental EMG, oronasal breathing, and digital plethysmography (at the index finger). In addition to standard paper recordings, data were digitally stored by means of locally developed software that was also used for the display and processing of the EEG signals (Rosa, 1989a, 1989b). The sampling frequency for acquisition and spectral analysis was 100 Hz. Sleep stages were classified using the Rechtschaffen and Kales criteria (1968). Scoring epochs were 20 s. In each group, the hypnograms were synchronized by the sleep onset (the first epoch of Stage 2).

Processing included the following parameters: (a) transition probabilities, that is, the probabilities of transition from i to j (in this case, they were estimated from awake (i) to any other stage (j), taking as reference the total number of transitions from i); and (b) transition rates from awake to other stages, computed for consecutive intervals of 15 min and estimated according to previous work (Kemp, 1987).

The spectral characteristics of the EEG were analyzed in selected epochs, taking spontaneous awakenings as benchmarks. For that, 10 subjects from each group were chosen randomly in order to select the spontaneous awakenings. In a total of 100 awakenings analyzed, 53 belonged to Nor and 47 to Dyst. The power spectra were computed by means of periodograms for epochs of 15 s. The epochs of occurrence of an awakening were considered to be time 0, and the analysis was performed backward and forward. Backward analysis included the 12 or 20 consecutive epochs preceding the awakening (negative time), and forward analysis included the 12 epochs following the end of the awakening (positive values in the time axis).

Awakenings were selected as follows: (a) occurring only in NREM sleep (2, 3, or 4 NREM); (b) having a stable preceding sleep period of at least 3 min; and (c) returning to a stable period of sleep of at least 3 min, during which epochs of 1 NREM were no longer than 1 min.

The average values per epoch of power spectra were divided into the conventional frequency bands: sigma (11.8–16.6 Hz), alpha (7.6–11.4 Hz), theta (4.4–7.2 Hz), and delta (0.4–4.2 Hz). This study was carried out on a small number of subjects selected randomly from both groups. A total of 100 awakenings was investigated, 53 belonging to normal subjects and 47 to dysthymics; their mean duration was 47.5 and 59.5 s, respectively.

RESULTS

The sleep parameters for the two groups are shown in Table 1. Patients have a higher percentage of awake, a lower sleep efficiency, and a reduced percentage of SWS, as well as a longer sleep latency and a higher proportion of awake. The number of awake epochs was similar in both groups; the respective values were Nor (21.5 ± 10.8) and Dyst (23.6 ± 12.7) ($F_{1,44}$ = 0.758; p = 0.386). Wake epochs in patients were, however, longer in duration; indeed, the mean duration in Nor was

Table 1

Sleep Parameters and Transitions from Awake

	Normal Ss		Dysthymic Ss			
	M	SD	M	SD	F test	P level
% Awake	5.3	4.5	9.1	7.8	8.13	0.0054*
% 1 NREM	10.8	7.8	12.9	6.2	1.65	0.2020
% 2 NREM	42.5	7.8	46.3	10.7	3.45	0.0670
% 3 NREM	7.4	5.3	10.8	5.5	8.81	0.0039*
% 4 NREM	19.8	6.0	8.6	7.5	59.29	0.0001*
% REM	18.9	5.5	18.6	5.0	0.04	0.8480
Sleep efficiencies	95.2	3.7	91.1	7.2	11.54	0.0010*
REM efficiencies	84.1	12.1	81.9	10.9	0.68	0.4110

NOTE: The sleep parameters are presented as percentages together with the sleep and REM efficiencies. One-way ANOVA used 44 degrees of freedom.

0.99 min $\pm$ 0.72; whereas in Dyst, the mean was 1.7 min $\pm$ 1.1 min ($F_{1,44}$ = 10.76; p = 0.0015).

The transition probabilities from wakefulness to all other sleep stages were as follows: Probabilities from W > 1 were the most frequent (Nor = 0.7243; Dyst = 0.7112; $F_{1,44}$ = 0.06, p = 0.806). Those from W > 3 and W > 4 were relatively rare; their values were, for W > 3, Nor = 0.0044; Dyst = 0.0013; $F_{1,44}$ = 1.38, p = 0.240; and for W > 4, they were nonexistent in both groups. The mean values were therefore similar in both groups, with the exception of the transition from W > 2, which was more frequent in Nor (Nor = 0.0626; Dyst = 0.0314; $F_{1,44}$ = 16.003, p = 0.0001).

The transition rates from wakefulness to all the other sleep stages in terms of their temporal evolution across the night are shown in Figure 1. It may be observed that there are no significant group differences in the transition W > 1. Transition W > 2 varied across time: It was low for both groups during the first 300 min; however, at the end of the night, there existed two distinct peaks in Dyst. Transition W > R was always very low in Dyst, but in Nor, three distinct peaks appeared, which delineate the third, fourth, and fifth sleep cycles.

The study of the EEG changes preceding an awakening was performed on the digitized data. Figure 2 shows the mean values of the frequency bands for the two groups; in all cases, the changes preceding (pre-W) and following (post-W) the awakening are considered separately. Table 2 shows the mean values and statistical results.

For the sigma band during pre-W, the mean values in Dyst are slightly higher, but the temporal evolutions were identical. In patients there was a transient post-W increase in the sigma band, which accounted for the difference in temporal evolution (p = 0.0001).

In the alpha band, a different pattern was observed, with patients having markedly higher mean values of alpha activity. The differences occurred mostly post-W and included diagnosis (p = 0.031), temporal evolution (p = 0.032), and their interaction (p = 0.03).

For the theta band, the mean values were always higher in Dyst, both before and after the awakening. Nor presented a clear increase in

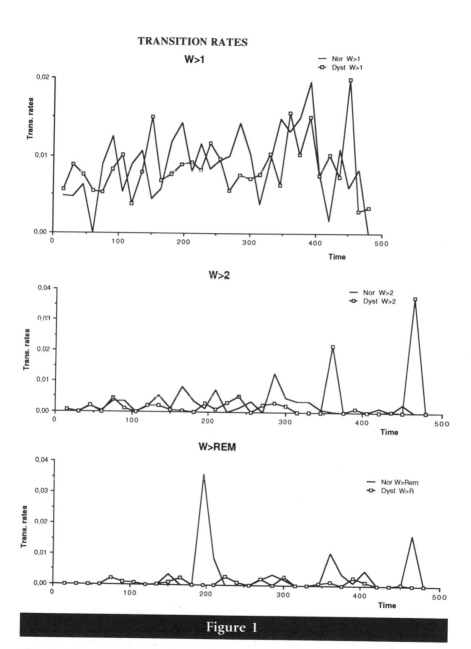

Figure 1

The transition rates from W to 1, 2, and REM are plotted for the total sleep period (time in minutes) to represent their temporal evolution. The only differences concern W > 2, with clear peaks in Dyst later in the night, and W > REM, with clear peaks in Nor according to the sleep cycles.

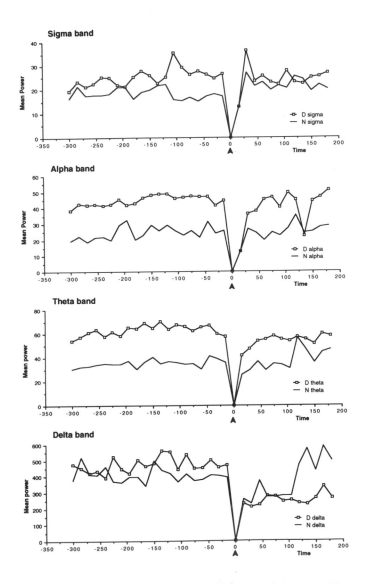

Figure 2

Mean spectral values for sigma, alpha, theta, and delta synchronized by the spontaneous awakenings. The horizontal axis is time, in seconds; D = dysthymic patients and N = normal subjects. The principal differences concern the alpha and delta bands.

Table 2

Spectral Values Pre- and Postawakenings

	Normals	Dysthymics	A(df = 1,98)		B(df = 1,11)		A × B (df = 1,11)	
	M	M	F	p	F	p	F	p
Pre-sigma	21.15	26.85	3.56	0.062*	0.70	0.739	2.00	0.025*
Post-sigma	26.62	23.07	0.69	0.406	3.79	0.0001*	1.10	0.355
Pre-alpha	25.24	46.34	18.02	0.0001*	1.42	0.156	0.53	0.887
Post-alpha	29.26	43.27	4.78	0.031*	1.93	0.032*	1.95	0.030*
Pre-theta	33.17	64.76	37.39	0.0001*	1.26	0.245	1.21	0.279
Post-theta	42.66	54.06	1.46	0.229	3.10	0.0004*	1.49	0.128
Pre-delta	356.24	489.66	4.06	0.047*	0.72	0.719	0.76	0.683
Post-delta	475.81	253.43	2.71	0.031*	2.36	0.007*	1.79	0.050*

NOTE: The mean values for each spectral frequency, pre-W and post-W, are presented, together with the results of a two-way ANOVA.

theta around 2 min post-W, and therefore the temporal evolution was significantly different ($p = 0.0004$).

The delta band presented the most striking differences. In pre-W, there were slightly higher values in Dyst with significant differences between the two diagnoses ($p = 0.047$); however, in the post-W period, Nor group showed, after 2 min, a clear increase in delta activity, which relates to the sleep reinitiation. This pattern was not observed in patients. The differences between groups concerned mainly the temporal evolution ($p = 0.007$) and its interaction with diagnosis ($p = 0.050$).

CONCLUSIONS AND DISCUSSION

Our work had two different objectives: determining the relation of awake to the other sleep stages and the EEG changes preceding and following an awakening. The following conclusions may be drawn concerning the interrelation between awake and the other sleep stages:

1. W > 1 is the most common transition in both groups, and transitions W > 3 and W > 4 occur very infrequently.
2. W > 2 is more frequent in normal subjects than in patients, showing the propensity of the former group to reinitiate sleep.
3. In each population, individual subjects can be synchronized by sleep onset.
4. There are rhythmicities in the evolution of stage transitions identical to the ones observed in sleep cycles, mainly W > R and W > 2, and these are different in normal and in dysthymic individuals.

In general, these findings are consistent with previous work with normal subjects (Gaillard, 1979; Kemp, 1987; Kemp & Kamphuisen, 1986; Merica & Gaillard, 1985). However, some new information was obtained regarding pathological sleep in patients with insomnia, which shows a pattern that is different from normal sleep in several details. A main feature of this difference concerns the temporal evolution of stage transitions. From the data obtained, it may be concluded that the temporal evolution of stage transitions contains information that is more detailed in several aspects than the one concealed in conventional sleep cycle analysis.

The second part of this work dealt with EEG changes related to spontaneous awakenings. It was observed that there were clear changes in the alpha and delta activities, and that these changes were more striking in the comparison of the two groups. Again, when using a short time base scale, two phenomena (already observed in all night recordings) were observed: that it was possible to synchronize several subjects of a given population, and that there were clear-cut rhythmicities in the spectral frequency bands.

More specifically, the following conclusions can be drawn:

1. The differences in pre- and post-awakenings concerned mostly the delta band. In both groups, there was a transient change after the awakening, but in normal subjects, a clear-cut increase was

observed after 1 min, showing the EEG slowing because of the reestablishment of sleep.

2. There were no significant differences pre- and post-awakening in alpha activity. The level of the alpha activity was, however, consistently higher in the patients, especially before the awakening.

3. The changes in the theta and sigma bands were less conspicuous and concerned mainly the temporal evolution after the awakening, suggesting again the propensity of normal subjects to restart the sleep process. There were increases in both bands after a few epochs.

The results obtained so far indicate that, in sleep recordings, there exist clear rhythmicities in several time scales and that such periodicities are more marked in normal sleep and partially lost in cases of pathological sleep. Other authors have described, in normal and pathological sleep, the existence of rhythmicities, for example, the cyclic alternating pattern (CAP; Terzano et al., 1985). The CAP phenomenon is more marked, however, in disturbed sleep. The time scale of CAP is nevertheless different from those in this work, either in what concerns the stage transition rates or in the spectral EEG changes, and therefore it may be said that we are dealing with different phenomena.

Thus, two hypotheses may be formulated: The first concerns normal sleep, composed of several periodicities with different periods in the time domain, which are interconnected and built upon each other; the second refers to pathological sleep, in which some of these periodicities are lost. Nevertheless, it must be said that the links between these phenomena, although envisaged (Terzano & Parrino, 1991), have not been fully demonstrated and that the appropriate analysis must be developed in future work.

REFERENCES

American Psychiatric Association. (1987). *Diagnosis and statistical manual of mental disorders—revised (DSM-III-R)*. Washington, DC: Author.

American Sleep Disorders Association. (1992). EEG arousals: Scoring rules and examples. The Atlas Task Force. *Sleep, 15,* 173–184.

Arriaga, F., Rosado, P., & Paiva, T. (1990). The sleep of dysthymic patients: A comparison with normal controls. *Biological Psychiatry, 27,* 649–656.

Beersma, D. G. M., van den Hoofdakker, R. H., & Dijk, D. J. (1987). Complaints about sleep quality. EMG-arousal and objective sleep continuity. *Clinical Neurology & Neurosurgery, 89-2* (Suppl. 1), 168–171.

Carskadon, M. A., & Dement, W. A. (1989). Normal human sleep: An overview. In M. H. Kryger, T. Roth, & W. C. Dement (Eds.), *Principles and practice of sleep medicine* (pp. 3–13). Philadelphia: W. B. Saunders.

Gaillard, J. M. (1979). Temporal organization of human sleep: General trends of sleep stages and their ultradian cyclic components. *L'Encéphale, 5,* 71–93.

Kemp, B. (1987). *Model-based monitoring of human sleep stages.* Doctoral dissertation, Twente University, The Netherlands.

Kemp, B., & Kamphuisen, H. A. C. (1986). Simulation of human hypnograms using a Markov chain model. *Sleep, 9,* 405–414.

Merica, H., Blois, R., & Gaillard, J. M. (1990). The intrasleep relationship between wake and stage 4 examined by transition probability analysis. *Physiology and Behavior, 46,* 929–934.

Merica, H., & Gaillard, J. M. (1985). Statistical description and evaluation of the interrelationships of standard sleep variables for normal subjects. *Sleep, 8,* 261–273.

Montagna, P., Sforza, E., Tinuper, P., Cirignotta, F., & Lugaresi, E. (1990). Paroxysmal arousals during sleep. *Neurology, 40,* 1063–1066.

Muzet, A., Schieberg, J. P., Ehrhart, J., & Lienhard, J. P. (1973). Les phases d'activation transitoire et les changements de stades electroencéphalographiques de sommeil [Transitory activation phases and electroencephalographic stage changes in sleep]. *Revue: Electroencéphalographie, Neurophysiologie Clinique, 3,* 219–222.

Paiva, T., Arriaga, F., Rosa, A., & Leitão, J. N. (1993). Sleep phasic events in dysthymic patients: A comparative study with normal controls. *Physiology & Behavior, 54,* 819–824.

Paiva, T., Arriaga, F., Wauquier, A., Lara, E., Largo, R., & Leitão, J. N. (1988). Effects of Ritanserin on sleep disturbances of dysthymic patients. *Psychopharmacology, 96,* 395–399.

Rechtschaffen, A., & Kales, A. (1968). *A manual of standardized terminology, techniques and scoring system for sleep stages of human subjects.* Washington, DC: U.S. Government Printing Office.

Rosa, A. C. (1989a). *AGX: Acquisition and real time display under MS-DOS* (Internal report CEEM, CAPS-INIC). Lisbon, Portugal: Technical University.

Rosa, A. C. (1989b). *CASES: Computer aided sleep event scoring* (Internal report CEEM, CAPS-INIC). Lisbon, Portugal: Technical University.

Terzano, M.G., Mancia, D., Selati, M. R., Costani, G., Decembrino, A., & Parrino, L. (1985). The cyclic alternating pattern as a physiologic component of NREM sleep. *Sleep, 8,* 137–145.

Terzano, M.G., & Parrino, L. (1991). Functional relationship between micro- and macrostructure of sleep. In M. G. Terzano, P. L. Halász, & A. C. Declerck (Eds.), *Phasic events and dynamic organization of sleep* (pp. 101–119). New York: Raven Press.

16

Are There Changing CNS Priorities in Sleepiness and Sleep? EEG and ERP Evidence

Robert D. Ogilvie, Robin A. Battye, and Iain A. Simons

W e wish to examine the microstructure of sleep onset and sleep by pairing and comparing brief samples of electroencephalogram (EEG) activity with nearly simultaneously obtained late components of auditory event-related potentials (ERPs). The purpose of these analyses is to determine whether the sensitivity of EEG and ERP measures to changes in sleepiness and in the S–W (sleep–wake) state can be attributed best to a single or to multiple (asynchronous) CNS arousal regulating mechanism(s). Two investigations will be summarized.

The relationship between the EEG measures of drowsiness and sleep has been studied for over 50 years: Davis, Davis, Loomis, Harvey, & Hobart (1937) discovered ERP changes related to sleep, and Williams, Tepas, and Morlock (1962) ushered in modern sleep–ERP investigation. Studies of behavioral degradation, sleepiness, and sleep loss have also been conducted for a considerable length of time (Davis et al., 1937; Wilkinson, 1969).

However, direct EEG–ERP comparisons have been rare, except for a series of studies by Basar (1980) and co-workers. Basar (1980) proposed a new metric that he called EEG–EPograms that involved computing a combination of the two procedures—the combined analysis procedure (CAP)—in an attempt to understand dynamic brain activity. To calculate EEG–EPograms, he recorded 1 s of prestimulus EEG plus the EP to auditory stimuli. He examined animal and human responses obtained primarily from subcortical and cortical structures, respectively, to determine the influence of the prestimulus EEG on single-trial EPs. Much of this work stressed the enhancement of certain EP components by specific prestimulus EEG frequencies. For example, Basar, Basar-Eroglu, Rosen, and Schutt (1984) studied the relationship between prestimulus EEG and P300 activity, finding that prestimulus delta and theta frequencies result in increased P300 amplitudes.

Recently, Mecklinger, Kramer, and Strayer (1992) varied demands on memory in an investigation of the electrophysiological changes accompanying increased cognitive complexity. They found that prestimulus theta power was related directly to cognitive demand, whereas P300 amplitude was linked inversely. Jasiukaitis and Hakerem (1988) detected higher amplitude P300s in the presence of high versus low prestimulus alpha levels.

Another tool that might facilitate sample-by-sample EEG–ERP comparisons is single-trial ERP analyses. Single-trial analyses of major ERP components like P300 and contingent negative variation (CNV) have already proven useful (e.g., Segalowitz, Unsal, & Dywan, 1992). This paradigm has not been carefully explored with regard to studying arousal level changes. In the two studies discussed here, the interaction between many nearly coincident EEG and ERP measures was studied during the transition from wakefulness to sleep (Study 1) and throughout sleep (Study 2).

Without simultaneous comparisons between EEG and ERP analyses in an arousal paradigm, it has not been possible to determine whether the sleep-related changes in EEG activity (Rechtschaffen & Kales, 1968) and the widely noted changes in ERP components at sleep onset (Campbell, Bell, & Bastien, 1992; Ogilvie, Simons, Kuderian, MacDonald, & Rustenburg, 1991; Williams et al., 1962) reflect a single underlying process or two or more independent arousal modulators. Recent work from this laboratory addresses this issue.

Ogilvie et al. (1991) assessed EEG and ERP component changes simultaneously during the sleep-onset period (SOP). They used behavioral response latency to define sleepiness and sleep (no response). EEG and ERP data were both ranked according to response latency and behavioral sleep. The rank-ordered, prestimulus EEG samples were subjected to fast Fourier transform (FFT) analysis, and poststimulus samples were used for ERP computation. The pretonal data revealed significant increases in RMS power for all standard frequency bands during the SOP as behavioral sleep onset (SO) was reached. Changes in the amplitude of all late ERP components, except P2, were significantly related to decreased responsivity. The authors interpreted the marked increase in EEG power and ERP amplitude changes associated with behavioral response cessation (sleep) as providing convergent evidence of a more precise SO process within the SOP, when behavioral rather than EEG criteria are used to locate SO.

Using a similar approach, the current studies involved a correlational (factor-analytic) technique in which EEG spectra and ERP components were sampled pre- and posttonally (in a within-subjects paradigm) throughout the SOP and continuing all night. Such an approach permitted the simultaneous monitoring of ongoing changes in EEG spectra and single-trial ERP components. These two important indices of arousal have not been compared in this manner during the SOP.

EXPERIMENT 1

In this first study, we predicted that a descriptive factor analysis would show that both the ERP components and FFT power spectrum changes would tend to load primarily on a single "sleepiness" factor during the transition into sleep (SOP).

Method

Subjects

Eleven university-aged, self-described light sleepers were paid to spend two nonconsecutive nights in the laboratory. Participants were selected if they were relatively normal (but light) sleepers based on the Sleep

Quality Questionnaire (SQQ) scores (Kuderian, Ogilvie, McDonnell, & Simons, 1991). All subjects were tested for normal hearing.

Apparatus

A 14-channel Nihon Kohden (model 4314B) electroencephalograph recorded all electrophysiological and behavioral parameters. All data were stored on-line using an AST Premium 386/25 computer with a 12-bit National Instruments A/D board (model AT-MIO-16) and the Microcomputer Quantitative Electrophysiology (MQE) acquisition and analysis program developed by Imaging Research, Inc. Data were backed up using a maximum-storage optical disk drive (model APX-5200). A Beltone audiometer was used for hearing assessment. Respiratory data were recorded on a Respitrace respiration monitor.

Behavioral Response System

A microcomputer with a custom-built clock/sound interface card was programmed to deliver faint 1000-Hz tones randomly to a walkman-like earphone taped in the subject's ear of choice (for details, see Ogilvie et al., 1991). Each subject was allowed to select a tone level that was minimally obtrusive and yet clearly audible.

Procedure

After a full orientation tour of the laboratory, signed consent was obtained. The subjects were then required to complete the SQQ (Kuderian et al., 1991) to ensure that they had normal sleep habits, and each underwent an audiometric test to verify normal hearing. Participants were then scheduled for two nonconsecutive nights in the laboratory. During the days scheduled for participation, the subjects were asked to avoid alcohol and daytime naps as well as to abstain from caffeine following supper. As electrodes were applied, each subject completed a presleep questionnaire designed to screen for daytime activities that might result in atypical sleep patterns.

The electrophysiological parameters recorded were two monopolar EEG channels (C3-A2, C4-A2), two electrooculographic (EOG) channels, one bipolar submental electromyographic (EMG) channel, and abdominal and thoracic respiration (Respitrace system).

Following electrode application, the button–switch was secured to the subject's preferred hand, the earphone was taped into the subject's ear of choice, and the behavioral response system's tone volume was set. In the morning, all subjects completed a postsleep questionnaire that provided a qualitative report of their night's sleep. Only data from night two were analyzed.

EEG Analyses

Ten-second samples of continuous EEG activity were obtained during the entire S–W session. The sampling rate for the A/D conversion was 9.77 ms per point; thus, a total of 1,024 samples per channel were taken during each sweep. During both EEG and ERP analyses, the trigger channel placed the onset of each tone in the center of the 10-s window. EEG analyses were conducted on the 5-s pretone sample, whereas ERP computations were based on 2-s samples of EEG immediately following the same tone onset. Each 5-s sample was individually subjected to FFT analysis. Power for each of the five EEG spectra was included: delta, .3–3 Hz; theta, 3–8 Hz; alpha, 8–12 Hz; sigma, 12–15 Hz; and beta, 15–25 Hz. FFT analyses were performed from a computer-calculated baseline, determined from the calibration data obtained before each recording session. A visual inspection of each 10-s window permitted artifact rejection.

The initial analysis consisted of sampling a maximum of 100 pretonal EEG samples per subject, in chronological order, from the beginning of the night (first tone) until approximately 1 to 3 min of failed responses (behavioral sleep) had occurred. Sleep was defined behaviorally as greater than four consecutive failed responses. As a result, the number of samples ranged from 30 to 100, with a mean of 67.3 ($SD = 23.7$). All sampling was initiated 5 s prior to stimulus onset, providing an index of the level of arousal immediately antecedent to (and uncontaminated by) each tone.

Single-Trial ERP Analyses

Single-trial ERP data were acquired during the first 2 s following tone onset (posttonally). As in the EEG/FFT analysis, the single-trial ERP samples consisted of sampling a maximum of 100 posttonal samples per subject. Amplitude was measured in microvolts from a 1,000-ms pretonal baseline. The component definitions were the following: N1 = lowest peak between 75 and 150 ms; P1 = highest peak between 150 and 250 ms; N2 = lowest peak between 250 and 350 ms; N3 = lowest peak between 500 and 750 ms; P3 = highest peak between 750 and 1,500 ms; and P300 = highest peak between 250 and 500 ms. The rationale for selection of these components is described in detail elsewhere (e.g., Ogilvie et al., 1991). P2 was omitted from the present analysis because of its failure to show any promise in that earlier work. Analyses were limited to trials in which both pre- and posttonal data met all inclusion criteria; thus, the number of posttonal ERP samples per subject was identical to that for the EEG/FFT analysis.

Results

For each subject, a correlation matrix was computed within and between all EEG/FFT and ERP components. Table 1 shows the average values for those matrices.

Upon initial examination of Table 1, it is clear that the predicted across-domain correlations were negligible compared to within-domain coefficients: None of the ERP components correlated highly with the EEG frequency bands. However, relatively high correlations within the EEG frequencies and among ERP components were apparent, providing evidence of the relative independence of ERP and EEG variables during the SOP.

To describe the relationship between the EEG and ERP components further, a principal components analysis with a Varimax rotation was performed on all single-trial EEG and ERP data separately for each subject. Only those factors with eigenvalues greater than 1 and showing some consistency across subjects were examined closely. Table 2 illus-

Table 1

Averaged Correlations for All Subjects and Variables

	N1	N2	N3	P1	P3	P300	Delta	Theta	Alpha	Sigma	Beta
N1	—	.25	.15	.27	.02	−.04	−.06	−.09	.04	.01	.09
N2	—	—	.22	.40	.06	.27	.02	.04	−.09	−.02	.03
N3	—	—	—	.11	−.01	.06	−.06	−.11	.04	.04	.04
P1	—	—	—	—	.13	.25	−.06	−.15	.10	.01	.11
P3	—	—	—	—	—	.30	.21	.11	−.09	−.04	−.20
P300	—	—	—	—	—	—	.17	.19	−.09	.01	−.20
Delta	—	—	—	—	—	—	—	.11	−.57	−.17	−.64
Theta	—	—	—	—	—	—	—	—	−.39	−.14	−.52
Alpha	—	—	—	—	—	—	—	—	—	.14	.25
Sigma	—	—	—	—	—	—	—	—	—	—	.07
Beta	—	—	—	—	—	—	—	—	—	—	—

NOTE: Correlations were transformed to z-scores, averaged across subjects, and transformed back to a Pearson's correlation coefficient. Although significance levels cannot be calculated strictly for averaged correlations, the r-values presented are based on 737 pairs of measures. If significance could be assessed, correlations $\geq r = .072$ would be significantly different from zero ($p < .05$), although no useful variance is accounted for by very low correlations.

trates two typical examples of the patterns of factor loadings for each subject's analysis. (Loadings below .30 were not included in the table.) The first example is typical of 8 of the 11 subjects. Here, it can be seen that the EEG/FFT components account for the most variance (23.2% to 34.5%, becoming Factor 1), whereas fewer ERP measures load on the slightly weaker second factor (accounting for 14.4% to 22.1% of variance). The second example shows that ERP intercorrelations (Factor 1) generally outweigh EEG loadings (Factor 2). For all subjects, the alpha and beta frequency bands loaded in the opposite direction from the delta and theta frequencies. All of the ERP components, however, loaded in a positive direction. Most important for this study was that intercorrelations between domains were rarely seen until Factor 3 had been extracted and, then, were not seen consistently.

Table 2

Factor Loadings Following Varimax Rotation of Two Typical Patterns

Variables	Factor loadings pattern A		Factor loadings pattern B	
	Factor 1	Factor 2	Factor 1	Factor 2
N1	—	—	—	—
P1	.63	—	.71	—
N2	—	.86	.79	—
N3	—	.83	.69	—
P3	—	−.83	.64	—
P300	—	—	.83	—
Delta	−.75	—	—	−.92
Theta	−.85	—	—	—
Alpha	.68	—	—	.78
Sigma	—	—	—	—
Beta	.89	—	—	—

NOTE: Dashes signify loadings below .30.

EXPERIMENT 2

Our initial prediction of a strong common relationship between EEG/FFT and ERP indices was not supported in Study 1. We decided, therefore, to look for secondary covariation between the two measurement domains and to look at factor patterns more closely. To do this with reasonable fidelity required increased within-subject sample sizes. (The first study was a replicated single-subject design.) The increased number of data points per subject was obtained by continuing to analyze information on near-simultaneous pairs of data points throughout the night. This approach permitted a comparison of EEG/FFT and ERP correlations within each sleep stage. We added one subject, changed our approach to FFT analysis in several ways (described later), and analyzed the entire night (including the presleep period of Study 1).

Method

EEG Analyses

Only differences from Study 1 will be reported. Sleep stages were scored normally, but again, epoch length was 5 s. Subsequently, individual pretonal C4-A2 EEG samples were subjected to FFT analysis to produce an amplitude spectrum from which the absolute and total power were determined for each of the following bandwidths: delta, .200 3.40 Hz; theta, 3.40–7.80 Hz; alpha, 8–11.80 Hz; sigma, 12–14.80 Hz; beta 1, 15–19.80 Hz; and beta 2, 20–29.80 Hz. The total number of data points obtained from each subject ranged from 664 to 958, with a mean value of 808 ($SD = 97.31$). Only the absolute measures for amplitude spectra were used in the analysis, to avoid problems with attenuation of data in the weaker bandwidths (typically upper) and to maintain independence of individual bandwidths.

Single-Trial ERP Analyses

ERP samples were based on the EEG immediately following tone onset (posttonally), corresponding one to one with the trials used in the EEG analysis. Using 1,000 ms of pretonal EEG as baseline, measures were taken based on expected ranges of typical ERP components in accordance with a single-trial paradigm discussed in Basar et al. (1984). Measures included the maximum and minimum values for amplitude (in microvolts) and peak latencies (in milliseconds) for the same components as in Study 1.

Results

The individual all-night correlation matrices were slightly variable, but across all S–W conditions, there were relatively small across-domain correlations between EEG/FFT and ERP variables. Those seen occurred mainly in the delta and beta 1 and 2 ranges. Although the across-domain correlations were relatively low, the within-domain correlations, although somewhat variable, were occasionally high ($>.70$) for physiological measures. All variable distributions proved to be relatively normal, except for a few Stage 4 samples that had a relatively low sample size.

The averaged correlation matrix (Table 3) illustrates the between-variable relations but shows lower correlations (because of averaging) and a weaker EEG–ERP interrelationship, with the exception of P3, which often correlated with an individual's EEG/FFT components.

Next, a series of principal components factor analyses with Varimax rotations was performed on each subject's data. Individual data were subdivided into the following arousal states: all night, presleep, post-

Table 3

Averaged Correlations of All Subjects and Variables for All Night Data

Averaged correlation matrix for EEG absolute power and ERP amplitude data for all subjects

	Delta	Theta	Alpha	Sigma	Beta 1	Beta 2	N1	N2	N3	P1	P3	P300
Delta	—	−.37	−.64	−.44	−.79	−.80	.16	.14	.06	.03	.38	.18
Theta	—	—	.07	.06	.08	−.01	−.06	−.06	−.01	−.04	−.12	−.04
Alpha	—	—	—	.36	.46	.40	−.09	−.09	−.03	−.01	−.25	−.11
Sigma	—	—	—	—	.27	.22	−.04	−.07	.00	−.01	−.10	−.04
Beta 1	—	—	—	—	—	.78	−.10	−.01	−.06	−.03	−.35	−.02
Beta 2	—	—	—	—	—	—	−.13	−.08	−.06	−.02	−.35	−.17
N1	—	—	—	—	—	—	—	.51	.28	.18	.14	.06
N2	—	—	—	—	—	—	—	—	.36	.18	.11	.21
N3	—	—	—	—	—	—	—	—	—	.01	.07	.04
P1	—	—	—	—	—	—	—	—	—	—	.17	.44
P3	—	—	—	—	—	—	—	—	—	—	—	.23
P300	—	—	—	—	—	—	—	—	—	—	—	—

NOTE: Correlations were transformed to z-scores, averaged across subjects, and transformed back to a Pearson's correlation coefficient ($N = 9,697$). As in Table 1, averaging prevents accurate reporting of significance levels for correlations. If significance could be assessed, correlations $\geq r = .02$ would be significantly different from zero, although r^2 serves as a reminder that no useful variance is accounted for by very low correlations.

sleep, wake, Stage 1, Stage 2, Stage 3, Stage 4, and REM. These analyses consistently produced at least three principal factors (eigenvalues > 1). The average percentage of variance accounted for in each of these factors was similar to that seen in Study 1. Factor 1 accounted for over 22% of the variance (22.15% to 34.05%), closely followed by Factor 2 (16.81% to 25.75%), whereas Factor 3 claimed 10% to 12%. The three factors combined to account for well over 50% of the variance in every arousal state. The components of the first two factors generated loadings to .97.

Table 4 shows that the first two factors contained the most clearly interpretable data, when examined across individual subjects and all-night, presleep, and postsleep conformations. The presence of specific within-domain components varied across S–W state, but at least 3 of 6 components within each domain loaded on each of the two primary factors. In some instances, across-domain loadings were observed; often P3 loaded on the EEG factor, but across-state variability in factor composition remained low in the single-subject analysis of the first two factors. As in Study 1, there were a few cases in which the ERP factor was more heavily weighted than the EEG factor. Factor 3 appeared to

Table 4

Averaged Percent of Variance Accounted for in Each Factor Analyzed for Different Levels of Arousal (Subjects: $n = 12$)

Factor	Sleep state								
	Presleep	Postsleep	All night	Wake	Stage 1	Stage 2	Stage 3	Stage 4	REM
Factor 1	23.91	34.05	33.27	26.68	22.96	23.28	27.64	28.99	22.2
Factor 2	17.46	16.81	16.49	19.88	21.93	20.11	21.76	18.78	25.8
Factor 3	12.21	10.28	10.30	12.50	12.67	11.97	12.96	11.94	11.9
Cumulative percentage	53.58	61.14	60.06	59.06	57.56	55.36	62.36	59.71	59.8

vary independently from the other two and, to some extent, to show different patterns in different people. In an attempt to resolve Factor 3 further, the remaining factor classifications were based on factor component loadings greater than .30.

To get a clearer picture of the emerging factor patterns, each subject's ($n = 12$) data were separated into individual arousal state measures and then combined for each factor, as shown in Figure 1.

Once again, the frequency of loadings on the Factors 1 and 2 illustrates the primary independence of the EEG and ERP variables, with very little cross-domain interrelationship.

The factor structure in Factor 3, however, when investigated across the different subjects and arousal states, oscillated across both measurement domains. Initially, in Stages Wake, 1, and 2, the frequencies of loadings were distributed somewhat evenly across Factor 3, but as Stages 3 and 4 commenced, the distribution became skewed toward the ERP domain. Conversely, stage REM looked "wakelike," describing another predominantly balanced EEG/FFT factor. The pattern in this factor did not seem random, yet the total frequency of loadings was low; as a result, interpretations must be made with caution. Progressing down the arousal continuum, the delta and beta components maintained their high frequency of loading, but the theta, alpha, and sigma components varied markedly. These measures started with a relatively low frequency of loading during wakefulness and continually increased to match the delta and beta loadings in Stages 3 and 4. REM sleep approximated the patterns found in Stage 1 sleep, but with more frequent loadings contributed by the sigma component.

From wake to Stage 3, the number of ERP factor loadings increased in a stepwise fashion in each group, with the exception of N3, which dropped in Stage 3. Stage 4 produced a notable drop in all the observed loadings, which is in contrast to REM, where each measure was observed in its highest rate of occurrence overall. There were no notable sustained, across-domain interrelationships, with the exception of a P3 peak in the EEG postsleep factor.

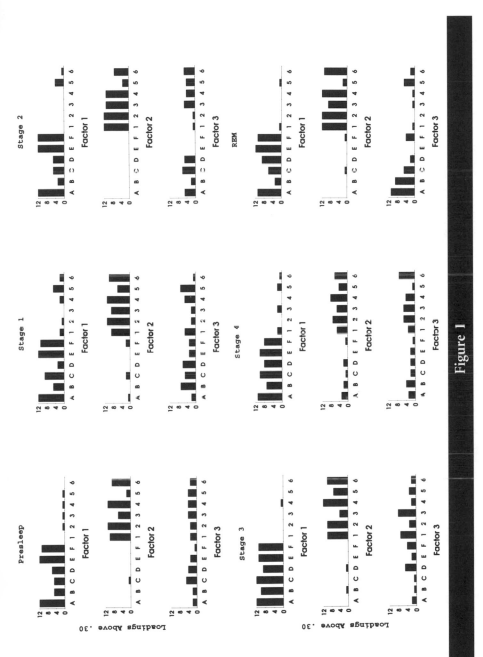

Figure 1

Number of subjects (0–12) showing factor loadings >.30 plotted separately for each factor (1–3) and sleep–wake stage. NOTE: A = delta area; B = theta area; C = alpha area; D = sigma area; E = beta 1 area; F = beta 2 area; 1 = N1; 2 = N2; 3 = N3; 4 = P1; 5 = P3; and 6 = P300.

DISCUSSION

We have attempted to describe the relationship between EEG spectra and ERP components as people become increasingly sleepy (Study 1) and as they sleep through the night (Study 2). Previous research (e.g., Ogilvie et al., 1991), which analyzed FFT and ERP data *separately*, found a marked increase in RMS power and ERP amplitudes during the SOP. It was hypothesized that the changes in FFT and ERP parameters during SO would reflect a unitary CNS process. That is, perhaps arousal components of the FFT and ERP variables are influenced by one and the same thing—the rapid reorganization and/or synchronization of brain frequencies during the onset of sleep (Study 1). As sleep unfolded throughout the night, arousal level shifts were expected to continue to produce correlated changes in FFT frequencies and ERP components (Study 2). The present data clearly fail to support that prediction. Beginning with the initial within-subject correlation matrices of Study 1, all subsequent matrices and factor analyses suggested that the EEG/FFT and ERP indices of arousal were measuring primarily different aspects of CNS processes during the SOP. These data show that the ERP and FFT variables are independent of each other, as indicated by the first two extracted factors. Instead of the predicted pattern of a mixture of FFT and ERP measures loading heavily on a single factor, the descriptive factor analyses consistently revealed two factors accounting for most of the variance. Within those two factors, the EEG/FFT spectra generally determined the first or largest factor, accounting for more variance than the ERP components. ERP variables tended to load heavily on the second factor. Occasionally, the most coherent factor would be composed of ERP intercorrelations, but only 1 of the 11 subjects in Study 1 showed the predicted heavy loading of both types of arousal indices on the primary factor. Study 2 was generally consistent with this pattern throughout all S–W stages, although a number of interesting stage differences emerged secondarily.

It is important to remember that the data in Study 1 were acquired during the rapid EEG fluctuations of the SOP, with its "waxing" and "waning" between alert wakefulness, drowsiness, lapses in performance (or microsleeps), and so forth. Sampling was terminated after greater than four failed responses; there were no instances in which subjects had failed to respond or had been asleep by behavioral definition for longer than 2–3 min. All data for Study 1 were thus obtained during the SO process where the electrophysiological oscillations between waking and sleeping were taking place. The EEG and ERP data were obtained from identical electrodes and recording conditions, almost simultaneously in both studies.

In Study 1, the P3 component was the only ERP variable to show any consistent relation to EEG variables across analyses (subjects); five analyses had a high loading for the P3 component. This relationship between P3 and prestimulus EEG is in line with reports by several authors (Basar, 1980; Basar et al., 1984; Mecklinger et al., 1992). The remaining ERP components loaded on the EEG factor infrequently and inconsistently across analyses.

The second factor, on the other hand, generally appeared to be an ERP factor. For the majority of the analyses, all ERP components tended to load in a positive direction. None of the FFT frequencies that loaded on this factor showed any reliable pattern across analyses (subjects).

Several of the analyses performed yielded high loadings (>.40) on only two or three variables. With a Varimax rotation, such factors are sometimes the result of artifacts of rotation. However, the present factors appeared to be stable, because oblique rotations (while not reported) produced results similar to those of the Varimax method. This stability was also supported by significant correlations between the variables within each factor and across subjects.

For Study 2, and beginning with presleep data and continuing throughout all sleep stages, the major relationships seen in Study 1 were confirmed. Here again, there were two large, stable factors that showed domain-dependent factor patterns. Again, the strongest factor across all S–W stages and replicated across most subjects was the FFT factor. Close behind in terms of variance accounted for was the ERP factor.

Consistent cross-domain loadings were infrequent; P3 loaded on the FFT factor in Stage 1 in 4 of 12 subjects, but no single FFT frequency loaded that consistently on the ERP factor in any stage. In Stage 4, however, the ERP factor was most influenced by FFT activity in that there was a total of 9 FFT loadings from all 12 subjects, where the maximum possible was 72 (Subjects × Bands).

As implied, FFT bands and ERP components contributed differentially to the factor structures across the six S–W states and stages. Delta and beta areas contributed consistently to the FFT factor across all stages in virtually all subjects, whereas changes in the number of subjects showing loadings above .30 across stages were observed in the alpha, theta, and sigma bands. In the ERP factor, N1 and N2 showed the most consistent high loadings across states.

The large increase in sampling points in Study 2 permitted a more detailed (but still tentative) examination of Factor 3. Figure 1 shows that, although the number of loadings greater than .30 was greatly reduced compared to the first two factors, there was a much more symmetrical pattern of loadings across domains. In fact, the pattern of loadings on Factor 3 was consistent with what had been predicted for the strongest factor. However, there was considerable between-subject variability in loading patterns for Factor 3.

Although the data from both studies reflect changing patterns of intercorrelation as a function of changes in arousal level or S–W state, it must be remembered that, within both measurement domains, there is a degree of dependence among variables. Changes in power within one EEG frequency band have some influence on the others. Similarly, the negativity or positivity of one ERP component influences the absolute voltage of subsequent components, just as shifting prestimulus baselines can. Thus, it is not surprising that a certain degree of within-method correlation can be found. What was not predicted was that that variance sometimes outstrips the one seen within and across domains, which results from their common sensitivity to changes in arousal. Sensitivity to arousal can also be seen, but it is somewhat blurred by within-method variance.

Looking at the distribution of factor loadings across all three factors, we find that, during sleep and wakefulness, EEG and ERP variation would appear to be interesting primarily *within* each of these domains. There are consistent changes within each domain as a function of S–W state, but cross-domain variance is clearly secondary to within-domain processes. It remains likely that the cross-domain variance represented by Factor 3 is due to a common influence on these parameters produced by changes in arousal level, but replication and more fine-grained analysis would need to be conducted before such a relationship could be established firmly. It is clear, however, that there are predictable changes among intercorrelations *within* FFT and ERP domains when wakefulness, sleep onset, and the standard sleep stages are traversed. We are continuing to explore changes in arousal at SO and during sleep, as reflected by simultaneous FFT and ERP measurement.

REFERENCES

Basar, E. (1980). *EEG–brain dynamics: Relation between EEG and brain evoked potentials*. Amsterdam: Elsevier/North-Holland Biomedical Press.

Basar, E., Basar-Eroglu, C., Rosen, B., & Schutt, A. (1984). A new approach to endogenous event-related potentials in man: Relation between EEG and P300-wave. *International Journal of Neuroscience, 24,* 1–21.

Campbell, K., Bell, I., & Bastien, C. (1992). Evoked potential measures of information processing during natural sleep. In R. J. Broughton & R. D. Ogilvie (Eds.), *Sleep, arousal, and performance* (pp. 88–116). Cambridge, MA: Birkhauser Boston.

Davis, H., Davis, P. A., Loomis, A. L., Harvey, E. N., & Hobart, G. (1937). Changes in human brain potentials during the onset of sleep. *Science, 86,* 448–450.

Jasiukaitis, P., & Hakerem, G. (1988). The effect of prestimulus alpha activity on the P300. *Psychophysiology, 25,* 157–165.

Kuderian, R. H., Ogilvie, R. D., McDonnell, G., & Simons, I. (1991). Behavioural response home monitoring of insomniac and normal sleepers. *Canadian Journal of Psychology, 45,* 169–178.

Mecklinger, A., Kramer, A. F., & Strayer, D. L. (1992). Event related potentials and

EEG components in a semantic memory search task. *Psychophysiology, 29,* 104–119.

Ogilvie, R. D., Simons, I. A., Kuderian, R. H., MacDonald, T., & Rustenburg, J. (1991). Behavioral, event-related potential, and EEG/FFT changes at sleep onset. *Psychophysiology, 28,* 54–64.

Rechtschaffen, A., & Kales, A. (1968). *A manual of standardized terminology, techniques and scoring system for sleep stages of human subjects.* Los Angeles: University of California Brain Research Institute.

Segalowitz, S. J., Unsal, A., & Dywan, J. (1992). Cleverness and wisdom in 12-year-olds: Electrophysiological evidence for late maturation of the frontal lobe. *Developmental Neuropsychology, 8,* 279–298.

Wilkinson, R. T. (1969). Sleep deprivation: Performance tests for partial and selective sleep deprivation. In B. F. Reiss & L. E. Abt (Eds.), *Progress in clinical psychology* (Vol. 8, pp. 28–43). New York: Grune and Stratton.

Williams, H. L., Tepas, D. I., & Morlock, H. C. (1962). Evoked responses to clicks and electroencephalographic stages of sleep in man. *Science, 138,* 685–686.

PART FIVE

ERP Changes

17

Stimulus Processing Awake and Asleep: Similarities and Differences in Electrical CNS Responses

Dean F. Salisbury

The electrical signals generated by the central nervous system (CNS) in response to stimuli deviating from a repetitive sequence have received considerable attention in the awake human, particularly the long-latency, *endogenous* or *cognitive* event-related potentials (ERPs), N2 and P3. These electrical signals reflect synchronous activity in cortical and subcortical areas and occur between 200 and 500 ms post-stimulation. These ERPs are of interest in that they seem to reflect complicated perceptual and memory processes in the subject rather than sensory aspects of the stimuli.

Stimuli presented to the sleeping human evoke electrical signals similar to those evoked in the awake human. These similar potentials are generally early in onset latency (≤ 200 ms). Stimuli presented during sleep also evoke signals distinctly different from those evoked in the awake subject. These sleep-specific potentials are generally of long onset latency (≥ 300 ms) and are typically referred to as the *K-complex*. The exact time point in stimulus processing during sleep (as reflected by CNS electrical activity) in which state-similar activity ends and sleep-specific activity begins remains unknown. Presumably, a high degree of similarity in an ERP between the awake and sleep states suggests that the processing reflected by that ERP is relatively automatic and preattentive, that is, independent of selective attention mechanisms.

The cognitive ERPs, N2 and P3, occur in the awake subject at a latency that, during sleep, is in the transition zone from state-similar to K-complex activity. The demonstration of N2 and P3 during sleep would suggest that the processes which they reflect might be less dependent on selective cognitive and perceptual analysis than previously reported. Deviant, low-probability stimuli presented to the sleeping subject evoke N2 and P3 potentials highly similar to those evoked in the awake subject, without concomitant K-complex activation. This demonstration suggests that the endogenous ERPs may be highly *exogenous*, or stimulus dependent, and that the sleeping brain monitors the environment for atypical events in a complex but automatic or obligatory fashion not much different from that of the awake brain.

THE EVENT-RELATED POTENTIAL

Averaging Principles

The EEG is an envelope reflecting the summed activity of all brain electrical activity at any point in time. With rare exceptions, this activity is the summation of dendritic postsynaptic potentials and reflects the portions of the field that are perpendicular to the scalp (for a thorough review, see Regan, 1989; Williamson & Kaufman, 1990). To visualize activity solely related to stimulus processing, averaging techniques must be used. These consist of multiple stimulus presentations and recording of the EEG for a specified time base after each presentation. These epochs are aligned at stimulus presentation and arithmetically averaged. Electrical activity related to stimulus presentation is time locked, because signals are propagated over a fixed distance (determined by head size and cortical location), and assuming that processing time in any neural area is relatively constant, postsynaptic potentials in each cortical area should occur at the same time after each stimulus presentation. On the other hand, the remainder of EEG activity is random with regard to stimulus presentation. As such, it should be equally positive or negative at any point in the epoch and normally distributed about the zero-potential line. Theoretically, time-locked stimulus-processing activity should remain in the average, whereas random activity approaches zero. In practice, the resolution of ERP averages improves as a function of the signal-to-noise ratio and the number of trials averaged (e.g., Möcks, Gasser, & Köhler, 1988; Picton & Hink, 1974). This effect is illustrated in Figure 1. As the number of traces in each average increases, the resolution of the electrical responses also increases against a background of alpha waves and other brain activities not related to the tones.

Event-Related Potential Types

ERPs occur in three general time ranges: short latency, midlatency, and long latency. Short-latency ($\leq$10 ms) potentials reflect the peripheral afferent activity in relay nuclei and along long axon bundles (the exception to the postsynaptic activity rule). Midlatency potentials (11–49 ms) most likely reflect brain-stem activity, thalamic activity, and primary cortical activation. Long-latency potentials ($\geq$50 ms) reflect cortical and limbic activation, particularly from secondary and tertiary cortical areas and medial temporal lobe structures. Long-latency activity is thought to reflect higher order cognitive processing in the awake human and is discussed in greater detail below under "Endogenous Potentials." Note that the time bases used to image the different classes of potentials are different; one may visualize a class of potentials, but usually at the expense of the other types of responses in that the temporal sensitivity necessary to see one group will be either too fine or too coarse to see the others.

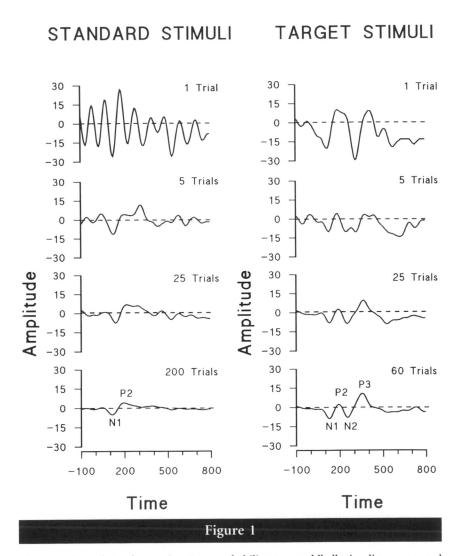

Figure 1

The procedure of signal averaging. Low-probability target oddball stimuli are presented in trains of standard stimuli. As the number of traces included in the average increases, the potentials more clearly emerge. Left traces are responses to highly probable standard stimuli. N1 and P2 are relatively small sensory potentials. Right traces are responses to oddballs. N2 and P3 are evident in these averages.

AUDITORY EVENT-RELATED POTENTIALS AWAKE AND ASLEEP

Exogenous Potentials

Exogenous potentials are by definition sensory. This means that their shape is defined by the physical characteristics of the evoking stimuli, not by any conscious mechanisms engaged by the subject. The short- and midlatency potentials are primarily exogenous, as are the earliest of the long-latency components. The morphology of the different exogenous potentials and the effect of state on their morphology follow.

Auditory Brain-Stem Responses (ABRs)

ABRs reflect activity of the eighth-nerve relay nuclei and ascending afferent pathways from the cochlea to the thalamus and perhaps also to the primary auditory cortex. They occur within the first 10–15 ms after stimulation and are evident as six potentials (Jewett & Williston, 1971). ABRs are routinely used to test the integrity of the peripheral neural pathways. A number of researchers have shown that ABR morphology is unaffected by sleep, with remarkably stable amplitudes and latencies of these waves regardless of the state of the subject (e.g., Amadeo & Shagass, 1973; Campbell & Bartoli, 1986; Picton, Hillyard, Krause, & Galambos, 1974). This suggests that auditory signals are processed identically along peripheral afferent pathways during wake and sleep states.

Midlatency Potentials

This series of five waves occurs roughly 10–40 ms after stimulation. These potentials arise most probably in the medial geniculate and polysensory nuclei of the thalamus, the ascending reticular activation system, and the primary auditory cortex. Like ABRs, they vary in latency and amplitude with stimulus parameters and have been demonstrated to be fairly independent of level of arousal, being largely unaffected during sleep (e.g., Erwin & Buchwald, 1986; Mendel et al., 1975; Picton et al., 1974). The lack of state effects on these midlatency potentials suggests that auditory signals may be processed identically as far as primary auditory cortex in wake and sleep states.

Long-latency Potentials

Three long-latency potentials appear to be highly sensory in nature: P1, a positive potential at roughly 50 ms; N1, a negative potential at 100 ms; and P2, a positive potential at 200 ms. All of these waves, and the classes already discussed, can be evoked by the presentation of one repetitious stimulus and have been shown to vary with stimulus intensity. P1 amplitude has been reported to increase during sleep (Williams, Tepas, & Morlock, 1962), although others have reported decreases in P1 as a function of sleep (Erwin & Buchwald, 1986; Kevanishvili & Von Specht, 1979). Still others have reported no changes in P1 (e.g., Weitzman & Kremen, 1965). Likewise, the effect of sleep on N1 and P2 amplitude have been variable. Most have reported no effect of sleep state (e.g., Picton et al., 1974; Ujszászi & Halász, 1988; Weitzman & Kremen, 1965), although there is some general feeling that N1 is reduced and P2 increased, at least in Stage 2 (e.g., Frühstorfer & Bergström, 1969; Mendel et al., 1975; Nielsen-Bohlman, Knight, Woods, & Woodward, 1991). It is unclear whether auditory processing is the same during wake and sleep states at this late level of processing. Much of the variability of long-latency potentials during sleep may be due to the activation of these potentials simultaneously with the K-complex.

Endogenous Potentials

Since its initial description by Sutton, Braren, Zubin, and John (1965), the P3 component, a positive potential occurring roughly 300 ms after stimulation, has received a great amount of study in awake subjects, particularly because it is thought to reflect higher order cognitive operations rather than sensory activation. Therefore, P3 and the negative potential preceding it at roughly 200 ms, N2, are referred to as *endogenous* in nature. Sutton et al. (1965) presented subjects with trains of one of two stimuli (light flashes or tone pips) in sequence. The subject had to guess what the next stimulus would be. Stimuli presented subsequent to the guess elicited the previously undescribed potentials, N2 and P3. Sutton et al. argued that the N2 and P3 potentials reflected the cognitive processes involved with the uncertainty of their guessing task.

Later research established that noncognitive stimulus factors were important in N2 and P3 generation. Tueting, Sutton, and Zubin (1971) demonstrated that low probability of occurrence of one of the two stimuli was a crucial factor. Squires, Wickens, Squires, and Donchin (1976) demonstrated that even with low a priori probability, high local probabilities (i.e., long sequences of targets without interspersed standards) would reduce P3, even with active target detection by the subject. Donchin (1981) suggested that P3 amplitude was a function of two factors: *subjective probability* of the target stimulus and *task relevance* of the stimulus. Johnson (1986) further defined dimensions involved in P3 generation and identified three main factors in his triarchic model of P3 amplitude: *subjective probability, stimulus meaning*, and *information transmission*. P3 generation can be considered a function of *externally* and *internally determined information*. Externally determined information resides in the stimulus pattern, namely subjective probability and, partly, information transmission (e.g., degraded stimuli are ambiguous). Internally determined information resides in the cognitive operations of the subject, namely stimulus meaning (how the stimuli relate to task instructions) and information transmission (whether the requisite information is extracted from the stimulus by the subject).

Because of the large effect of probability, N2 and P3 are typically evoked using the *oddball paradigm*, wherein a subject must detect, either by pressing a button or mentally counting, a deviant target stimulus in a train of standard stimuli. P3 is generally associated with the mental counting aspect of the task and is typically used as a probe of *selective attention*, that is, the conscious allocation of volitional attention, or in Johnson's (1986) scheme, *internally determined information*. In general, if a subject is presented tones in a "counting" condition, the attended oddball will evoke N2 and P3. If the subject is presented the same tones in an "ignore" condition, the nonattended oddball will not evoke N2 and P3. This suggests that the internally determined factors in P3 generation are more important than the externally determined information factors. However, if the oddball stimuli are sufficiently intrusive (e.g., loud), N2 and P3 will be evoked, even if the subject is not actively detecting them. For example, Polich (1989) presented subjects with blocks of 10 tones. The 7th, 8th, 9th, or 10th tone of the sequence was a deviant. Deviant tones elicited P3, even when subjects daydreamed or did a word-finding puzzle. N. K. Squires ascribed a passively evoked P3 to highly discrepant oddball stimuli. The oddball tones elicited P3, even when subjects were reading a book. The demonstration that P3 can be evoked when subjects are not attending the tones, or are actively engaged in another task, suggests that attention to the task is not crucial for N2–P3 generation. That is, attention to task may enhance N2–P3 amplitudes, but it may be unnecessary for engaging the processes reflected in N2–P3. If so, this effect suggests that externally determined information in the stimulus pattern is more important in P3 generation than internal factors. Perhaps N2–P3 activation with passive paradigms reflects an orienting response with subsequent passive drawing of the subject's selective attention to the intrusive stimulus. In this case, selective attention would still be necessary for eliciting N2–P3, and internal factors once again take precedence over external factors. Alternatively, N2 and P3 may reflect an automatic orienting response to highly deviant stimuli, and the attention effects may reflect an overallocation of attentional resources. Externally determined information may be all that is necessary for N2–P3 generation, but selective attention, when directed to the stimulus pattern, may allow for greater sensitivity. One way to examine whether the passively elicited P3 is automatic or controlled and secondary to an orienting response is to present subjects with passive paradigms while they are asleep, when active, conscious counting of oddball stimuli does not occur.

During sleep, the ERP is dominated by a large negative potential and a large positive potential. These waves reflect the slow potential of the K-complex but have been interpreted as large increases in the amplitude and latency of N2 and P3. It is doubtful that these potentials are truly analogous with the N2 and P3 evoked in the awake subject for a number of reasons: They appear during sleep as repetitive stimuli, their latencies are longer and amplitudes disproportionately larger, and they have different scalp distributions. We term these large, frontally distributed sleep waves *N3* and *P4*. There have been reports of two different negative waves that overlap during sleep (e.g., Weitzman & Kremen, 1965). Recently, Ujszászi and Halász (1986, 1988) examined this biphasic negative event during sleep and concluded that the earlier peak (at roughly 350 ms) might be an analogue of the N2 seen in awake subjects, whereas the later negative peak (at roughly 500 ms) reflected the slow component of the K-complex (N3). Similarly, there may be two different positive potentials in the long-latency range during sleep: one with a latency of roughly 400 ms, which may be analogous to the P3 seen in awake subjects, and another large positive wave with a latency of 900 ms, presumably reflecting K complex activity. The possibility arises that the N2–P3 complex seen in the awake subject may in fact be evoked during sleep, which would suggest that this complex reflects an automatic orienting process but is superimposed on the slow component of the K-complex, a sleep-specific response. Two different processes may be activated during sleep after P2. One is the same as that in awake subjects and generates N2 and P3. The other is the sleep-specific K-complex, which generates a large negative and a large positive potential (termed here *N3* and *P4*). These two different processes would be "smeared" together in the ERP average.

THE TWO-SYSTEM HYPOTHESIS

The two-system hypothesis proposes that two processes are evoked by stimulation during non-rapid eye movement (NREM) sleep. The morphology of the ERP evoked during sleep can be explained by the arithmetic summation of the distinct activity of these two systems. This hypothesis is graphically presented in Figure 2. If the activity of the awake ERP with an N2–P3 complex is superimposed on the activity of the sleep-specific K-complex system, comprising one large negative po-

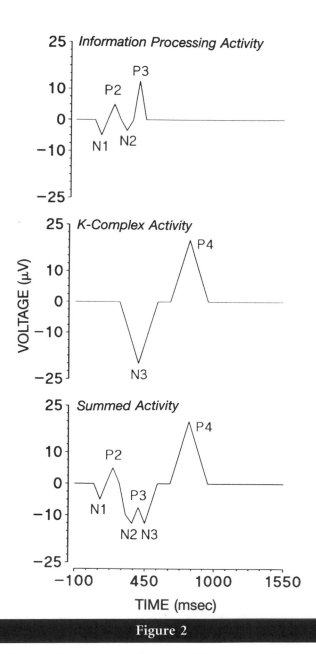

Figure 2

Schematic diagram of the two-system hypothesis. When auditory information analysis signals overlap with K-complex activity, the result is a biphasic negative wave, with artifactual decrease in N3 amplitude and increase in N3 latency.

tential and one large positive deflection, the result is a waveform similar to that of the sleep ERP, namely a biphasic negative peak in the long-latency range. A second observation is that the latency of the negative slow component of the K-complex is artifactually prolonged when there is simultaneous N2–P3 activity. This is a result of the positive activity of P3 reducing the negative activity of N3 when both are active.

THE ODDBALL PARADIGM DURING SLEEP

To examine whether the N2–P3 complex could be evoked during sleep and dissociated from the K-complex, Nancy K. Squires and I, along with Stu Ibel and Tom Maloney, tested sleeping subjects with the paradigm described above, which evoked N2 and P3 in awake subjects during nonattending conditions. The tones used were extremely disparate in both frequency (pitch) and intensity (loudness). The standard tone, presented 90% of the time, was 250 Hz, 40 dB normal hearing level (NHL), whereas the target (oddball) tone, presented 10% of the time, was 3 kHz, 60 dB NHL. Even when awake subjects read and ignored the tones, N2 and P3 were evoked, albeit of smaller amplitude than when targets were actively detected.

The difference in the physical characteristics of the stimuli used in nonattending tasks is crucial for evoking N2 and P3 in awake subjects when their attention is not focused on the tones. Presumably, differences in stimulus characteristics are also crucial during sleep, which seems more logically analogous to an awake nonattending state than an awake attending state. Obviously, one cannot count rare tones while asleep, although the tones might wake one up. There are low-level cognitive mechanisms monitoring the environment during sleep, but information about the environment is not processed by the higher order perceptual mechanisms associated with waking consciousness.

Other researchers have also tried to elicit N2 and P3 during sleep using oddball paradigms, but most of those studies used stimuli that were not highly disparate and would not evoke N2 and P3 in awake subjects unless they were actively counting the target stimuli. For instance, Paavilainen et al. (1987) presented 1000-Hz standard tones and 1050-Hz target tones at 75 dB. They were unable to detect any long-latency components during sleep. Similarly, Harsh, Voss, Hull, Schrepfer, and Badia (1994) reported the absence of the N2–P3 complex during Stage 2 sleep when subjects were presented 1500-Hz targets interspersed among 1000-Hz standards. Using an even wider pitch separation, Dijk (1990) presented 1-kHz standard tones and 2-kHz targets. Even at this level of stimulus disparity, N2 and P3 were not observed in sleeping subjects. However, using the highly disparate stimuli previously described, our group was able to detect fairly well defined N2–P3 complexes during Stage 2 sleep (Salisbury, Squires, & Ibel, 1992; Salisbury, Squires, Ibel, & Maloney, 1992). Examples of these waveforms are presented in Figure 3. A positive potential with similar latency

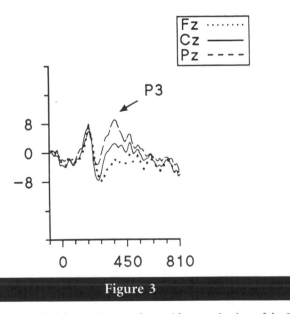

Figure 3

N2 and P3 potentials evoked during Stage 2 sleep without activation of the K-complex. Average of 20 evoked responses to low-probability, highly disparate oddball tone from 1 subject.

and amplitude distribution as the P3 seen in awake subjects can be observed during sleep without activation of the K-complex.

K-Complex Entrainment

One of the most striking effects of using two-tone oddball paradigms during sleep is K-complex entrainment. Because most studies of K-complex behavior used one repetitious tone, this probability sensitivity of the K-complex remained unknown. This effect was reported by Salisbury, Squires, and Ibel (1992), Salisbury, Squires, Ibel, and Maloney (1992), and Dijk (1990) and is illustrated in Figure 4. In Panel A, K-complexes can be observed in the raw EEG when oddball stimuli are presented but are not evoked by the standard stimuli. When stimuli of unequal probability are presented during sleep, the K-complex will fire only to the rarer of the stimuli. This effect has potentially great ramifications, particularly for evoked response audiometry (ERA), in that sleep audiometry was abandoned largely due to the variability of the K-complex to repetitious tones. For example, Osterhammel, Davis, Wier, and Hirsh (1973) measured thresholds to different-frequency tone pips while subjects were awake and then presented pips during sleep. Whereas the ERPs in awake subjects typically showed vertex potentials within 10 dB of threshold, the sleep records were quite different. The sensory potentials were smaller, and the most prominent potentials were the K-complex. The sleep waveforms were highly variable, with highly unreliable patterns in the long-latency ranges. The authors advised clinicians to perform ERA in awake subjects. As demonstrated in Figure 4, Panel B, electrical responses during sleep to the standard, high-probability stimulus contain very little N2 and P3 or K-complex activity. We suspect that these stable responses are excellent candidates for sleep audiometry.

Stimulus Parameter Effects

Because N2 and P3 could be evoked sporadically during sleep without K-complex contamination using highly disparate stimuli, we were in-

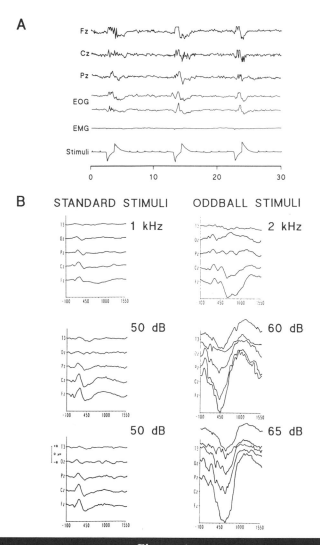

Figure 4

(A) When oddball, but not standard, stimuli are presented to the sleeping subject (larger notches in the stimuli trace), K-complexes are elicited. Note that time is in seconds. EOG = electrooculogram, EMG = electromyogram. (B) K-complex entrainment is also evident in the averaged responses. Responses to the frequently presented standard stimuli show little K-complex contamination. Responses to the oddball stimuli show K-complex activity. Note that time is in milliseconds, responses reflect averages from individual subjects, and there were approximately 180 standard stimuli and 20 rare stimuli in each pair.

terested in testing whether we could find a level of disparity that could more reliably evoke N2 and P3, but not the K-complex, and whether the N2–P3 complex could be evoked during Stage 4 sleep. Ujszászi and Halász (1986, 1988) had demonstrated that N350 (the putative N2 analogue) and N500 (the K-complex potential) responded differently to changes in stimulus intensity. We proposed that parametric manipulations of the disparity in pitch and loudness between the two tones in the oddball paradigm might identify a reliable difference when N2 and P3 were activated but the K-complex was not. Because the K-complex presumably reflects a mechanism associated with behavioral arousal from sleep, it is possible that there is a disparity threshold for engaging the arousal system that is greater than the disparity evoking the N2–P3 complex, in that arousal and loss of sleep are consequences of activation of the K-complex system.

N2 and P3 could be evoked in individual subjects during Stage 2 and Stage 4 sleep without K-complex activation. These potentials show a posterior distribution like the P3 seen in awake subjects and are presented in Figure 5. Grand averaged responses, averaged across subjects, are presented in Figure 6. Although we could not identify a disparity level where the K-complex was not activated, we were able to demonstrate that the K-complex was sensitive to stimulus parameters and was larger and earlier during Stage 4. The results of these parametric manipulations, namely a larger and earlier N2–P3 complex in Stage 2 and a larger and earlier K-complex in Stage 4, are predicted by the two-system model, which may explain the variable morphology of the ERP during sleep.

SUMMARY

Our data suggest that a high degree of information processing occurs during NREM, as reflected in N2 and P3. Furthermore, the demonstration that N2 and P3 can be evoked at all in the sleeping subject suggests that the processes reflected by these ERPs, although modifiable

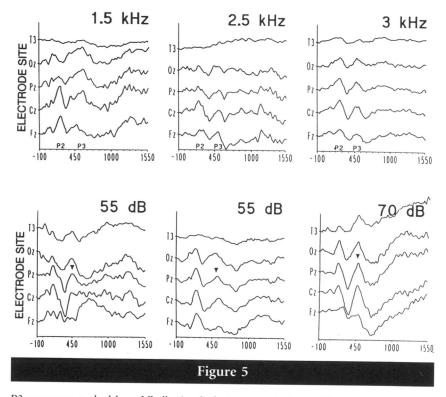

Figure 5

P3 responses evoked by oddball stimuli during stage 2 sleep without K-complex activation. Top three traces reflect averaged oddball response from individual subjects to a tone pitched differently from a 1-kHz standard. P2 and P3 are labeled. Note that P3 is larger posteriorly. Lower three traces reflect averaged oddball response from individual subjects to a tone louder than a 50-dB standard. Arrowheads indicate P3 at parietal electrode site.

by active selective attention, are in themselves automatic in nature. In Johnson's (1986) terminology, externally determined information is all that is necessary for the generation of N2 and P3, provided that the stimuli are sufficiently disparate. Cognitive mechanisms may provide for greater sensitivity (i.e., larger P3 amplitude to smaller stimulus differences) but may not be necessary for generating P3.

The two-system hypothesis also explains some of the variability of the responses during sleep reported in earlier studies. The presence of

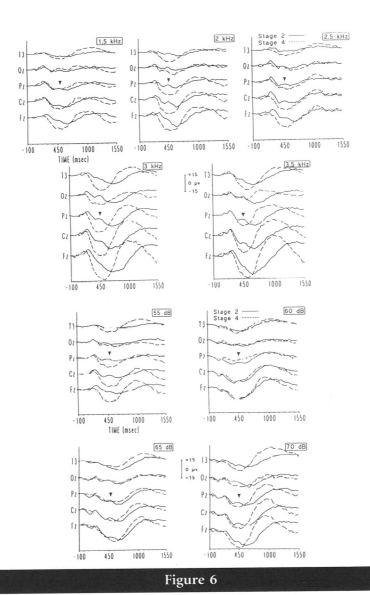

Figure 6

Grand averaged responses, collapsed across all subjects, during Stages 2 and 4 of sleep. Top five traces reflect grand averaged responses to oddball stimuli pitched differently from a 1-kHz standard. Bottom four traces reflect grand averaged responses to oddball tones louder than a 50-dB standard. Arrowheads in all traces point to small P3 potential. Note that P3 appears in Stage 2 but is virtually absent in Stage 4 and that the slow component of the K-complex (N3) has a shortened latency and larger amplitude in Stage 4.

two separate systems simultaneously active and with different response properties would lead to great variability in different studies that use different methodologies. Future examination of the sleep ERP must take into account the differential activation of the evoked electrical responses, which presumably reflects the differential activation of two dissimilar systems.

In summary, activity from two separate systems can be elicited during NREM sleep: One reflects information processing remarkably similar to the potentials seen in the awake subject; the other reflects the K-complex. These systems are generally activated simultaneously, but through the use of multistimulus tasks, they can be demonstrated to have different response properties.

The presence of N2 and P3 in NREM sleep suggests that the sleeping brain can process information to a high degree, with information reaching tertiary cortical and limbic areas. On the other hand, the presence of N2 and P3 in sleep suggests that the processes reflected in N2 and P3 may be somewhat more automatic than previously suspected and, as such, may not be true markers of the highest levels of cognitive–perceptual mechanisms.

REFERENCES

Amadeo, M., & Shagass, C. (1973). Brief latency click evoked potentials during waking and sleep in man. *Psychophysiology, 10,* 244–250.

Campbell, K., & Bartoli, E. (1986). Human auditory evoked potentials during natural sleep: The early components. *Electroencephalography and Clinical Neurophysiology, 65,* 142–149.

Dijk, J. G. van (1990). Auditory event-related potentials using an oddball paradigm during sleep. In A. M. L. Coenen (Ed.), *Sleep/wake research in the Netherlands* (p. 31). Leiden, The Netherlands: Dutch Society for Sleep/Wake Research.

Erwin, R., & Buchwald, J. (1986). Midlatency auditory evoked responses: Differential effects of sleep in the human. *Electroencephalography and Clinical Neurophysiology, 65,* 383–392.

Frühstorfer, H., & Bergström, R. (1969). Human vigilance and the auditory evoked responses. *Electroencephalography and Clinical Neurophysiology, 27,* 346–355.

Harsh, J., Voss, U., Hull, J., Schrepfer, S., & Badia, P. (1994). ERP and behavioral changes during the wake/sleep transition. *Psychophysiology, 31*, 244–252.

Jewett, D., & Williston, J. (1971). Auditory-evoked far fields averaged from the scalp of humans. *Brain, 94*, 681–696.

Johnson, R. (1986). A triarchic model of P3 amplitude. *Psychophysiology, 23*, 367–384.

Kevanishvili, Z., & Von Specht, H. (1979). Human slow auditory evoked potentials during natural and drug-induced sleep. *Electroencephalography and Clinical Neurophysiology, 47*, 280–288.

Mendel, M., Hosick, E., Windman, T., Davis, H., Hirsh, S., & Dinges, D. (1975). Audiometric comparison of the middle and late components of the adult auditory evoked potentials awake and asleep. *Electroencephalography and Clinical Neurophysiology, 38*, 27–33.

Möcks, J., Gasser, T., & Köhler, W. (1988). Basic statistical parameters of event-related potentials. *Journal of Psychophysiology, 2*, 61–70.

Nielsen-Bohlman, L., Knight, R., Woods, D., & Woodward, K. (1991). Differential auditory processing continues during sleep. *Electroencephalography and Clinical Neurophysiology, 79*, 281–290.

Osterhammel, P., Davis, H., Wier, C., & Hirsh, S. (1973). Adult auditory evoked vertex potentials in sleep. *Audiology, 12*, 116–128.

Paavilainen, P., Cammann, K., Alho, K., Reinikainen, K., Sams, M., & Näätänen, R. (1987). Event-related potentials to pitch changes in an auditory stimulus sequence during sleep. *Electroencephalography and Clinical Neurophysiology, 40*, 246–254.

Picton, T., Hillyard, S., Krause, H., & Galambos, R. (1974). Human auditory evoked potentials: I. Evaluation of components. *Electroencephalography and Clinical Neurophysiology, 36*, 179–190.

Picton, T., & Hink, R. (1974). Evoked potentials: How? What? and Why? *American Journal of EEG Technology, 14*, 9–40.

Polich, J. (1989). P300 from a passive auditory paradigm. *Electroencephalography and Clinical Neurophysiology, 74*, 312–320.

Regan, D. (1989). *Human brain electrophysiology: Evoked-potentials and evoked magnetic fields in science and medicine*. New York: Elsevier.

Salisbury, D., Squires, N. K., & Ibel, S. (1992). A P300-like potential evoked during sleep. *International Journal of Neuroscience, 63*, 242.

Salisbury, D., Squires, N. K., Ibel, S., & Maloney, T. (1992). Auditory event-related potentials during Stage 2 NREM sleep in humans. *Journal of Sleep Research*, *1*, 251–257.

Squires, K. C., Wickens, C., Squires, N. K., & Donchin, E. (1976). The effect of stimulus sequence on the waveform of the cortical event-related potential. *Science*, *193*, 1142–1146.

Sutton, S., Braren, M., Zubin, J., & John, E. R. (1965). Evoked potential correlates of stimulus uncertainty. *Science*, *150*, 1187–1188.

Tueting, P., Sutton, S., & Zubin, J. (1971). Quantitative evoked potential correlates of the probability of events. *Psychophysiology*, *7*, 385–394.

Ujszászi, J., & Halász, P. (1986). Late component variants of single auditory evoked responses during NREM Sleep Stage 2 in man. *Electroencephalography and Clinical Neurophysiology*, *64*, 260–268.

Ujszászi, J., & Halász, P. (1988). Long latency evoked potential components in human slow wave sleep. *Electroencephalography and Clinical Neurophysiology*, *69*, 516–522.

Weitzman, E., & Kremen, H. (1965). Auditory evoked responses during different stages of sleep in man. *Electroencephalography and Clinical Neurophysiology*, *18*, 65–70.

Williams, H., Tepas, D., & Morlock, H. (1962). Evoked responses to clicks and electroencephalographic stages of sleep in man. *Science*, *138*, 685–686.

Williamson, S., & Kaufman, L. (1990). Theory of neuroelectric and neuromagnetic fields. In F. Grandori, M. Hoke, & G. Romani (Eds.), *Auditory evoked magnetic fields and electric potentials* (pp. 1–39). Basel, Switzerland: Karger.

18

Event-Related Potential Changes During the Wake-to-Sleep Transition

John R. Harsh

Phasic changes in electroencephalographic (EEG) activity recorded on the human scalp in the first few hundred milliseconds following a stimulus event are related to the physical and to the psychological characteristics of the event and also to the state of the subject. The electrical signals are sometimes less than one microvolt in amplitude but can be resolved using signal-averaging techniques. The averaged signal consists of a series of positive and negative peaks (components) that are designated often by their polarities and peak latencies and also possess characteristic scalp distribution and morphology. The components of most interest to psychologists are referred to as *event-related potentials (ERPs)* because of their sensitivity to the psychological, as opposed to the physical, characteristics of an event. Because ERPs reflect central processes and can be recorded without requiring behavioral responses, they can be used in the study of information processing in states of reduced behavioral responsiveness, such as during sleepiness and sleep (see Campbell, Bell, & Bastien, 1992; Kutas, 1990).

This research was supported in part by US Army contract DAMD17-84-C-8016 34125.

The emphasis of this chapter is on sleep-related changes in components of ERPs known as P300 (also known as P3) and N350. The P300 is a probe of selective attention. It is studied most often in alert subjects and is thought to reflect specific cognitive events in the attention-dependent processing of task-relevant stimuli (e.g., Donchin, Karis, Bashore, Coles, & Gratton, 1986). The few studies of the effects of sleep on P300 have produced mixed results. Some investigators report that P300 disappears during sleep (e.g., Campbell et al., 1992); others report that P300 can be found in sleep (e.g., Bastuji, Garcia-Larrea, Franc, & Mauguiere, 1990; Nielsen-Bohlman, Knight, Woods, & Woodward, 1992; Salisbury, Chapter 17, this volume; Salisbury, Squires, Ibel, & Maloney, 1992; Wesensten & Badia, 1988).

The N350 is a prominent negative-going waveform that appears in association with sleepiness and sleep (e.g., Campbell et al., 1992; Ornitz, Ritvo, Carr, LaFranci, & Walter, 1967). This component is less well understood than P300. It is presumably a variant of vertex waves described as occurring in deep drowsiness (Niedermeyer, 1987). The N350 was chosen for analysis here because of its relationship to sleep onset, because it may reflect information processing (Campbell et al., 1992; Ujszászi & Halász, 1988), and because it has maximum amplitude in the same period as P300 and, thus, may be associated with the sleep-related changes in P300.

The research to be described had two main objectives. The first was to document P300 changes during the sleep-onset period using a research protocol allowing a description of P300 variation related to sleep onset as indexed by sleep stage, reduced behavioral responsiveness, and the emergence of the sleep-related N350 waveform. The second was to assess cognitive and behavioral factors related to N350. The protocol involved first collecting behavioral and ERP data from fully awake subjects performing an oddball task. Additional data were then collected following instructions to the subjects to continue performing the task but to allow themselves to go to sleep. Manipulation of task and subject variables permitted the comparison of relationships obtained in wakefulness with those obtained during sleepiness and sleep.

P300 IN WAKEFULNESS AND SLEEP

Key Determinants of P300 in Awake Subjects

The P300 is typically studied using a task involving serial presentation of two brief visual or auditory stimuli, with one stimulus presented less frequently than the other. Subjects are instructed to respond to or to count the occurrences of the oddball or target stimuli. Conclusions about the close link between the P300 and information processing are based on ERP data collected as instructional set and task features are varied while subject state is held constant. Figures 1 and 2 illustrate important and well-known relationships. These data were obtained from sleep-deprived but awake subjects tested in our laboratory (Harsh, Voss, Hull, Schrepfer, & Badia, 1994; Hull & Harsh, 1994b). Shown in Figure 1 are grand averages of 1,350-ms EEG recordings beginning 150 ms prior to rare target and frequent nontarget stimuli. Subjects in the attend condition ($n = 7$) were instructed to signal the occurrence of the target with a fingerlift response. Subjects in the ignore condition ($n = 8$) were presented the same stimulus sequence but with instructions to ignore the stimuli. The stimuli were high- and low-pitched 45-ms pure tones (60 dB) presented 2 s apart in a Bernoulli sequence with the probability of the rare stimulus equal to .2 ($p = .2$). Stimuli were presented to each subject while awake and sitting in a chair until a total of 25 target stimuli had been delivered. Figure 1 shows that P300 is a prominent positivity at the parietal recording site and that maximum P300 amplitude occurs some 300 ms after onset of the rare target stimulus when subjects attend but not when they ignore the stimulus events (cf. Duncan-Johnson & Donchin, 1977).

Figure 2 shows that P300 is dependent on both the task relevance and the probability of a stimulus event. These data were also obtained using an oddball task (Hull & Harsh, 1994b). The subjects ($n = 10$) were tested three times, once with target probability of .2 (probability of the nontarget stimulus was .8), once with target probability of .5 (nontarget probability was also .5), and once with target probability of

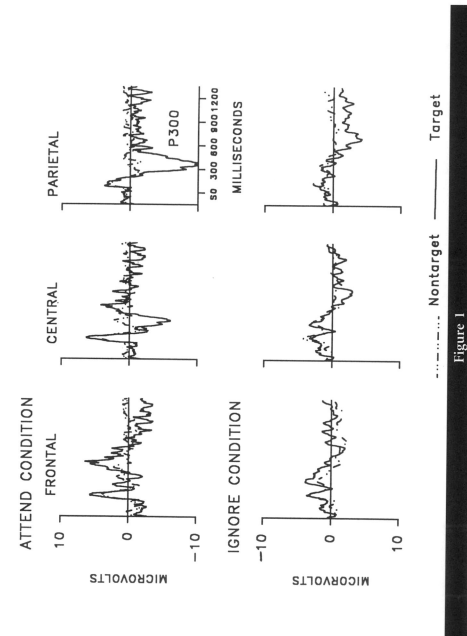

Grand ERP averages recorded at Fz, Cz, and Pz following target ($p = .20$) and nontarget ($p = .80$) stimuli. Subjects were awake and were instructed to lift their finger in response to targets (attend condition) or instructed to ignore the stimuli (ignore condition)

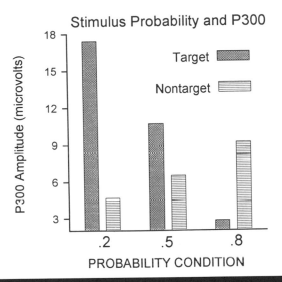

Figure 2

Mean amplitude of P300 following both target and nontarget stimuli from subjects tested under three target probability conditions. Target probabilities of .2, .5, and .8 resulted in nontarget probabilities of .8, .5, and .2.

.8 (nontarget probability was .2). As shown, the P300 was maximal following the stimulus with the lowest probability, whether the stimulus was designated as target or nontarget. When target and nontarget probabilities were the same (the .5 condition), P300 was again largest following the target. The findings shown in these two figures establish that P300 in these studies is an attention-dependent, parietally maximal positivity that is inversely related to stimulus probability and directly related to task relevance (cf. Duncan-Johnson & Donchin, 1977).

P300 During the Wake-to-Sleep Transition

We examined changes in P300 in relation to the EEG and behavioral changes that occur as subjects move from alert wakefulness to sleep. Subjects whose data are shown in Figures 1 and 2 were tested while lying in bed after being told to continue to lift their finger to target stimuli but not to fight off sleep. (The subjects were tested in afternoon naps following 2- to 3-hr reduction in sleep the prior night.)

Figure 3 contains grand-average ERPs in relation to stages of sleep. Averages at Fz, Cz, and Pz for target and nontarget stimuli are presented for Stage Awake, Stage 1A (50–80% alpha), Stage 1B (conventional Stage 1), Stage 2A (first 5 min of Stage 2) and Stage 2B (first 5 min of Stage 2, preceded by 5 min of uninterrupted Stage 2). Sleep stages were scored for 30-s EEG epochs. Each subject was presented a minimum of 15 target stimuli. As can be seen, the P300 was smaller in Stage 1B sleep and not evident in Stages 2A and 2B sleep. These data were obtained from the attend condition of the Harsh et al. (1994) study. Similar findings were reported by Hull and Harsh (1994b), with target stimulus probabilities of .2, .5, and .8. This outcome suggests that P300 is dependent on the subjects maintaining wakefulness.

It is also apparent from Figure 3 that in late Stage 1 and Stage 2 sleep, there is a marked change in ERP morphology. There are several peaks in the sleep-related ERP, and peak amplitudes are sometimes much higher than in wakefulness. We have labelled the peaks of the sleep-related ERP according to their polarity and approximate latency (see bottom left of Figure 3).

Inspection of individual subject averages and individual trials (sweeps) indicated that the transition from an ERP dominated by a parietal P300 to the sleep-related ERP was closely tied to behavioral responding. Figure 4 describes data obtained from a subject who responded either quickly or not at all and who stopped responding, but then restarted several (nine) times during the transition to sleep. This pattern of responding permitted averaging ERPs before and after response cessation. Shown on the left side of Figure 4 are averaged ERPs for target presentations, resulting in a behavioral response, that were followed by target presentations not resulting in a behavioral response. The averaged ERPs for the latter are shown on the right side of the figure. It can be seen that the change in ERP morphology was related to behavioral response cessation. For this and other subjects, an ERP

ATTEND CONDITION

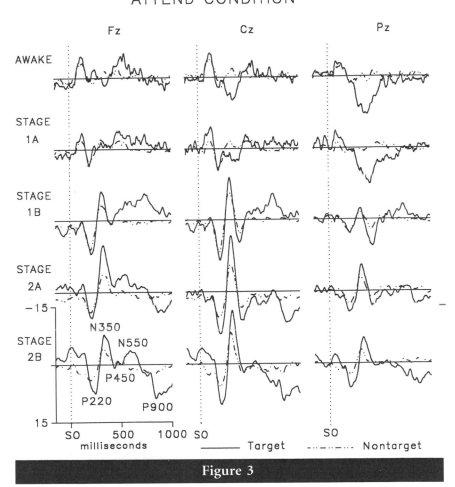

Figure 3

Grand ERP averages recorded at Fz, Cz, and Pz under the attend condition during Stage Awake and each sleep stage (SO = stimulus onset). (Adapted from Harsh et al., 1994.)

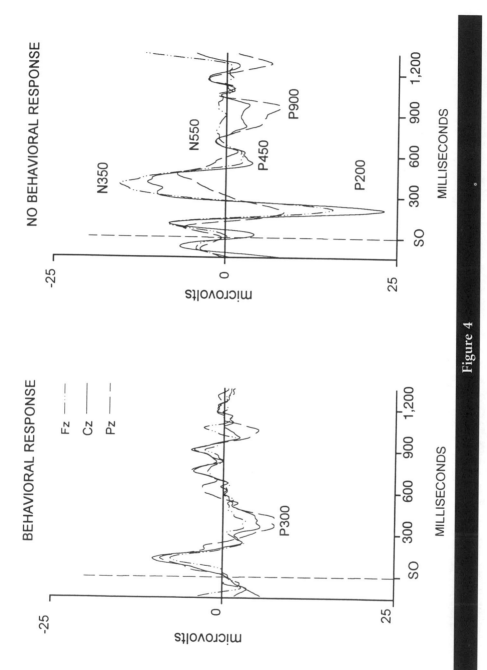

Figure 4

Averaged ERPs (one subject) for targets resulting in behavioral responses (left) that were followed by targets not resulting in behavioral responses (average on right) (SO = stimulus onset).

dominated by parietal P300 followed targets accompanied by short latency responses, and the sleep-related ERP was evident whenever responding failed to occur. For subjects whose responding ceased gradually rather than suddenly, intermediate response latencies resulted in an ERP that appeared to be a composite of the P300 and sleep-related ERP (see Harsh et al., 1994; cf. Ogilvie, Simons, Kuderian, MacDonald, & Rustenburg, 1991).

The finding that disappearance of the P300 coincided closely with emergence of the sleep-related ERP raises an important measurement issue; that is, the sleep-related changes in P300 might be attributable, in part or entirely, to emergence of sleep-related potentials in the same time frame. The processes underlying P300 may be activated in sleep, but the cortical manifestation of this activity may be different. One of the ways to address this possibility is by identifying the determinants of the components of the sleep ERP.

Our own analysis (Harsh et al., 1994; Hull & Harsh, 1994b) suggests that the sleep positivities P220, P450, and P900 seen in Figure 3 cannot be taken for P300. In addition to having different morphology and scalp distribution (they are frontal or frontocentral as opposed to parietal), these positivities (a) could be seen following both target and nontarget stimuli, (b) were not dependent on instructions to attend to the stimuli, or (c) had amplitudes inversely related to task relevance (the opposite relationship is found for P300). The last piece of evidence seems to be the most critical. To conclude that a waveform in sleep reflects the same processes as P300 in wakefulness would seem to require, at minimum, evidence that the sleep waveform is sensitive to the same variables (especially task relevance and stimulus probability) as the waking P300.

Is There a P300 in Sleep?

Analysis of our data provided no evidence of P300 in established (Stage 2) sleep. Other laboratories have also reported diminished P300 amplitude with sleepiness (Aguirre & Broughton, 1987; Harsh & Badia, 1989) and absent P300 in NREM sleep (Bastuji et al., 1990; Campbell et al., 1992). It is not yet clear how these findings are to be reconciled with those of investigators who report P300 in sleep (Nielsen-Bohlman et al., 1992; Salisbury, chapter 17, this volume; Salisbury et al., 1992; Wesensten & Badia, 1988). Our conclusions are based on data obtained from subjects performing a routine task while going into NREM sleep. It may be that P300 is present in NREM sleep when especially intrusive stimuli are used (see Salisbury, chapter 17, this volume). The P300 may be present in REM sleep (cf. Bastuji et al., 1990). A further possibility is that positivities being described as P300 are actually instances of waveforms described here as P220, P450, and P900. These waveforms may reflect more elemental, noncognitive processes as opposed to the higher order processing associated with P300 (Donchin et al., 1986). Further study is needed of the sleep-related changes in P300 and the implications of these changes for cognitive and behavioral events.

SLEEP-RELATED ERPs: N350

The nomenclature used to describe sleep-related ERPs varies considerably. In our research, N350 refers to the maximum negativity occurring between 250 and 450 ms following onset of a stimulus presented during the transition from wakefulness to sleep. The N350 has an unknown relationship with the processing negativities studied in alert wakefulness and is different from, but may be related to, the frontal negativity associated with the K-complex (Campbell et al., 1992; Ujszászi & Halász, 1986).

Earlier research has shown N350 to have constant morphology and scalp distribution (maximal at Cz) across stimulus modalities (e.g., Goff, Allison, Shapiro, & Rosner, 1966; Williams, Tepas, & Morlock, 1962). It is a potential that emerges after repetitive presentation of simple stimuli (e.g., Williams et al., 1962) and is, thus, not dependent on a stimulus being novel, task relevant, or behaviorally significant. Ornitz et al. (1967) found this negativity to be maximal near sleep onset. Our data (see Figures 3 and 4) indicate that, for subjects performing a behavioral task, N350 emerges in association with diminished P300 and reduced behavioral responsiveness. Taken together, these observations suggest that N350 is an index of a general process activated following stimulus detection at or near sleep onset that is related closely to diminished cognitive and behavioral functioning. It seems reasonable to consider that N350 reflects tonic or phasic inhibitory mechanisms that reduce a drowsy individual's ability to process stimulus-bound information and to initiate unlearned (orienting) or learned motor responses.

We examined the relationship between N350 and task variables to assess how the presumably general process reflected by N350 might be altered by information-processing activity. Figure 5 shows mean N350 amplitudes following target and nontarget stimuli presented in Stage Awake through Stage 2B. One group of subjects was instructed while awake to respond (fingerlift response) to targets but not to nontargets (attend condition). A second group of subjects was presented the same stimuli with instructions to ignore the stimuli (ignore condition). These are the attend/ignore groups for whom data on P300 are presented in Figure 1. It can be seen in Figure 5 that N350 was larger in the attend condition in Stages 1B, 2A, and 2B. This effect suggests that the characteristics of ERPs during sleep are related to presleep instructions, but do not necessarily indicate that N350 is altered by stimulus evaluation processes under the attend condition, because this condition may have resulted in a general increase in responsiveness to stimulation.

A more relevant finding shown in Figure 5 is that, under both the attend and ignore conditions during Stages 1B, 2A, and 2B, there was a larger N350 following the rare (target) relative to the frequent (nontarget) stimulus. This replicates and extends the work of Nielsen-Bohlman et al. (1991), who also demonstrated that N350 is sensitive to stimulus novelty. This provides evidence that the N350 is an index of, at least, a low level of information processing.

Examination of Figure 5 further reveals that the rare–frequent stimulus differences were larger under the attend relative to the ignore condition, suggesting an effect specific to task relevance. The effect was not statistically reliable, however. To pursue further the role of task relevance, we examined N350 under three conditions during which the

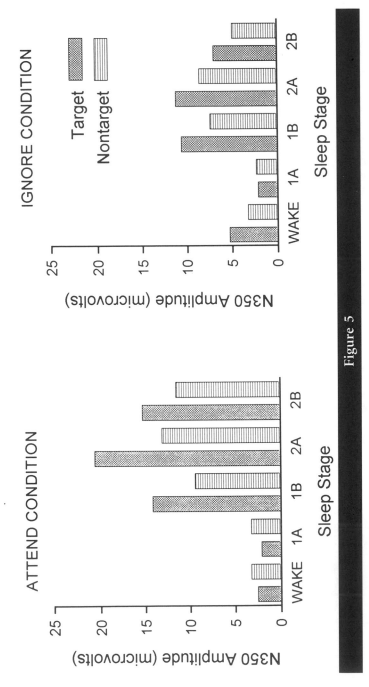

Figure 5

Mean N350 amplitudes following target and nontarget stimuli during the wake–sleep transition (see text) under attend and ignore conditions.

probability of the target and nontarget stimuli varied. Twelve subjects were tested with target probabilities of .2, .5, and .8 (nontarget probabilities for the three conditions were .8, .5, and .2, respectively). These are the conditions for which P300 data are presented in Figure 2. The N350 amplitude data obtained are shown in Figure 6. It can be seen that, as expected, the amplitude of N350 for both targets and nontargets was inversely related to stimulus probability. Rarer stimuli elicited larger N350s. With regard to the task-relevance effect, with equally probable targets and nontargets (the .5 condition), the N350 following the target was reliably smaller than following the nontarget. (Counterbalancing ruled out differences related to the physical characteristics of the experimental stimuli.) This outcome suggests that amplitude variations of the N350 component reflect higher order information processing in sleepiness and sleep.

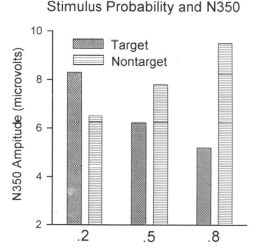

Figure 6

Mean amplitude of N350 following both target and nontarget stimuli from subjects tested under three target probability conditions. Target probabilities of .2, .5, and .8 resulted in nontarget probabilities of .8, .5, and .2.

Interestingly, the amplitudes of both N350 and P300 vary with stimulus rarity and task relevance. The inverse relationship between task relevance and N350 amplitude is, however, the opposite of the direct relationship found between task relevance and P300 amplitude (see Figure 2). This finding, and others reviewed earlier, make it evident that N350 and P300 involve different underlying mechanisms. The nature of these differences remains a matter of speculation; however, it would appear that P300 is a correlate of specific cognitive events, whereas N350 reflects a nonspecific process that is altered by activation of stimulus evaluation resources. Our interpretation is that N350 is a cortical manifestation of a general state of central inhibition that is prerequisite for the natural progression of sleep onset. Specifically, occurrence of the N350 reflects blocking of cortical activation (arousal) following stimulus presentation. Stimulus evaluation mechanisms determine the amount and timing of activation and also produce cortical potentials that cooccur with N350.

SUBJECT VARIABLES AND SLEEP-RELATED ERPS

The hypothesis that N350 reflects a mechanism that gates stimulus-related activation resulted in studies assessing subject differences in sleep ERPs. Voss and Harsh (1994) compared ERPs during the wake–sleep transition of subjects grouped by information-processing style. The Miller Behavioral Style Scale (Miller, 1987) was selected to identify groups of young adult subjects differing in coping strategies used in threatening settings. The scale assesses Monitoring, which describes sensitivity to threat-relevant information, and Blunting, which refers to the tendency to avoid or transform threat-relevant information. Behavioral and ERP data were recorded from eight subjects identified as high monitors and low blunters (Monitors) and eight subjects identified as low monitors and high blunters (Blunters). The experimental protocol was the same as that in the studies described earlier, except that the stimuli were equiprobable presentations of the subjects' own name, another name, and a neutral tone. The subjects were instructed to lift their finger whenever they heard their own name but to allow themselves to go to sleep. We predicted that Blunters would be better able to "block out" the experimental stimuli and would go to sleep more readily. This prediction was confirmed. Furthermore, as shown in the graph at the top of Figure 7, Blunters had reliably larger N350s during sleep. We suggested that these findings are consistent with the view that N350 reflects blocking of stimulus-related activation, an important process in the initiation of sleep.

One additional experiment to be reported also relates to the functional significance of N350. The graph at the bottom of Figure 7 presents data from an experiment by Hull and Harsh (1994a) involving Good sleepers (reported nightly sleep-onset latencies less than 5 min) and Poor sleepers (reported sleep-onset latencies greater than 30 min and reduced daytime functioning). The experimental protocol was the same as that in the studies described earlier. The findings were not so clear cut as those in the Voss and Harsh study; however, Poor sleepers did have reliably smaller N350 amplitudes in Stage 2B sleep. We concluded that the Poor sleepers' smaller N350 (and their sleep initiation difficulties) was due to their lesser ability to inhibit the activation resulting from stimuli presented during the sleep-onset period.

SUMMARY

The data presented here provide further understanding of the changes in ERPs that occur in relation to sleepiness and sleep. It would appear that the cognitive events reflected by P300 are not readily evoked during sleepiness and sleep. The close association between reduced behavioral responsiveness, the disappearance of P300, and the emergence of the sleep-related ERP suggests specific sleep-onset related processes that are actively linked to reduced cognitive and behavioral functioning.

The finding that the amplitude of the N350 component of sleep-related ERPs varies with stimulus novelty, task relevance, and personal

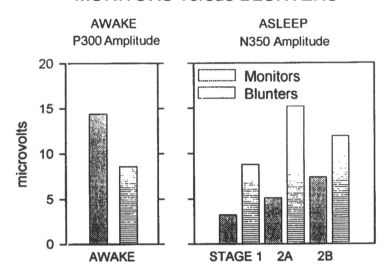

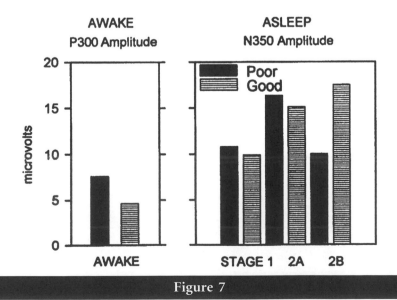

Figure 7

P300 amplitudes (awake) and N350 amplitudes (Stages 2A and 2B sleep) for Monitors and Blunters (top) and Good and Poor sleepers (bottom).

significance indicates the value of this measure as a tool for the study of information processing during sleep. Our hypothesis that N350 reflects an inhibitory process that is modulated by activation of stimulus evaluation resources is tentative but helps to organize existing data.

REFERENCES

Aguirre, M., & Broughton, R. J. (1987). Complex event-related potentials (P300 and CNV) and MSLT in the assessment of excessive daytime sleepiness in narcolepsy–cataplexy. *Electroencephalography and Clinical Neurophysiology, 67,* 298–316.

Bastuji, H., Garcia-Larrea, L., Franc, C., & Mauguiere, F. (1990). Sleep-related modifications of auditory cognitive potentials. In *Abstracts of the 10th Congress of the European Sleep Society,* 379.

Campbell, K., Bell, I., & Bastien, C. (1992). Evoked potential measures of information processing during natural sleep. In R. J. Broughton & R. D. Ogilvie (Eds.), *Sleep, arousal, and performance* (pp. 88–116). Boston: Birkhäuser.

Donchin, E., Karis, D., Bashore, T. R., Coles, M. G. H., & Gratton, G. (1986). Cognitive psychophysiology and human information processing. In M. G. H. Coles, E. Donchin, & S. W. Porges (Eds.), *Psychophysiology: Systems, processes, and applications* (pp. 244–267). New York: Guilford Press.

Duncan-Johnson, C. C., & Donchin, E. (1977). On quantifying surprise: The variation of event-related potentials with subjective probability. *Psychophysiology, 14,* 456–467.

Goff, W. R., Allison, T., Shapiro, A., & Rosner, B. S. (1966). Cerebral somatosensory responses evoked during sleep in man. *Electroencephalography and Clinical Neurophysiology, 21,* 1–9.

Harsh, J., & Badia, P. (1989). Auditory evoked potentials as a function of sleep deprivation. *Work and Stress, 3,* 79–91.

Harsh, J., Voss, U., Hull, J., Schrepfer, S., & Badia, P. (1994). ERP and behavioral changes during the wake–sleep transition. *Psychophysiology, 31,* 244–252.

Hull, J., & Harsh, J. (1994a). Behavioral and ERP changes during the transition to sleep in good and poor sleepers. Manuscript submitted for publication.

Hull, J., & Harsh, J. (1994b). ERP changes during the wake–sleep transition: Probability and task relevance effects. Manuscript submitted for publication.

Kutas, M. (1990). Event-related brain potential (ERP) studies of cognition during sleep: Is it more than a dream? In R. R. Bootzin, J. F. Kihlstrom, & D. L. Schacter (Eds.), *Sleep and cognition* (pp. 43–57). Washington, D.C.: American Psychological Association.

Miller, S. M. (1987). Monitoring and blunting: Validation of a questionnaire to assess styles of information seeking under threat. *Journal of Personality and Social Psychology, 52,* 345–353.

Niedermeyer, E. (1987). Sleep and EEG. In E. Niedermeyer and F. Lopes da Silva (Eds.), *Electroencephalography* (pp. 93–105). Baltimore: Urban & Schwarzenberg.

Nielsen-Bohlman, L., Knight, R. T., Woods, D. L., & Woodward, K. (1991). Differential auditory processing continues during sleep. *Electroencephalography and Clinical Neurophysiology, 79,* 281–290.

Ogilvie, R., Simons, I., Kuderian, R., MacDonald, T., & Rustenburg, J. (1991). Behavioral, event-related potential, and EEG–FFT changes at sleep onset. *Psychophysiology, 28,* 54–64.

Ornitz, E. M., Ritvo, E. R., Carr, E. M., LaFranci, S., & Walter, R. D. (1967). The effect of sleep onset on the auditory average evoked response. *Electroencephalography and Clinical Neurophysiology, 23,* 335–341.

Salisbury, D., Squires, N. K., Ibel, S., & Maloney, T. (1992). Auditory event-related potentials during Stage 2 NREM sleep in humans. *Journal of Sleep Research, 1,* 251–257.

Ujszászi, J., & Halász, P. (1986). Late component variants of single auditory evoked response during NREM sleep Stage 2 in man. *Electroencephalography and Clinical Neurophysiology, 64,* 260–268.

Ujszászi, J., & Halász, P. (1988). Long latency evoked potential components in human slow wave sleep. *Electroencephalography and Clinical Neurophysiology, 69,* 516–522.

Voss, U., & Harsh, J. (1994). Semantic processing during the transition from wakefulness to sleep in Monitors and Blunters. Manuscript submitted for publication.

Wesensten, N. J., & Badia, P. (1988). The P300 component in sleep. *Physiology and Behavior, 44,* 215–220.

Williams, H. L., Tepas, D. I., & Morlock, H. C. (1962). Evoked responses to clicks and EEG stages of sleep in man. *Science, 138,* 685–686.

19

Modification of the Multiple Sleep Latency Test

Paul Naitoh and Tamsin L. Kelly

A proper identification of sleep onset plays an important role in the diagnosis of sleep disorders. Sleep onset terminates a transitional state when wakefulness is being replaced by sleep. This switching from wakefulness to sleep takes a finite period of time, as suggested by the concept of a sleep-onset period (SOP; Ogilvie & Wilkinson, 1984). Earlier, Davis stated that sleep onset could not be located at one time point because the process of transition from wakefulness to sleep is continuous (Davis, Davis, Loomis, Harvey, & Hobart, 1937)

Sleep onset is not explicitly specified in the sleep-staging manuals (Agnew & Webb, 1972; Rechtschaffen & Kales, 1968). Most often, sleep onset is placed in a 30-s sleep-record epoch, in which the electroencephalographic (EEG) alpha activities appear in less than 50% of the epoch (i.e., Sleep Stage 1). In sleep medicine, sleep onset and sleep latency are usually determined by the Multiple Sleep Latency Test (MSLT), or "nap opportunity" test, to unmask underlying sleepiness. After all-night polysomnography, the patient lies on a bed in a quiet, dark room and is told to go to sleep or nap for 20 min. This nap test is repeated at 2-hr intervals beginning 1.5 to 3 hr after wake-up (Carskadon et al., 1986). For example, an initial session starting at 0930 hr is followed by five more tests at 2-hr intervals, with the last test at 1930 hr (Carskadon & Dement, 1992). Sometimes, the MSLT is given under the constant routine (Carskadon & Dement, 1992). All of these procedural cares in administering the MSLT are aimed at obtaining a reliable measure of sleep onset and of sleep latency. The test–retest reliability of the four-test MSLT was reported at the .97 level over 4- to 14-month test–retest intervals (Zwyghuizen-Doorenbos, Roehrs, Shaefer, & Roth, 1988). Such a high reliability is necessary in sleep medicine for the unambiguous diagnosis of pathological excessive sleepiness in patients, which is defined as a sleep-onset latency of less than 5 min. However, this 5-min criterion may need to be reevaluated as to its validity in light of the report of a group of normal, healthy, sleepy subjects whose sleep latency averaged 3.8 min (Roth, personal communication, June 13, 1993).

Sleep Stage 1 is critical in defining sleep onset in the MSLT (Carskadon & Dement, 1992; Carskadon et al., 1986; Roehrs & Roth, 1992). Richardson et al. (1978) defined sleep latency as the interval from the start of each MSLT to the first epoch of NREM (usually Stage 1 sleep) or REM sleep. In the latest proposal by the Standards of Practice Committee of the American Sleep Disorders Association (Roehrs & Roth, 1992; Thorpy, 1992), sleep onset for the MSLT was defined as the first 30-s epoch of any sleep stage, including Stage 1. Earlier in 1982, Mitler, Gujavarty, and Browman (1982) defined a research version of sleep onset in the MSLT as (a) three consecutive 30-s epochs of Sleep Stage 1 or (b) any single 30-s epoch of Sleep Stage 2, 3, 4, or REM. Both MSLT sleep-onset criteria differ from the typical definition of nocturnal sleep onset, using the first epoch of Stage 2 or of REM SOREMP (sleep-onset REM period). In our multiple 20-min nap study (Naitoh, Kelly, & Babkoff, 1992, 1993), we used Stage 2 as sleep onset because it offered clearer conservative signs of sleep. However, sleep onset can certainly be detected during Stage 1 (Hayashi, Morikawa, & Hori, 1989; Ogilvie, Wilkinson, & Allison, 1989).

Webb (chapter 4, this volume) enumerated many factors that could affect sleep onset and sleep latency. As Webb suggested, sleep latency will be affected by prior hours of wake–sleep, that is, by sleep demands (Carskadon & Dement, 1979, 1981). MSLT results are influenced by a circadian rhythm mechanism, as exemplified by core body temperature (Clodore, Benoit, Foret, & Bouard, 1990; Nakagawa, Sack, & Lewy, 1992; Richardson, Carskadon, Orav, & Dement, 1982). Although the circadian rhythm of the sleep–wake system can be internally desynchronized from that of core body temperature, suggesting that they have independent rhythmic mechanisms (Wever, 1979), sleep latency, sleep duration, and spontaneous awakening normally are highly circadian controlled (Czeisler, Zimmerman, Ronda, Moore-Ede, & Weizman, 1980; Winfree, 1983). More precisely, the MSLT can be described to show a circasemidian rhythm, exhibiting two distinct periods of increased sleepiness: one around the midafternoon and the other around very late night and early morning (Broughton, 1992; Gander, Graeber, Connell, & Gregory, 1991; Lavie & Shulamit, 1989). However, increased afternoon sleepiness may be absent in the preadolescent. This maturational, age-related exception (Carskadon, 1979; Carskadon & Dement, 1992) was that the 10- to 12-year-old preadolescents had optimal sleep, sleeping about 9 hr at night and, hence, had no increased tendency to fall asleep in the daytime.

Light, noise, and ambient temperature in a sleep room are other factors that can influence the MSLT, but they are controlled to create a soporific environment during the test. Recumbency, hunger, thirst, and other physiological states, such as fullness of bladder, can influence the MSLT. These physical and physiological conditions in patients are also controlled during the test. However, two behavioral components, attention–excitement–anxiety and learned ability to unmask sleepiness, appear to influence the results of the MSLT, yet they are mostly ignored and typically not controlled. This lack of control over the mental state before and during the MSLT appears to weaken the validity of the test as a measure of sleepiness. Wilkinson (1992) pointed out these methodological flaws in the MSLT.

We agree with Wilkinson and feel that the one methodological flaw is that the patient's mental state is assumed to be relaxed, sleepy, and free from worrying and compulsive thoughts because of the soporific physical environment created for the MSLT. This assumption may be reasonable for narcoleptics but may not be for others, for example, those who suffer from insomnia. A second methodological flaw is that the MSLT cannot distinguish the ability to fall asleep from degree of sleepiness. Some individuals have short sleep latencies, not necessarily because they are more sleepy, but because they have learned how to fall asleep quickly in any sleep environment.

In this chapter, we address the first flaw. In the MSLT, the decision was made to exclude all stimuli from the 20-min nap opportunity. All visual, auditory, and other stimuli were excluded during the MSLT because they were thought to interfere with the normal process of falling asleep. But this leaves no way to measure a patient's mental arousal state and, worse, no way to ensure that the arousal level during the MSLT is low across all patients.

Wilkinson (1992) argued that performance tasks could provide better measures of sleepiness than the MSLT because they controlled the mental state by "channeling mental activity into execution of task" (p. 257). We would argue that the combination of the MSLT procedure with a simple performance task might provide an optimal sleepiness measure and an attractive alternative to the current practice of leaving a patient to his or her own device, such as "counting sheep."

We propose that the MSLT be modified to include a simple, minimally arousing task to channel a patient's attention and to displace other mental activity that might cause excitement and anxiety. There are many tasks that would be suitable for channeling mental activity without causing undue arousal. Wilkinson (1992) discussed a variant of event-related potentials (ERPs), that is, contingent negative variation (CNV) as a psychophysiological measure of sleepiness, and we propose to incorporate the CNV into the MSLT. In a CNV paradigm, patients receive a warning "get ready" stimulus ($Stim_1$) followed shortly by another "go" stimulus ($Stim_2$) to which they are instructed to make a simple response. In the context of the MSLT, patients would be instructed to respond to $Stim_2$ as long as possible, but not to resist letting sleepiness take over.

The CNV paradigm offers an attractive option as a channeling task because, along with controlling the mental state, it provides additional measures of sleepiness and sleep onset during the MSLT. Unlike other evoked potentials techniques, the CNV paradigm provides a better time resolution because the CNV magnitude is relatively large and does not require averaging across many trials. Table 1 shows the results from six studies and one review article on sleepiness and CNV.

With the exception of the first two studies (Aguirre & Broughton, 1987; Broughton & Aguirre, 1987), the CNV has been uniformly found to be reduced by increased sleepiness. Figure 1 shows an example of the CNV from a subject in our studies published in 1971 and 1974. In these studies, subjects had a CNV session once in the morning of each experimental day. There were 4 baseline days (B_1, B_2, B_3, and B_4; B_1 and B_2 data are not shown), 2 days of total sleep loss (D_1 and D_2), 2 days of partial sleep recovery treatment (R_1 and R_2; not shown), and 2

Table 1

Sleepiness and Contingent Negative Variation (CNV)

Authors	n	Findings and comments
Aguirre and Broughton (1987)	12 controls 12 narcoleptics	CNV amplitudes of untreated narcoleptics were the same as the matched controls.
Broughton and Aguirre (1987)	12 narcoleptics	REM sleepiness caused a total suppression of the slow negative component of the CNV.
Gauthier and Gottesmann (1983)	19 normals	After a period of 48 hr of sleep loss, the CNV amplitude was reduced.
Naitoh, Johnson, and Lubin (1971)	8 normals	One night of sleep loss decreased the CNV; 2 nights of sleep loss abolished the CNV.
Naitoh, Johnson, and Lubin (1973)	14 normals	One night of sleep loss attenuated the CNV.
Wilkinson (1992)	(Review paper)	The CNV was suggested as a good measure of sleepiness.
Yamamoto, Saito, and Endo (1984)	6 normals	CNV amplitude decrease is a nonspecific aftereffect of disturbed sleep.

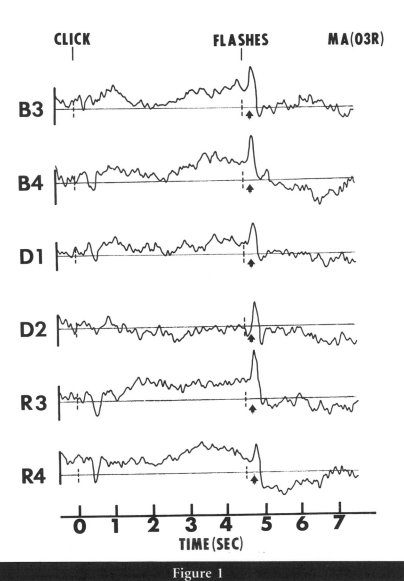

Figure 1

Drowsiness and the contingent negative variation (CNV). CNV was observed in a single subject during baseline (B_3/B_4), after 2-day total sleep deprivation (D_1/D_2), and after recovery sleep (R_3/R_4). Vertical bar = 50 μV. The arrows indicate the average response time to turn off photo flashes. This figure shows the negativity up and the CNV (the surface negative wave) defined by the waves above the baseline zero-voltage line, as indicated by a horizontal line. The CNV of this subject disappeared after 2 days of total sleep loss. MA(03R) = coded subject's name, SEC = seconds.

days of complete recovery sleep (R_3 and R_4). The partial sleep recovery treatment consisted of either REM sleep or Stage 4 sleep deprivation to determine whether sleep without REM or Stage 4 would be as powerful as uninterrupted complete recovery sleep in restoring impaired performance caused by total sleep loss. The subject in Figure 1 was deprived of REM sleep. The CNV paradigm consisted of presenting a warning click ($Stim_1$), which was followed in 4.5 s by light flashes ($Stim_2$), which were terminated when the subject closed a hand-held switch. The EEG responses to the pair of stimuli were averaged across 12 trials to capture the surface negativity between $Stim_1$ and $Stim_2$. The intertrial interval was 30 s. To avoid excessive eye-movement artifacts on the EEGs, the subjects were asked to fix their gaze toward the imagined position of photo flashes through closed eyelids. This subject clearly developed an increasing surface negativity from the time of the click to that of the flashes, that is, CNV that was resolved (ended) with a motor response. The evoked potentials to the photo flashes ($Stim_2$) are also clearly present. Sleep loss of one night reduced the CNV magnitude. Two nights of sleep loss abolished the CNV altogether, although the motor response to terminate photo flashes was intact, and the visual evoked potentials to photo flashes remained unaffected. Only those trials with background EEGs indicating a waking state and a reaction time of less than 1 s were used in the analysis, to ensure that each trial represented a sleepy but not completely asleep state. Increasing sleepiness appeared to reduce the surface negativity preceding $Stim_2$ (photo flashes), perhaps reflecting a psychological state in which a subject could no longer be ready to respond. Although the subject can still respond to $Stim_2$, $Stim_1$ no longer can provide a warning of the imminent demand for action. Ultimately overcome with sleep, a subject will stop responding to $Stim_2$. This CNV paradigm is almost as simple as "counting sheep," yet it provides physiological as well as behavioral indicators on whether one can maintain a low-level response readiness. Incorporating a CNV paradigm does not add to the cost of the MSLT because a patient is already prepared for sleep recording. The only extra recording requirement is the need for a longer time constant to capture slow EEG changes.

Can a patient fall asleep while performing a CNV task? How much does a CNV task interfere with the process of falling asleep? No data exist in which a CNV paradigm has actually been used during MSLT, but we do have an example showing that an experimental subject started to fall asleep while performing a CNV task. Figure 2 shows a subject who is working under the same CNV paradigm on a morning after a full nocturnal sleep.

In the first CNV record, which was obtained 5 min before lights out, the subject was instructed to listen to the click and to watch for photo flashes, but not to perform any motor response. Under this condition, no CNV was seen. At Time 0, the subject was asked by an experimenter to "try hard" to turn the photo flashes off quickly so as to generate a large CNV. After the Time 0 session, the subject was told to go to sleep, to attend to the click–flash event, and to turn the photo flashes off *but without really trying hard*. The subject was told that, if he became sleepy, it would be all right not to respond to photo flashes. After this instruction, the click–flashes pairs were given every 30 s for the remainder of a 40-min experiment. The subject was fully awake 13 min after lights out, with a well-defined CNV and moderately fast reaction time of 0.23 s. At 38 min after lights out, the CNV disappeared, but the subject continued to respond to photo flashes, although with somewhat reduced speed. Unfortunately, the CNV session was terminated before the subject stopped responding to photo flashes. However, on the basis of the previously discussed sleep-deprivation research, the loss of the CNV would appear to define the onset of deep sleepiness in this subject.

We would like to propose the addition of a CNV (and perhaps other ERPs) procedure to the MSLT. Development of such a modified protocol would require extensive testing to establish normal ranges for the various measures. The duration of testing sessions might need to be lengthened, perhaps on the order of the Maintenance of Wakefulness Test (Mitler et al., 1982), that is, 40 min per session. This modification

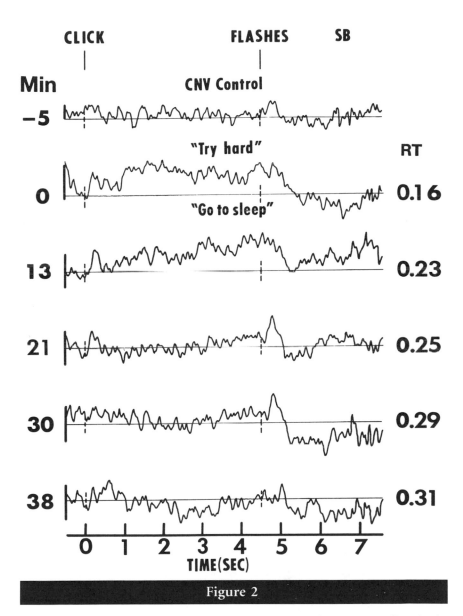

Figure 2

Sleep loss and the contingent negative variation (CNV). The CNV paradigm is the same as in Figure 1, except that this subject was told to fall asleep but to continue to respond to photo flashes as long as possible without "fighting to stay awake." After being on the bed in a dark room for 38 min, the subject was still able to respond to the photo flashes at the response time of 0.31 s. However, the CNV was significantly attenuated after the subject was on the bed for 13–21 min in a dark, soporific environment. RT = reaction time, SB = coded subject's name, SEC = seconds.

would provide a more valid and a more valuable test of sleepiness, sleep onset, and sleep latency.

REFERENCES

Agnew, H. W., & Webb, W. B. (1972). *Sleep stage scoring. JSAS: Catalog of Selected Documents in Psychology, 56,* 2. (Ms. No. 293)

Aguirre, M., & Broughton, R. J. (1987). Complex event-related potentials (P300 and CNV) and MSLT in the assessment of excessive daytime sleepiness in narcolepsy–cataplexy. *Electroencephalography and Clinical Neurophysiology, 67,* 298–316.

Broughton, R. J. (1992). Qualitatively different states of sleepiness. In R. J. Broughton & R. D. Ogilvie (Eds.), *Sleep, arousal, and performance* (pp. 45–59). Cambridge, MA: Birkhauser Boston.

Broughton, R. J., & Aguirre, M. (1987). Differences between REM and NREM sleepiness measured by event-related potentials (P300, CNV), MSLT and subjective estimate in narcolepsy. *Electroencephalography and Clinical Neurophysiology, 67,* 317–326.

Carskadon, M. A. (1979). *Determinants of daytime sleepiness: Adolescent development, extended and restricted nocturnal sleep* (p. 224). Unpublished doctoral dissertation, Stanford University, CA.

Carskadon, M. A., & Dement, W. C. (1979). Effects of total sleep loss on sleep tendency. *Perceptual and Motor Skills, 48,* 495–506.

Carskadon, M. A., & Dement, W. C. (1981). Cumulative effects of sleep restriction on daytime sleepiness. *Psychophysiology, 18,* 107–113.

Carskadon, M. A., & Dement, W. C. (1992). Multiple Sleep Latency Tests during the constant routine. *Sleep, 15,* 396–399.

Carskadon, M., Dement, W. C., Mitler, M. M., Roth, T., Westbrook, P. R., & Keenan, S. (1986). Guidelines for the Multiple Sleep Latency Test (MSLT): A standard measure of sleepiness. *Sleep, 9,* 519–524.

Clodore, M., Benoit, O., Foret, J., & Bouard, G. (1990). The Multiple Sleep Latency Test: Individual variability and time of day effect in normal young adults. *Sleep, 13,* 385–394.

Czeisler, C., Zimmerman, J. C., Ronda, J. M., Moore-Ede, M. C., & Weizman, E. D. (1980). Timing of REM sleep is coupled to the circadian rhythm of body temperature in man. *Sleep, 2,* 329–346.

Davis, H., Davis, P. A., Loomis, A. L., Harvey, E. N., & Hobart, G. (1937). Changes in human brain potentials during the onset of sleep. *Science, 86*, 448–450.

Gander, P. H., Graeber, R. C., Connell, L. J., & Gregory, K. B. (1991). *Crew factors in flight operations: VIII. Factors influencing sleep timing and subjective sleep quality in commercial long-haul flight crews.* NASA Technical Memorandum, 103852 (p. 37). Moffett Field, CA: National Aeronautics and Space Administration, Ames Research Center.

Gauthier, P., & Gottesmann, C. (1983). Influence of total sleep deprivation on event-related potentials in man. *Psychophysiology, 20*, 351–354.

Hayashi, M., Morikawa, T., & Hori, T. (1989). Topographic mapping of EEG with the variation of sleepiness (in Japanese). *Memoirs of the Faculty of Integrated Arts and Sciences III, 13*, 61–71.

Lavie, P., & Shulamit, S. (1989). Twenty-four-hour structure of sleepiness in morning and evening persons investigated by the ultrashort sleep–wake cycle. *Sleep, 12*, 522–528.

Mitler, M. M., Gujavarty, K. S., & Browman, C. P. (1982). Maintenance of wakefulness test: A polysomnographic technique for evaluating treatment efficacy in patients with excessive somnolence. *Electroencephalography and Clinical Neurophysiology, 53*, 658–661.

Naitoh, P., Johnson, L. C., & Lubin, A. (1971). Modification of surface negative slow potential (CNV) in the human brain after total sleep loss. *Electroencephalography and Clinical Neurophysiology, 30*, 17–22.

Naitoh, P., Johnson, L. C., & Lubin, A. (1973). The effect of selective and total sleep loss on the CNV and its psychological and physiological correlates. *Electroencephalography and Clinical Neurophysiology* (Suppl. 33), 213–218.

Naitoh, P., Kelly, T. L., & Babkoff, H. (1992). Napping, stimulant, and four-choice performance. In R. J. Broughton & R. D. Ogilvie (Eds.), *Sleep, arousal, and performance* (pp. 198–219). Cambridge, MA: Birkhauser Boston.

Naitoh, P., Kelly, T., & Babkoff, H. (1993). Sleep inertia: Best time not to wake up? *Chronobiology International, 10*, 109–118.

Nakagawa, H., Sack, R. L., & Lewy, A. J. (1992). Sleep propensity free-runs with the temperature, melatonin and cortisol rhythms in a totally blind person. *Sleep, 15*, 330–336.

Ogilvie, R. D., & Wilkinson, R. T. (1984). The detection of sleep onset: Behavioral and physiological convergence. *Psychophysiology, 21*, 510–520.

Ogilvie, R. D., Wilkinson, R. T., & Allison, S. (1989). The detection of sleep onset: Behavioral, physiological, and subjective convergence. *Sleep, 12,* 458–474.

Rechtschaffen, A., & Kales, A. (1968). *A manual of standardized terminology, techniques and scoring system for sleep stages of human subjects.* Washington, DC: U.S. Government Printing Office.

Richardson, G. S., Carskadon, M. A., Flagg, W., Van den Hoed, J., Dement, W. C., & Mitler, M. M. (1978). Excessive daytime sleepiness in man: Multiple sleep latency measurement in narcoleptic and control subjects. *Electroencephalography and Clinical Neurophysiology, 45,* 621–627.

Richardson, G. S., Carskadon, M. A., Orav, E. J., & Dement, W. C. (1982). Circadian variation of sleep tendency in elderly and young adult subjects. *Sleep, 5,* S82–S94.

Roehrs, T., & Roth, T. (1992). Multiple Sleep Latency Test: Technical aspects and normal values. *Journal of Clinical Neurophysiology, 9,* 63–67.

Thorpy, M. J. (1992). Report from the American Sleep Disorders Association. The clinical use of the Multiple Sleep Latency Test. *Sleep, 15,* 268–276.

Wever, R. A. (1979). *The circadian system of man: Results of experiments under temporal isolation.* Berlin: Springer-Verlag.

Wilkinson, R. T. (1992). The measurement of sleepiness. In R. J. Broughton & R. D. Ogilvie (Eds.), *Sleep, arousal, and performance* (pp. 254–265). Boston: Birkhäuser.

Winfree, A. T. (1983). Impact of a circadian clock on the timing of human sleep. *American Journal of Physiology, 245,* R497–R504.

Yamamoto, T., Saito, Y., & Endo, S. (1984). Effects of disturbed sleep on contingent negative variation. *Sleep, 7,* 331–338.

Zwyghuizen-Doorenbos, A., Roehrs, T., Shaefer, M., & Roth, T. (1988). Test–retest reliability of the MSLT. *Sleep, 11,* 562–565.

20

Mismatch Negativity in Sleep

Risto Näätänen and Heikki Lyytinen

One of the most fascinating issues in sleep research involves the amount and quality of information processing that a sleeping human being is capable of. For obvious reasons, there are many advantages to using a psychophysiological research methodology instead of a purely behavioral one in dealing with this issue. On the other hand, physiological measures suffer, in general, from a validity problem, at least when used as indices of information processing. With regard to the majority of these physiological measures, it is unclear what the measured responses mean in purely informational terms (Näätänen, 1992).

However, one electrophysiological measure, the mismatch negativity (MMN; Näätänen, Gaillard, & Mäntysalo, 1978) of the event-related potential (ERP), is a clear exception, providing a good measure of automatic sensory processing in audition (see Näätänen, 1990). The MMN is a negative ERP component usually peaking at 150–200 ms from stimulus onset, which is elicited by any discriminable change in a repetitive stimulus, even in the absence of attention. Because of this attention-independent elicitation, the MMN appears to represent a pre-perceptual discrimination of stimulus change. One might, with good reason, wonder whether this automatic change-detection process occurs even in sleep.

MMN IN SLEEPING ADULTS

Paavilainen, Cammann, Alho, Reinikainen, Sams, and Näätänen (1987) were the first to study the occurrence of the MMN in sleep. Their subjects were young adults whose ERPs were recorded first while reading and, then, during a gradual transition (via drowsiness) to sleep in the late evening hours and at midnight. Figure 1 presents data from this experiment, in which standard stimuli were tones of 1000 Hz interspersed with deviant tones of 1050 Hz occurring randomly at a probability of 10%. It can be seen that although there is a clear MMN during reading and during drowsiness, it seems to vanish at sleep onset (see also Nielsen-Bohlman, Knight, Woods, & Woodward, 1991).

One reason for the MMN disappearance in this study (Paavilainen et al., 1987) might be the small magnitude of stimulus deviation used. Indeed, Campbell, Bell, and Bastien (1991) obtained an MMN kind of negativity in response to 2000-Hz deviants interspersed with 1000-Hz standards, even though the probability of their deviant stimuli was very high (40%). This negativity, which was of low amplitude and of unusually short latency, emerged during late Stage-2 and REM sleep in the second half of the night.

Sallinen, Kaartinen, & Lyytinen's (in press) very recent study further illuminates the conditions of MMN elicitation in Stage-2 sleep. By averaging all responses to deviant stimuli (tones of 1200 Hz, standards of 1000 Hz) together, they could see no clear MMN. However, when only those trials at which the K-complex was elicited were included, it was possible to observe an early negative wave resembling the MMN found with the same subjects during reading (Figure 2). In these trials, the K-complex was clearly preceded by a significant ($p < .001$ at Fz and Cz) MMN-like deflection at peak latency of about 150 ms (see thick line in Figure 2). No MMN-like response was found in trials in

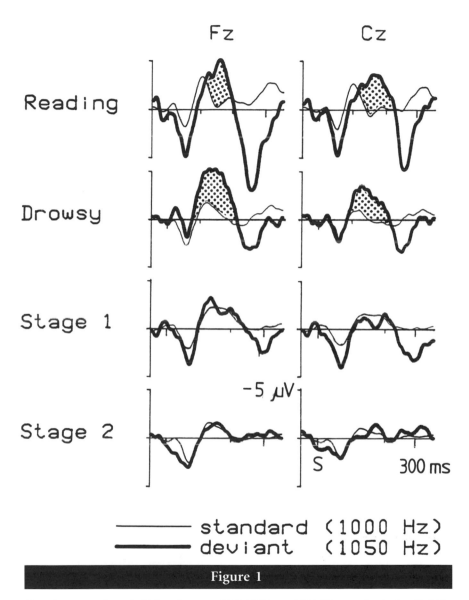

Figure 1

Grand-average frontal (Fz) and vertex (Cz) ERPs to 1000-Hz standard stimuli (thin line) and 1050-Hz deviant stimuli (thick line) during reading (top row), drowsiness (second row), Stage-1 sleep (third row), and Stage-2 sleep (bottom row). The cross-hatched area indicates the mismatch negativity (MMN). From Paavilainen et al. (1987). Adapted with permission.

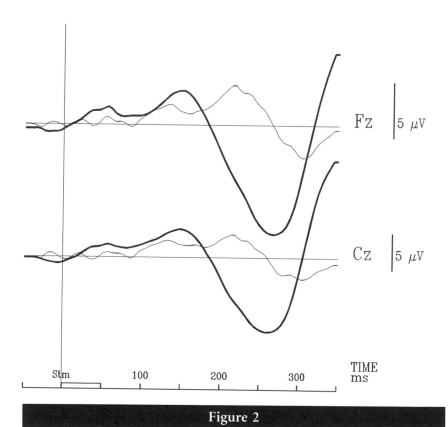

Figure 2

Grand-average frontal (Fz) and vertex (Cz) ERPs (6 subjects) from K-complex trials of Stage-2 sleep (thick line) and from reading condition (thin line) to pitch-deviant (1200 Hz, 2%) tones presented among 1000-Hz standard tones. Tones were presented at an intensity of 45 dB SPL; negativity up. From Sallinen et al. (in press). Reprinted with permission.

which another type of late response or no response at all was elicited (thin and dotted lines in Figure 3).

No comparable negative wave was elicited at the K-complex (or other) trials by the same deviants presented with no intervening standards in a subsequent control condition (Figure 4, thick line). Thus, the negative wave observed to precede the K-complex, in response to

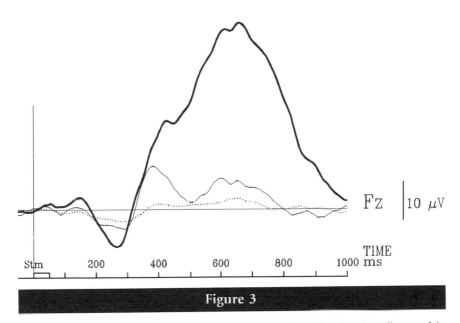

Fz $\quad$ 10 μV

TIME

Stim $\qquad$ 200 $\qquad$ 400 $\qquad$ 600 $\qquad$ 800 $\qquad$ 1000 ms

Figure 3

Grand-average frontal (Fz) ERPs to the deviant tones from the situation illustrated in Figure 2, but separately for trials classified as K-complex trials (thick line) according to the Rechtschaffen and Kales (1968) criteria, for trials showing an observable deflection but no clear K-complex (thin continuous line), and for trials with no observable EEG responses; negativity up. From Sallinen et al. (in press). Reprinted with permission.

deviants presented among standards, appears to correspond to the notion of the MMN.

MMN IN SLEEPING INFANTS

It appears that the MMN is easier to obtain in sleeping infants than in sleeping adults. Alho, Sainio, Sajaniemi, Reinikainen, and Näätänen's (1990) subjects were 1- to 4-day-old infants whose ERPs were recorded in slow-wave sleep (SWS). Standard stimuli were tones of 1000 Hz, deviant stimuli ($p = .1$) being 200 Hz higher in frequency. A large MMN kind of negativity was obtained in response to these deviant stimuli (Figure 5). The interpretation of this negativity in terms of the MMN is supported by the very different midline distribution of such

343

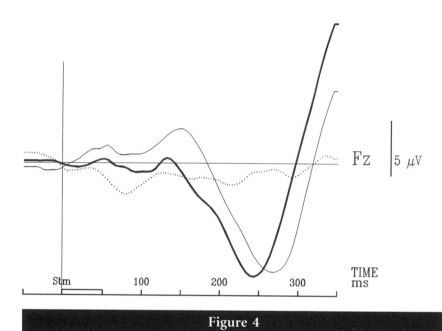

Fz |5 μV

Figure 4

Grand-average frontal (Fz) ERPs to infrequent tones presented with (thin line) and without (thick line) interspersed standard tones as well as to these standard tones (dotted line). The data are from experiments illustrated in Figures 2 and 3; negativity up. From Sallinen et al. (in press). Reprinted with permission.

negativity in comparison with that of the negativity elicited by these deviant stimuli when presented with no standard stimuli (Figure 5).

Also, a phonetic change seems to elicit the MMN in sleeping newborns. This was shown (Figure 6) by Cheour-Luhtanen et al. (in press), who presented the Finnish vowels /y/ and /i/ as their standard and deviant ($p = .1$) stimuli, respectively, to newborns 2 to 5 days of age who were in quiet sleep.

MMN IN SLEEPING ANIMALS

The MMN of a cat to a frequency change was demonstrated by Csépe, Karmos, and Molnár (1987). The MMN was also obtained in SWS

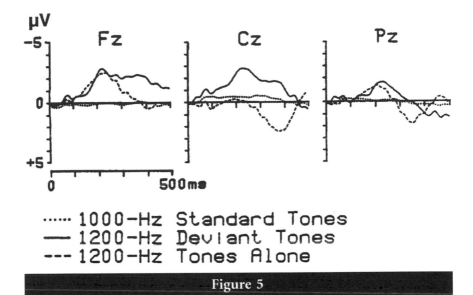

Figure 5

Grand-average frontal (Fz), vertex (Cz), and parietal (Pz) ERPs of sleeping newborns to 1000-Hz standard tones (dotted line), to 1200-Hz deviant tones (solid line), and to these 1200-Hz infrequent tones when presented with no intervening standard tones (dashed lines). From Alho et al. (1990). Adapted with permission.

(Csépe et al., 1987; Csépe, Karmos, & Molnár, 1988, 1989) when its latency was longer and its cortical area less widespread than in wakefulness. Interestingly, Csépe et al. (1989) found an MMN, although at a low amplitude and only from a very limited cortical area, even during anesthesia.

WHY IS THE MMN ATTENUATED IN AMPLITUDE IN SLEEP?

The results reviewed suggest that the MMN amplitude is smaller in sleep than in wakefulness, at least in adult humans and animals. The explanation appears to be activational in nature. The MMN amplitude is known, on the basis of psychopharmacological studies, to depend on the level of cortical arousal. Born and his colleagues (Born, Fehm-

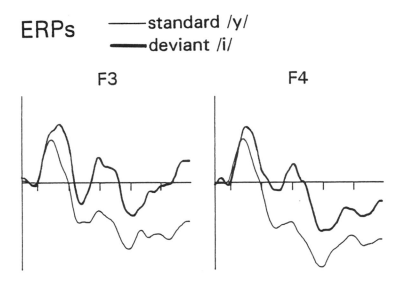

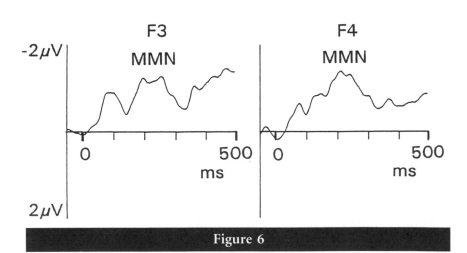

Figure 6

Left (F3) and right (F4) frontal ERPs of sleeping newborns to phonetic stimuli /y/ (standard) and /i/ (deviant; $p = .1$; upper curves) and the corresponding deviant minus standard difference waves (lower curves). From Cheour-Luhtanen et al. (in press). Reprinted with permission.

Wolfsdorf, Lutzenberger, Voigt, & Fehm, 1986; Born, Bothor et al., 1987; Born, Bruninger et al., 1987) showed that, whereas activating drugs enhance the MMN amplitude, sedative ones attenuate it. Furthermore, Lang, Mikkola, Rinne, and Eerola (1994) obtained results suggesting the dependence of the MMN amplitude on the functional state of the brain. These authors recorded the reading speed of subjects throughout the night without allowing them to nap and found that the momentary reading speed correlated with the MMN amplitude. In addition, this correlation was strengthened by including trials with slow eye movements, indicative of increased drowsiness.

So, it appears that the MMN amplitude is attenuated in sleep because of reduced cortical activation. This is also supported by the apparently easier MMN elicitation in Stage-2 and REM sleep than in SWS (Campbell et al., 1991; Sallinen et al., in press). Does this mean, then, that auditory sensory processing is deteriorated in sleep, so that there would be less and more inaccurate information in the brain about our acoustic environment than during wakefulness? No definite answer can be provided, but two alternative interpretations offer themselves: An attenuated MMN process might well result from weaker and less accurate stimulus representations in the neural-trace system underlying sensory memory (because of dampened sensory processing), but it might also result from a reduced activational support to the mismatch process itself, in which case sensory processing, as estimated in informational terms, might have remained unaffected. Näätänen (1991) suggested that two types of neuronal populations are involved in MMN generation: (a) computational neurons, that is, highly sensitive neurons that discriminate stimulus change, and (b) amplifying neurons, that is, interneurons that do not participate in the change detection itself but rather amplify the initially weak change-detection signal provided by the computational neurons. It is possible that sleep, apparently because of the decrease in cortical arousal, dampened the amplifying system of the MMN generation suggested, leaving the informational subsystem unaffected.

One might also ask why, in contrast with adults, a large MMN can apparently be recorded in newborns. This might point to a different role and functional significance of sleep in newborns: It is the predominant state; newborns sleep 17 to 18 hr a day and, therefore, might be closer to the waking state than sleeping adults are. With maturation, however, wakefulness becomes, presumably, the dominant state, and sleep gradually shifts toward an adult-type sleep that is very clearly different from wakefulness.

REFERENCES

Alho, K., Sainio, K., Sajaniemi, N., Reinikainen, K., & Näätänen, R. (1990). Event-related brain potentials of human newborns to pitch change of an acoustic stimulus. *Electroencephalography and Clinical Neurophysiology, 77,* 151–155.

Born, J., Bothor, R., Pietrowsky, G., Fehm-Wolfsdorf, G., Pauschinger, R., & Fehm, H. L. (1987). Influences in vasopressin and oxytocin in human event-related brain potentials in an attention task. *Journal of Psychophysiology, 4,* 351–360.

Born, J., Brüninger, W., Fehm-Wolfsdorf, G., Voigt, K. H., Pauschinger, R., & Fehm, H. L. (1987). Dose-dependent influences on electrophysiological signs of attention in humans after neuropeptide ACTH 4-10. *Experimental Brain Research, 67,* 85–92.

Born, J., Fehm-Wolfsdorf, G., Lutzenberger, W., Voigt, K. H., & Fehm, H. L. (1986). Vasopressin and electro-physiological signs of attention in man. *Peptides, 7,* 189–193.

Campbell, K., Bell, I., & Bastien, C. (1991). Evoked potential measures of information processing during natural sleep. In R. Broughton & R. Ogilvie (Eds.), *Sleep, arousal and performance* (pp. 88–116). Cambridge, MA: Birkhauser Boston.

Cheour-Luhtanen, M., Alho, K., Kujala, T., Sainio, K., Renlund, M., Reinikainen, K., Aaltonen, O., Eerola, O., & Näätänen, R. (in press). An auditory brain response to a phonetic change in newborns. *Hearing Research.*

Csépe, V., Karmos, G., & Molnár, M. (1987). Evoked potential correlates of stimulus deviance during wakefulness and sleep in cat: Animal model of mismatch negativity. *Electroencephalography and Clinical Neurophysiology, 66,* 571–578.

Csépe, V., Karmos, G., & Molnár, M. (1988). Evoked potential correlates of sensory mismatch process during sleep in cats. In W. P. Koella, F. Obal, H. Schulz, &

P. Visser (Eds.), *Sleep '86* (pp. 281–283). Stuttgart, Germany: Gustav Fisher Verlag.

Csépe, V., Karmos, G., & Molnár, M. (1989). Subcortical evoked potential correlates of early information processing: Mismatch negativity in cats. In E. Basar & T. H. Bullock (Eds.), *Spring series in brain dynamics 2* (pp. 279–289). Berlin, Germany: Springer-Verlag.

Lang, A. H., Mikola, H., & Eerola, O. (1994). *Slight fluctuations of alertness affect the mismatch negativity.* Manuscript submitted for publication.

Näätänen, R. (1990). The role of attention in auditory information processing as revealed by event-related potentials and other brain measures of cognitive function. *Behavioral and Brain Sciences, 13,* 201–288.

Näätänen, R. (1991). Mismatch negativity outside strong attentional focus: A commentary on Woldorff et al. (1991). *Psychophysiology, 28,* 478–484.

Näätänen, R. (1992). *Attention and brain function.* Hillsdale, NJ: Erlbaum.

Näätänen, R., Gaillard, A. W. K., & Mäntysalo, S. (1978). Early selective attention effect on evoked potential reinterpreted. *Acta Psychologica, 42,* 313–329.

Nielsen-Bohlman, L., Knight, R. T., Woods, D. L., & Woodward, K. (1991). Differential auditory processing continues during sleep. *Electroencephalography and Clinical Neurophysiology, 79,* 281–290.

Paavilainen, P., Cammann, R., Alho, K., Reinikainen, K., Sams, M., & Näätänen, R. (1987). Event-related potentials to pitch change in an auditory stimulus sequence during sleep. *Electroencephalography and Clinical Neurophysiology* (Suppl. 40), 246–255.

Rechtschaffen, A., & Kales, A. (1968). *A manual of standardized terminology, techniques and scoring system for sleep stages of human subjects.* Washington, DC: U.S. Government Printing Office.

Sallinen, M., Kaartinen, J., & Lyytinen, H. (in press). Is the appearance of mismatch negativity during Stage 2 sleep related to the elicitation of K-complex? *Electroencephalography and Clinical Neurophysiology.*

21

Attentional Allocation and Capacity in Waking Arousal

Sidney J. Segalowitz, Diana Velikonja, and
Jane Storrie-Baker

SLEEP ONSET, AROUSAL, AND ATTENTION

Sleep onset by definition involves a change in arousal, usually a gradual change, leading to a cessation of behavioral response and systematic changes in electroencephalogram (EEG) and event-related potentials (ERPs; Ogilvie, Simons, Kuderian, MacDonald, & Rustenberg, 1991; Ogilvie & Wilkinson, 1984; Segalowitz, Ogilvie, & Simons, 1990). The changes in the primary ERP components that appear with sleep onset are straightforward, whether using either behavioral cessation or EEG patterns as operational definitions of sleep onset (Broughton, 1988; Segalowitz et al., 1990). However, the interpretation of these patterns with regard to information processing is more difficult (Campbell, Bell, & Bastien, 1992). The focus of this chapter is the nature of these difficulties.

Cognitive and physiological psychologists bring different interpretations to studies of arousal and ERPs. A cognitive psychologist sees ERPs as a way of tracking information processing in the brain and devises ways to alter ERP components by manipulating stimulus parameters or by changing the way in which the subject processes the stimuli. By contrast, physiological psychologists see ERPs as a reflection of broader factors in information processing that are highly sensitive to an alteration in the resting level of cortical activation and, therefore, notice how a change in arousal levels can alter ERP components. We think that both approaches are correct and that the different interpretations reflect the basic experimental confounding factors in studies of arousal and ERPs.

The literature integrating arousal and attentional approaches to information processing has been complicated by the many meanings attributed to each term. In general, arousal as an experimental variable is manipulated in one of three ways: (a) by waiting for subjects to change state in a naturalistic fashion (sleep and sleepiness studies); (b) by increasing arousal level by introducing noise, social tension, or cognitive load (cognitive intervention); and (c) by administering drugs known (or assumed) to change cortical activation (physiological intervention). These methods may produce arousal change with different consequences for attentional processes.

We begin by describing two recent studies from our laboratory on this issue. Segalowitz et al. (1990) presented data on the systematic changes in the late ERP components as subjects fell asleep (Figure 1). The changes in the N1, P2, N2, and P3 components were found to be gradual, with large amplitude increases in the P2 and N2 components and with considerable reduction in the N1 and P3 as subjects dropped off to sleep, followed by a large K-complex. There were also small but statistically significant latency increases in all four components. We wanted to examine the generality of these results by reversing the procedure, when subjects were first waking up in the morning, with the help of their first cup of coffee (Velikonja & Segalowitz, 1992, 1993). In this study, we controlled for caffeine dose per body weight (3 mg/ kg), caffeine reactivity (moderate), diurnal rhythm, age, expectations (blind administration), lifestyle (university students), and time of day (early morning testing only). We found that contrary to our expectations, caffeine produced no changes in the amplitudes of the four ERP

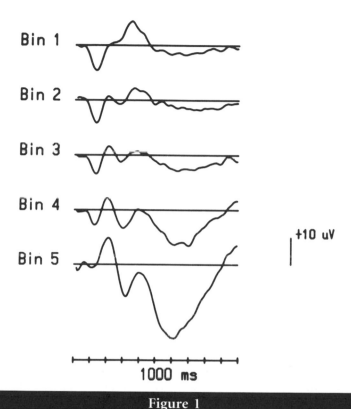

Figure 1

Group-averaged ERPs for each arousal bin during a sleep onset period, from Bin 1 = fastest 25% reaction times (fully awake) to Bin 4 = slowest 25% reaction times and Bin 5 = first no-response period (Stage 1 or 2 sleep). The negative and positive fluctuation seen during the first 400 milliseconds, most easily visualized in Bins 3 and 4, systematically change with sleep onset. From Segalowitz et al. (1990). Reprinted with permission.

components in an auditory oddball paradigm (Figure 2). Also, there was no change in the amplitude of the contingent negative variation (CNV; Figure 3), a measure reflecting the subjects' sustained attention in a vigilance task. However, there were systematic reductions in the latencies of every component of the auditory ERP (see Figure 2) that mirrored the increases in the latency of the components as subjects were falling asleep. There was also an interaction with diurnal rhythm

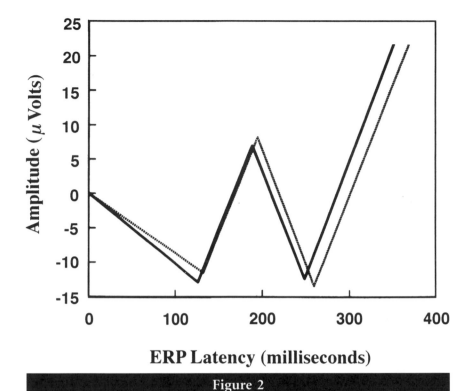

ERP Latency (milliseconds)

Figure 2

Schematic of auditory ERP peaks N1, P2, N2, and P3, averaged over subjects in a repeated-measures design for caffeine (solid line) and no-caffeine (dotted line) conditions. ERP peak values are taken from single-trial scoring and are amplitude adjusted for the 100 milliseconds prestimulus baseline. From Velikonja and Segalowitz (1993).

in which morning types showed a much larger latency enhancement with caffeine than did evening types (Figure 4).

The dissociation of the amplitude and latency of the ERP suggested that perhaps we had some factors to disentangle, these factors being attentional allocation and arousal. In our original sleep-onset study, not only were the subjects becoming drowsy, but they probably were also attending to stimuli less and less because the drowsiness reduced their ability or desire to allocate attention to the stimuli. If a drowsy subject does not process the stimulus, then we should not expect to find the ERP reflecting that processing. Unfortunately, it is impossible to know

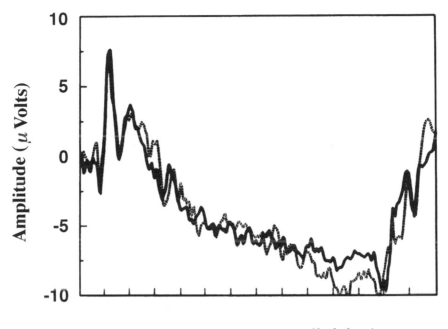

Time (200 msec per division)

Figure 3

Contingent negative variation ERPs taken during caffeine (solid line) and no-caffeine (dotted line) conditions, averaged over subjects. The first stimulus (at 0 milliseconds) allows the subject to anticipate the onset of the second stimulus (at 2,300 milliseconds). Each waveform is adjusted to a baseline of 200 milliseconds of EEG before the first stimulus. From Velikonja and Segalowitz (1993).

from such a study whether the change in arousal or the change in attention accounted for the changes in ERPs. If our caffeine study had similarly found an amplitude change, we also would not have been able to discuss a dissociation. The fact that caffeine altered neither ERP amplitudes nor the amplitude of CNVs suggests that although caffeine may affect arousal, it does not necessarily affect attentional processes, despite its normal use by the student volunteers in the study for just that purpose.

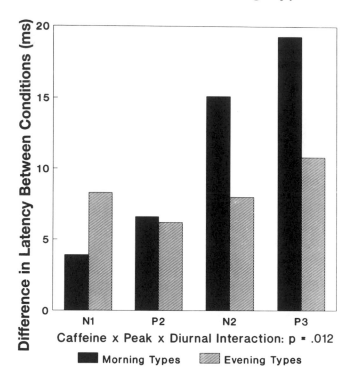

Amount of Speedup with Caffeine for Morning vs Evening Types

Difference in Latency Between Conditions (ms)

Caffeine x Peak x Diurnal Interaction: p = .012

■ Morning Types   ▨ Evening Types

(N1 and P2 at Cz, N2 and P3 at Pz)

Figure 4

Degree of speedup during the caffeine condition of the latencies for the N1, P2, N2, and P3 ERP peaks, showing the significant interaction for morning versus evening types. From Velikonja and Segalowitz (1993).

SOME DEFINITIONS

For our purposes here, *arousal* refers to a physiological state involving the level of activation of the nervous system, which for human cognitive functions means cortical activation. *Attention* refers both to the global capacity to focus mental processes on some experience, whether endogenous or exogenous, and to the process of allocating this infor-mation-processing capacity. Presumably, each nervous system has some capacity limit and some mode of allocating the available attentional resource. Despite the common usage of these terms in many areas of psychology, the relationship between arousal and attention is not simple.

As a starting point, we take Kahneman's (1973) summary of the classic capacity model of the attention–arousal relationship. In this model, arousal is the level of cortical activation driven from the retic-ular activating system and is considered to be a "low-level" process. It cycles during the night and during the day, with wide individual dif-ferences in the diurnal rhythms of "morningness" versus "eveningness" (Wegman, et al., 1986). The level of arousal, used here synonymously with the level of cortical activation, also accounts for the total atten-tional capacity (= attentional resources) available to the person (Figure 5). By this definition, a low arousal level produces a low level of total attentional resources. With regard to performance, however, very high arousal produces a curvilinear relationship such that there is some op-timal level of arousal. The drop in performance with very high arousal (the top end of the classic inverted-U relationship) may be due to attention being focused beyond the point of efficient task solution (Kahneman, 1973) or to overarousal being associated with distractibility (Naatanen, 1975; Tecce, 1976). In addition, the arousal level can be influenced by motivational factors on the part of the subject. When faced with an interesting task, increasing effort can by itself increase the arousal level, just as a boring or monotonous task can reduce effort, with a subsequent drop in arousal level (Hockey, 1984).

The subject is capable of allocating attention differentially to vari-ous ongoing events. Some events or activities normally require less at-tentional resources and some events require more. Measuring the de-gree of attentional allocation in any particular instance is, of course, much more complicated than getting a correlate of arousal level, but it can be manipulated by the experimental design. Dual-task paradigms are a popular method when manipulation of the difficulty of the pri-

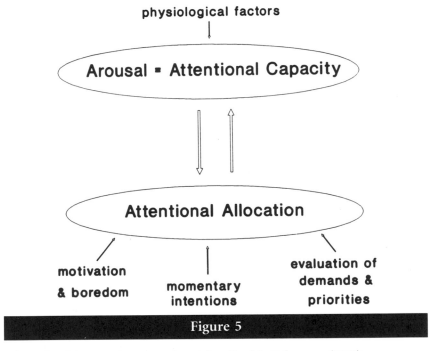

Figure 5

Schematic of the attention–arousal model outlined in Kahneman (1973).

mary task alters the performance on the secondary task, presumably, because fewer resources of the total attentional capacity remain available for it (Kramer & Spinks, 1991). In Kahneman's model, tasks that consume virtually no attentional resources—those that run mechanically or unconsciously—are considered to be "automatic" as opposed to "controlled" processes. Whereas some tasks can be automatized by the removal of any conscious decision-making or at ention-consuming algorithm (e.g., memorizing multiplication tables to substitute for mental calculations), others involve controlled processes permanently because the task does not permit rote performance (e.g., reading unfamiliar words backwards). Contemporary views on this dichotomy suggest more of a continuum than a clean distinction (Cohen, Dunbar, & McClelland, 1990). This classic capacity model of the arousal–attention relationship assumes that arousal and attentional capacity are, respectively, physiological and information-processing aspects of the same phenomenon of cortical activation. The model separates the process of attentional allocation from capacity.

Before we continue with electrophysiological correlates of each of these aspects of the model, we should point out that there are two research difficulties. First, individual subjects may differ from each other in how well they function at a given level of arousal. Some persons' high level of arousal (i.e., cortical activation) may be associated with their maximal level of attentional capacity. However, what might be maximal for them would perhaps be lower than the attentional capacity available to some other persons. To control for such individual differences, it is necessary to use within-subject research designs when mapping some other variable onto changes in the arousal-capacity dimension. Second, in the normal course of events, increases in arousal and, hence, in capacity mean that the subject has more resources to allocate and that the allocation can proceed more efficiently. A drop in arousal is accompanied by a drop not only in available resources but also in the ability to allocate the resources that remain. Because of this confounding factor, much of the literature has treated arousal, alertness, and attention as synonymous. We suggest that this is neither necessary nor useful.

ELECTROPHYSIOLOGICAL CORRELATES OF AROUSAL VERSUS ATTENTION

The arousal–attention model has a simplicity about it that has lent itself to the search for electrophysiological correlates of its various components. To date, evidence suggests that cortical arousal is reflected in the degree of fast-frequency EEG activity relative to slow-frequency activity. This distinction has a long history, which is based to a large extent on the clear differences in fast- versus slow-wave EEG in the extremes of wakefulness and sleep, although the same can be seen in various levels of waking arousal (Ogilvie & Wilkinson, 1984).

In general, the changes associated with reduced arousal are a slowing of the dominant alpha frequency (Davis, Davis, Loomis, Harvey, & Hobart, 1938; Erwin, Somerville, & Radtke, 1984) and an increase in theta and delta with a decrease in beta (Carriero, 1977; Davies, 1965; Gale, Haslum, & Penfold, 1971; Kornfield & Beatty, 1977; Morrell, 1966; Ogilvie & Simons, 1992; O'Hanlon & Beatty, 1977), and there is some controversy about alpha amplitude, with some subjects showing increased and others, decreased amounts (Santamaria & Chiappa, 1987). For example, we used a procedure (caloric stimulation) designed to increase temporarily the arousal level in a patient who had suffered a serious right hemisphere stroke. Increased arousal was manifested as increased beta and reduced alpha, theta, and delta, with the largest relative changes in theta (Storrie-Baker, Segalowitz, Black, McLean, & Sullivan, 1993).

Changes in waking arousal have strong and well-documented effects on various ERP components. The literature is far too large to be summarized here and mostly confirms the general pattern indicated earlier. However, the paradigms used do not systematically control for the attentional allocation aspect of the tasks; therefore, the two are usually confounded.

ERP correlates have also been suggested, with the N1 reflecting total capacity (and, thus, arousal in the Kahneman model) and the P3 amplitude reflecting attentional allocation (Kramer & Spinks, 1991). Studies of ERP changes during sleep onset and changes in waking arousal have traditionally confounded processes of arousal and attention because they have not separated attentional capacity (arousal) from attentional allocation. As indicated earlier, the ERP peak changes in the standard auditory oddball (or auditory ERP) paradigm while subjects are falling asleep include a reduction in the N1 and the P3 and a dramatic increase in the P2 and N2 amplitude (Broughton, 1988; Campbell et al., 1992). These changes are easily attributed to the drop in cortical activation associated with the drop in arousal, leading to the conclusion that the P3 amplitude is a reflection of the level of arousal of the subject. However, as subjects fall asleep, they may also allocate less of the available attentional resource to external events. Without systematically varying this allocation component, we cannot know to which aspect we should attribute the change. Such studies are not standard in the field, but could be made so. Unconfounding arousal and attentional allocation can be achieved in two ways: by examining ERP effects when allocation is varied, but arousal is held constant, and vice-versa.

UNCONFOUNDING AROUSAL AND ATTENTION

There is, of course, an extensive electrophysiological literature that varies the attentional allocation while keeping arousal levels constant by testing subjects within a relatively short period of time (see Jennings & Coles, 1991; Picton & Hillyard, 1988; Regan, 1989). The experimenter compares the ERPs to stimuli that draw on differing allocations of attention by varying the target stimulus frequency, the number of distractors, and other similar factors within a test session. For example, one method of varying attentional allocation is to bias the subject toward explicitly allocating more as opposed to less attention to a particular stimulus or task. The stimulus that is specially targeted for attention produces a larger P3, everything else being equal. Similarly, when one task receives more attention than others in a multiple-task paradigm, those stimuli also produce larger P3s (see Kramer & Spinks, 1991, for a review). Another method is to vary the probability of occurrence of the stimulus. The rarer it is, the larger the P300 associated with it (Duncan-Johnson & Donchin, 1977). In both methods, the targeted stimulus is associated with a certain amount of attentional allocation reflected in the amplitude of the P300 (see Picton & Hillyard, 1988, for a review).

Consider the three methods outlined earlier (sleepiness vs. cognitive intervention vs. drug use). As described earlier, the sleep and sleepiness studies do not usually separate out effects of arousal change from those of attentional allocation. An exception to this is the one reported by John Harsh (chapter 18, this volume), who uses the stimulus-probability method. Subjects show just as much sensitivity to stimulus probability in Stage-2 sleep as they do during wakefulness, albeit with a different ERP component (see also Harsh, Voss, Hull, & Schrepfer, 1994). Considering that the processing of the stimulus information cannot be the same, this change in ERP component is not surprising. What is impressive is that the sensitivity to the stimulus is still present in sleep (cf. Segalowitz, Ogilvie, Janicki, Simons, & Buetow, 1991, who report P300 effects during slow-wave sleep).

The second technique, using distress or motivation to alter activation levels, may not involve arousal in the sense used with regard to sleep onset because it relates to arousal by means of the interaction between psychological and physiological states, which complicates the paradigm considerably. Extraneous noise can, after all, change the information processing of the stimulus directly, not just through changing the arousal level.

The third method involves relatively mild stimulant drugs that are current in our mainstream culture, which will be reviewed very briefly here.

Mild Stimulant Drugs

To consider the changes in attention associated with arousal manipulation that may relate to normal waking performance, it is important to keep within some normal levels of arousal. Common drug stimulants are good candidates for two reasons: (a) The stimulating effects can easily be kept within normal levels for waking arousal, and (b) the subjects are more likely to be aware of their individual sensitivity to the drug because of its availability, allowing control for intersubjective variation in sensitivity. Stimulants present a picture that is consistent with the standard view of cortical firing and EEG (increases in arousal leading to an increased firing rate of single cells and a shift from slower to faster spectral frequencies). The results are less clear with regard to ERPs.

None of these studies, however, clarifies the possible differential effects on arousal and attention, and, unfortunately, most of the effects are plagued by the wide individual differences that subjects have in sensitivity to the drugs. The results for caffeine, nicotine, and amphetamines are very similar. There are wide individual difference in reactivity to and metabolism rates of caffeine (James, 1991; Münte, Heinze, Kunkel, & Scholz, 1984) and nicotine (e.g., Brown, 1973; Mangan & Golding, 1984; Remond, Izard, Martinerie, & Grob, 1979; Remond, Martinerie, & Baillon, 1979), and amphetamines are well known for their paradoxical effects on attention in subgroups of children with attention deficit hyperactivity (ADH) syndrome (Klorman, 1991; Naylor, Halliday, & Callaway, 1985).

There is a major problem of interpretation of the data on the electrophysiological effects of stimulant drugs. First, the results are inconsistent, in general. Part of the problem is that there are pharmacological interactions among the common drugs and possibly different mechanisms for their effects on arousal or attention. Second, there are no clear effects on subjects' ability to allocate attention, despite the well known stimulant mechanisms and the corroboratory evidence from EEG (i.e., reduction of slow-wave activity in favor of higher frequencies). The one exception is that methylphenidate and caffeine improve ADH children's ability to focus, consistent with the increase in P3 amplitude reflecting the increase in attentional allocation, without the ERP latency decrease associated with the arousal change expected with normal individuals.

The lack of stable effects in studies with normal subjects may be due to individual differences without within-subject experimental designs. Results may be influenced by subjective expectations, by the emotional and cognitive context, by individual differences in the level of baseline and of tonic arousal, by range effects, by individual differences in reactivity to the drugs, and by the drug doses used (some studies controlled for total dose, as opposed to administering a specific dose per body weight). For example, our significant interaction with diurnal rhythm may not have been detectable if we had not controlled for many other factors that are often left free to vary.

IMPLICATIONS FOR RESEARCH DESIGN

A shortcoming of past studies is the failure of the experimental design to address the attention–arousal confounding factor. As indicated earlier, most researchers who speak of the issue assume that arousal and attention are equivalent in their paradigms (instead of simply confounded). We suggest that, to unconfound them, we should not keep attentional requirements constant in psychophysiological studies of arousal, because doing so produces ambiguous results. For example, if we present target stimuli at one level of stimulus probability while collecting data at more than one level of arousal, we have controlled the attentional requirements of the task. However, if the subject's allocation of attention varies with the arousal change, we are left with the confounding factor.

As a research strategy, then, we suggest that attentional allocation can be inferred from the amplitude of various ERP peaks, *but only insofar as these amplitudes reflect a change related to some stimulus manipulation.* This is rarely done, although Harsh's studies clearly showed that attentional allocation is an active process in sleep. This manipulation of stimulus probability is critical, without which we are left with arousal and attentional allocation being confounded. As subjects fall asleep, they allocate less of their attentional resources to external events. Other methods of manipulating allocation of attention may be difficult in sleepiness paradigms—it is hard to get subjects to do dual tasks or attend to stimuli differentially when they are sleepy. However, these paradigms are more sensible with drug stimulation paradigms.

Cognitive electrophysiologists normally unconfound arousal and attentional allocation by varying the degree of attentional allocation within one test session and counterbalancing to avoid fatigue effects. Thus, standard ERP studies do not confound arousal and attention when attention is manipulated. However, when arousal is manipulated, this advantage is not available. We cannot simply keep attentional allocation demands constant, because the subject changes them without permission. Firmer control is needed over the allocation process. In other words, from a research design perspective, the relationship is not symmetrical.

SUMMARY

Electrophysiological studies of arousal normally confound attentional factors unintentionally. A review of the literature of EEG and ERP effects of sleep-onset studies and of arousal manipulation by mild stimulant drugs indicates that there is too little consensus to determine whether attentional allocation changes with alteration in arousal level. Many of the interpretation problems in the drug studies stem from inadequate control over individual differences, such as reactivity to the drugs, diurnal rhythm, and other major physiological factors, and from inadequate experimental manipulation of the stimulus parameters necessary to examine attentional allocation independently of arousal. Studies are needed that include standard paradigms for multiple levels of attentional allocation while manipulating the arousal level. An occasion when such studies could be conducted would be during the sleep-onset period.

REFERENCES

Broughton, R. (1988). Evoked potentials and sleep–wake states in man. In J. Horne (Ed.), *Sleep '88* (pp. 6–10). Stuttgart, Germany: Gustav Fischer Verlag.

Brown, B. B. (1973). Additional characteristic EEG differences between smokers and non-smokers. In V. H. Winston (Ed.), *Smoking behavior: Motives and incentives* (pp. 136–157). New York: Winston.

Campbell, K., Bell, I., & Bastien, C. (1992). Evoked potential measures of information processing during natural sleep. In R. Broughton & R. Ogilvie (Eds.), *Sleep, arousal and performance: A tribute to Bob Wilkinson* (pp. 88–116). Cambridge, MA: Birkhauser Boston.

Carriero, N. J. (1977). Physiological correlates of performance in a long duration repetitive visual task. In R. R. Mackie (Ed.), *Vigilance theory, operational performance and physiological correlates* (pp. 307–331). New York: Plenum.

Cohen, J. D., Dunbar, K., & McClelland, J. L. (1990). On the control of automatic processes: A parallel distributed processing account of the Stroop effect. *Psychological Review, 97*, 332–361.

Davies, D. R. (1965). Skin conductance, alpha activity and vigilance. *American Journal of Psychology, 78*, 304–306.

Davis, H., Davis, P. A., Loomis, A. L., Harvey, E. N., & Hobart, G. (1938). Human brain potentials during the onset of sleep. *Journal of Neurophysiology, 1*, 24–38.

Duncan-Johnson, C. C., & Donchin, E. (1977). On quantifying surprise: The variation of event-related potentials with subjective probability. *Psychophysiology, 14*, 456–467.

Erwin, C. W., Somerville, E. R., & Radtke, R. A. (1984). A review of electroencephalographic features of normal sleep. *Journal of Clinical Neurophysiology, 1*, 253–274.

Gale, A., Haslum, A., & Penfold, V. (1971). EEG correlates of cumulative expectancy and subjective estimates of alertness in a vigilance task. *Journal of Experimental Psychology, 23*, 245–254.

Harsh, J., Voss, U., Hull, J., & Schrepfer, S. (1994). Behavioral and ERP changes during the wake/sleep transition. *Psychophysiology, 31*, 244–252.

Hockey, R. (1984). Varieties of attentional state: The effects of environment. In R. Parasuraman & D. R. Davies (Eds.), *Varieties of attention* (pp. 449–483). Orlando, FL: Academic Press.

James, J. E. (1991). *Caffeine and health.* London: Academic Press.

Jennings, J. R., & Coles, M. G. H. (Eds.). (1991). *Handbook of cognitive psychophysiology.* New York: Wiley.

Kahneman, D. (1973). *Attention and effort.* Englewood Cliffs, NJ: Prentice Hall.

Klorman, R. (1991). Cognitive event-related potentials in attention deficit disorder. *Journal of Learning Disabilities, 24*, 130–140.

Kornfield, C. M., & Beatty, J. (1977). EEG spectra during a long-term compensatory tracking task. *Bulletin of the Psychological Society, 10*, 46–48.

Kramer, A., & Spinks, J. (1991). Capacity views of human information processing. In J. R. Jennings & M. G. H. Coles (Eds.), *Handbook of cognitive psychophysiology* (pp. 179–249). New York: Wiley.

Mangan, G. L., & Golding, J. J. (1984). *The psychopharmacology of smoking.* Oxford, England: Cambridge University Press.

Morrell, L. K. (1966). EEG frequency and reaction time: A sequential analysis. *Neuropsychologia, 4,* 41–48.

Münte, T. F., Heinze, H. J., Kunkel, H., & Scholz, M. (1984). Personality traits influence the effects of diazepam and caffeine on CNV magnitude. *Neuropsychobiology, 12,* 60–67.

Näätänen, R. (1975). Selective attention and evoked potentials in humans: A critical review. *Biological Psychology, 2,* 237–307.

Naylor, H., Halliday, R., & Callaway, E. (1985). The effect of methylphenidate on information processing. *Psychopharmacology, 90,* 522–527.

Ogilvie, R. D., & Simons, I. A. (1992). Falling asleep and waking up: A comparison of EEG spectra. In R. Broughton & R. Ogilvie (Eds.), *Sleep, arousal and performance.* Cambridge, MA: Birkhauser Boston.

Ogilvie, R. D., Simons, I. A., Kuderian, R., MacDonald, T., & Rustenberg, J. (1991). Behavioral, event-related potential, and EEG/FFT changes at sleep onset. *Psychophysiology, 28,* 54–64.

Ogilvie, R. D., & Wilkinson, R. T. (1984). The detection of sleep onset: Behavioral and physiological convergence. *Sleep, 8,* 146–154.

O'Hanlon, J. F., & Beatty, J. (1977). Concurrence of electroencephalographic and performance changes during a simulated radar watch and some implications for the arousal theory of vigilance. In R. R. Mackie (Ed.), *Vigilance theory, operational performance and physiological correlates* (pp. 189–201). New York: Plenum.

Picton, T., & Hillyard, S. (1988). Endogenous event-related potentials. In T. Picton (Ed.), *Human event-related potentials* (pp. 361–425). Amsterdam: Elsevier.

Regan, D. M. (1989). *Human brain electrophysiology.* Amsterdam: Elsevier.

Remond, A., Izard, C., Martinerie, J., & Grob, R. (1979). The action of smoking on visual evoked potentials, biofeedback, EEG changes and autonomous responses. In A. Remond and C. Izard (Eds.), *Electrophysiological effects of nicotine* (pp. 89–98). Amsterdam: Elsevier.

Remond, A., Martinerie, J., & Baillon, J.-F. (1979). Nicotine intake compared with other psychophysiological situations through quantitative EEG analysis. In A. Remond & C. Izard (Eds.), *Electrophysiological effects of nicotine* (pp. 61–87). Amsterdam: Elsevier.

Santamaria, J., & Chiappa, K. H. (1987). *The EEG of drowsiness.* New York: Demos Publications.

Segalowitz, S. J., Ogilvie, R. D., Janicki, M., Simons, I., & Buetow, C. (1991). ERP evidence for the paradox of REM sleep: Attention and distraction while awake and while asleep. *Sleep Research, 20,* 159.

Segalowitz, S. J., Ogilvie, R. D., & Simons, I. A. (1990). An ERP state measure of arousal based on behavioral criteria. In J. Horne (Ed.), *Sleep '90* (pp. 23–25). Stuttgart, Germany: Gustav Fischer Verlag.

Storrie-Baker, H. J., Segalowitz, S. J., Black, S. E., McLean, J. A. G., & Sullivan, N. (1993). Improvement of hemispatial neglect with cold-water calorics: An electrophysiological investigation. *Journal of Clinical and Experimental Neuropsychology, 15,* 110.

Tecce, J. J. (1976). Contingent negative variation and the distraction-arousal hypothesis. *Electroencephalography and Clinical Neurophysiology, 41,* 277–286.

Velikonja, D., & Segalowitz, S. J. (1992, October). *The effects of caffeine on cortical arousal.* Paper presented at the meeting of the Society for Neuroscience, Anaheim, CA.

Velikonja, D., & Segalowitz, S. J. (1993). The effects of caffeine on electrophysiological indicators of cortical arousal. *Journal of Clinical and Experimental Neuropsychology, 15,* 109–110.

Wegman, H., Grundel, A., Nauman, M., Samel, A., Schwartz, E., & Vejvoda, M. (1986). Sleep, sleepiness, and circadian rhythmicity in air crews operating on trans-Atlantic routes. *Aviation and Environmental Medicine, 57,* B53–B64.

Author Index

Numbers in italics refer to listings in the reference sections.

Subject Index

About the Editors

Robert D. Ogilvie, PhD, is professor of psychology and director of the Sleep Research Laboratory at Brock University, St. Catharines, Ontario, where he has taught psychology and studied sleep for over 20 years. He was chairman of the Department of Psychology during 1988–1991. He is coeditor of *Sleep, Arousal, and Performance: Problems and Promises* (1992) and has published many papers and book chapters on sleep and sleep onset. Dr. Ogilvie was coorganizer (with coeditor Dr. John R. Harsh) of the Sleep Onset Processes Conference (1993) and of the Sleep Arousal and Performance Conference (1990). He is past president of the Canadian Sleep Society.

John R. Harsh, PhD, is professor of psychology and director of the Sleep Research Laboratory at the University of Southern Mississippi. He received his doctoral degree in experimental psychology from Bowling Green State University in 1975. His most recent work has focused on the effects of sleepiness and sleep on cognitive and behavioral capacity.